If we can imagine God as one body, then we are like different cells and parts of that body of God. When any part of that body hurts, the whole body hurts. Similarly, when we hurt any other person, we hurt ourselves as well. We must treat each other with love and care in order to preserve the whole. Love is the most powerful source in the universe. When we give love we also receive it and as it moves back and forth, it grows and provides the healing for everybody involved. Only love can heal, and it is the only thing which really matters.

Also by Shakuntala Modi, M.D.

Memories of God amd Creation

REMARKABLE HEALINGS

A Psychiatrist Discovers Unsuspected
Roots of Mental and Physical Illness

SHAKUNTALA MODI, M.D.

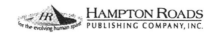

HAMPTON ROADS
PUBLISHING COMPANY, INC.

Cover design by Mayapriya Long

Hampton Roads Publishing Company, Inc.
Charlottesville, VA 22902
www.hrpub.com

Library of Congress Catalog Card Number: 98-072108

ISBN 978-1-57174-079-3

Printed in Canada
TCP
10 9 8 7 6 5

REMARKABLE
HEALINGS

Dedication

I dedicate this book first to my brother, Jawaharlal Chaudhari, whose sacrifice made it possible for me to be a doctor. We both wanted to become doctors. Due to financial problems, when he was told that only one of us could go to medical college, he selflessly stepped aside so that I could be a doctor. I am eternally grateful to him because without his love, support, and sacrifice I would not be a doctor today writing this book.

Also to my uncle, Bansilal Chaudhari, who provided financial support and encouraged me to become a doctor during a time when none of the girls in our family went to college.

Next, to my patients, through whom I was privileged to receive this knowledge. Their trust and perseverance and their willingness to explore and share the joy are greatly appreciated.

To all the angels, heavenly guides, and all the other Light beings for their never-ending attendance, assistance, protection, education, and enthusiastic participation.

Ultimately, I humbly dedicate this book to God, the giver of the Light and the knowledge, for the privilege of receiving and participating in the discovery of this knowledge.

Acknowledgments

In recognizing those who have been of great assistance to me in preparing for this book, I must begin with all my patients who have helped me in the quest for this knowledge. Without them there would be no subject matter about which to write.

My sincere thanks to my typists, Charlotte Hawk and Dorothy Kovacik, for their hours and hours of patient, tedious typing and retyping of several revisions.

I also thank my local editors, Milton Ronsheim and Jane Dulaney, for their careful reading, corrections, and suggestions.

I am grateful to everyone at Hampton Roads Publishing Company for editing, designing, producing, and promoting this book.

Ultimately, I must acknowledge God, the heavenly angels, guides, and all the other Light beings for their protection, guidance, and education and their gift of this book.

Contents

Chapter V   Possession or Attachment by Demon Spirits (Entities) and Other Spirits / 285

A Patient's Foreword

Looking for the Key

I looked within myself to find the answers
Because I knew although I can't say how,

That deep inside me the truth awaited me
So, fearlessly, I opened the door to eternity,

And walked in.

—Jane

Plagued by a myriad of acute and chronic ailments, I marched myself faithfully to the doctors for years. Despite the fact that they were, for the most part, good and caring doctors, my ailments persisted; and all I was able to do was to use the treatment provided by the doctors, which worked as a Band-Aid, and go on.

It was quite by accident, or so I thought, that I stumbled on spirit releasement and past life regression therapy. I felt a strong need, a drive, to find someone who could do this process for me. You've heard the expression, "This is the first day of the rest of your life." This saying took on a new dimension the day I met Dr. Modi.

I have always had a sixth sense about people. Nervous, excited, and emotional (I came to understand this emotional turmoil later), I entered Dr. Modi's office for the first time. She looked up from her desk, took one look at me, and asked, very solicitously, "Are you all right?" I thought my front was pretty good; I have always been good at hiding. But she saw clear through my assurances. From that moment, I knew I had come to the right person. Little did I know then just what a life-altering adventure I had begun and what a keenly perceptive, knowledgeable guide I had in Dr. Modi.

Dr. Modi led me gently through the processes of spirit releasement, explaining the concepts thoroughly beforehand. How reassuring it was to learn that so many of the feelings, problems, thoughts, and illnesses I had harbored were not mine alone. How exciting it was when, one by one, we released these unhappy souls and they happily left and took their problems with them.

Sickly as I had always been, I never felt I was a hypochondriac. Consequently, I never understood why it seemed I could never get well and stay well. Suddenly my problems began to leave with their proper owners. It seemed that all my acute presenting symptoms were spirit-owned, and as the entities left, so did the symptoms. And being a caring, nurturing, empathetic person, I was burdened with many of these entities.

When we moved into past life therapy, I began to find the clues to lifelong dreams as well as the answers to lifelong puzzles. I found places I have "seen" in dreams all my life. I found reasons for my fears and aversions, for recurring nightmares, and for certain of my personality characteristics and life patterns. I found not only the answers to many unanswered questions and healing for certain illnesses, but also the resolve and the courage to face some difficult changes I would never otherwise have been strong enough to make.

I also saw Satan and his demons firsthand! I watched as they pulled and tugged and manipulated my soul by holding soul parts and by using devices and other obstacles to interfere with my communication with God and cause me emotional, physical, and relationship problems.

I learned how easy it is for us to lose pieces of our souls, innocently enough, but lose them nevertheless in moments of weakness caused by strong emotions: fear, anger, grief, and even joy. Even though musicians toss out the idea of lovers sharing their souls, I found out how dangerous that notion can be, and that many of my problems were not really mine, but of those people whose soul parts I was harboring. When we lose those soul parts, we lay ourselves open, as darkness quickly takes over the empty spaces left by the lost soul parts.

I found angels. Do you know we have angels? And they are there at our bidding. Angels can do anything, as they are beings of the Light, untainted by mortal living. All we have to do is basically what our mothers taught us: say "Please" and "Thank you" and they will do anything for us.

I found heaven and met Jesus and God firsthand. What an unspeakable joy it is to know, really know, that God is always there, always loving, always concerned, and always on our side no matter what we do. God does not interfere with our free will but will help us if we ask. How reassuring it is to know that we are always connected to God through a silver cord that comes from God to our souls. That intangible, immortal essence that empowers and drives us—is our piece of the Divine. From God we came, and to God one day we all will return.

I found the kind of knowledge that makes a lifelong difference. Going to the Light (heaven) and viewing life as we know it from a heavenly perspective, rearranges one's priorities. Suddenly the little nagging worries in which we entangle ourselves seem unimportant. Knowing that God and the angels are always there to help us, we can go through our daily activities free from the stresses we cause ourselves through constant worry.

This has been a medical, psychological, and spiritual miracle for me. I have been freed of most of my psychological and physical problems. Thanks to Dr. Modi, I have been privileged to learn about healing, about living (and living again), about dying without fear, about Light (heaven), about what Elton John has so aptly termed "The Circle of Life." Dr. Modi's knowledge, persistence, courage, and steadfastness have made it possible for me to heal, to learn wonderful lessons, to place all my trust in God, and to live each day fully, free from fears and worries. Though I still occasionally fall into my old habits of "sweating the small stuff," it is never long before I catch myself. Now I realize that it is often due to the demonic influences, so I ask the angels to remove them, ask God for help, and get on with life.

Finally, I have learned that prayers are most important. God meant for us to communicate with Him through our silver cord, which is connected to God. God hears and answers all prayers. Although the answer is not always the one we were seeking, "there is a reason for that." I'd like to have a dollar for every time I heard Dr. Modi say that. I could probably start a nice little retirement fund.

It is comforting to know that God is there and he hears our prayers. Life is a long adventure, and this life is only one stop along the way and death is but another door to pass through. I was raised a Christian, and a Christian I remain. This experience has strengthened my faith in God, in Light, in Jesus, in angels, in love, and in the innate goodness that is at the center of us all.

Thank you, Dr. Modi, for transforming my life.

Jane

Chapter I

Introduction

Introduction

The Beginning

When I was doing my psychiatric residency, there were times when I felt very discouraged because there was no single treatment which worked for every patient. Medication works, but not in every patient; and it can make some patients more dysfunctional because of the side effects. Traditional talk therapy helps only a small percentage of patients. I saw patients who suffered for years, going from doctor to doctor and from hospital to hospital, searching for relief from their symptoms.

During my residency, I strived to learn different types of available treatment methods. I learned individual psychotherapy, family therapy, group therapy, psychodrama, transactional analysis, hypnosis, and hypnotherapy so I could use these various techniques with different patients to suit their needs for healing.

Medication, in some cases, does correct the chemical imbalance in the brain; in other cases, however, it just pushes the problems back into the subconscious and covers them up. The patient feels better temporarily but the problems continue to surface. More and more medication is required over a long period, restricting patients' day-to-day functioning. In some cases, patients become addicted to these medications, creating additional problems.

With talk therapy, whether individual, family, or group, patients deal with only the conscious mind. They relate to the reasons of which they are aware, consciously and intellectually. As a result, months and years of talk therapy can work to some extent, but this is only a Band-Aid approach. The problems keep recurring.

Traditional talk therapy has its successes; it also has its failures. Unfortunately, the number of failures in any given period far exceeds the number of successes. Even when augmented by psychotropic medications, the success rate of traditional talk therapy remains low.

Dismayed by the lack of success of traditional talk therapies, I decided to utilize other techniques, especially hypnotherapy, in combination with the traditional talk therapies. Hypnosis allows patients to uncover the underlying subconscious reasons for their emotional and physical problems. The unresolved problems are brought from the subconscious mind to the conscious mind. By recalling, reliving, releasing, understanding, and resolving the unresolved traumas and issues, patients can be freed from their longstanding problems in just a few sessions. Very little or no medication is required and the time involved is relatively short. I have used hypnosis effectively for insomnia, anxiety, habit control, pain control, positive suggestions for day-to-day functioning, and in hypnotherapy to uncover the underlying problems to help people.

Over the years of my psychiatric practice, I always felt good about the quality of my work and the results I had with my patients. I was able to help people with combinations of treatment modalities depending on the patients' needs. But still, at times, there were patients for whom I could not do much except use medications and supportive psychotherapy. I continued to search for ways to help my patients.

My Accidental Discovery of a Past Life

About eleven years ago, I saw **Martha**, a thirty-four-year-old housewife and mother of three children who was suffering from a longstanding claustrophobia, which crippled her daily life. The problem was getting worse and as a result she was becoming severely depressed and at times suicidal.

She had severe panic attacks, several times a day, every day. During these panic attacks she had difficulty breathing, palpitations, dizziness, feelings of intense fear and apprehension, and fear of dying. I began to treat her with medication and traditional talk therapy. These helped her to some extent, but her claustro-phobia and panic attacks continued.

During a session, I asked her about the last time she had a panic attack. All of a sudden she became anxious and said, "Doctor, I am having one right now," and she started to gasp for breath.

I asked her to close her eyes, focus on her emotional and physical feelings, and allow those feelings to take her back to another time, to the source of her problems when she felt the same way. Martha slipped into a self-induced trance state. I thought she would probably remember a childhood incident when she was being locked in a closet, attic, bathroom, or other small room from where she could not get out.

Instead, she said she was in a different time, different life, and in a different body as a young girl. "I am in a coffin," Martha cried. "They think I am dead! They are closing the lid. I am afraid to die but what if they close the lid of the coffin and I do not die? Then what am I going to do?"

I was taken by complete surprise, but I let her continue the story and release the emotions associated with it. When she came out of this self-induced trance, she looked puzzled but relaxed. I did not know what to make of that session. To my surprise, her panic attacks disappeared right after the session. In the next session she reported that she was free of her crippling claustro-phobia, depression, and panic attacks.

I was pleasantly surprised. I had not had such a miraculous result before. Many thoughts went through my mind. I wondered if any other psychiatrist or psychologist had similar occurrences where a patient spontaneously regressed to a past life and had such dramatic results.

None of my patients had ever before regressed to another life. I had heard of an accidental regression into a past life during a hypnosis conference and had seen a person being regressed to a past life on TV. I found the concept interesting, but I had not thought of utilizing it in the treatment of my patients.

I was impressed with Martha's cure. I started to search for literature on the subject of past life regression. To my surprise, there were many books written on the subject. There were many psychologists, psychotherapists, hypnotherapists, and a few psychiatrists who were using what they called "Past Life Regression Therapy."

I was upset with myself, thinking, "Where was I all this time? Why didn't I find out about it before?" I began to utilize this method in combination with other traditional therapies, often with fast and dramatic success in relieving patients' crippling symptoms.

What amazed me even more was that later, while working with other patients with claustrophobia, "being buried alive" is one of the most common themes presented by my patients and by recalling, reliving, releasing, and understanding the event, they were free of their symptoms too.

I realized that past life regression is an extension of age regression, only it takes the patient back into another life to a traumatic event that caused the problems in the current life.

Another patient, **Connie**, suffered from asthma. She also could not stand anything close to her neck. Under hypnosis, I asked her to move back in time to the source of her problems. She instantly found herself regressed to the time of her birth. The cord was wrapped around her neck and she could not breathe.

During the next session, Connie told me that her asthma was better but she still could not wear anything around her neck. I asked her, again under hypnosis, to go to the source of her problem and she found herself in another time and another life, when she was a man who was hanged. After releasing the emotions and the physical feelings associated with being hanged, she was completely free of her asthma and was able to wear necklaces and button her blouse all the way up to her neck.

I found that when I ask patients, under hypnosis, to "go to the source of the problem," they find themselves going to a trauma in the present life at a younger age or at the time of birth or in the womb. At other times they find themselves regressing to another time and another life. I realized that a person's subconscious mind often has the answers to his or her problems and if I allow the patient to recall, relive, release, and resolve it, he or she can be free of the symptoms.

This realization marked the beginning of an exciting journey, looking deep into the subconscious and seeking the reasons for mental illnesses. I began to understand that there are several sources of patients' problems, i.e., present-life traumas, including birth traumas and traumas in the womb, and also traumas from one or more past lives. The process is like an onion: we need to remove the reasons for the problems layer by layer.

My Discovery of the Earthbound Spirit (Entity)

After Martha was regressed into her past life to find the source of her claustrophobia, I began to use past life regression therapy effectively for treating patients with emotional and physical problems.

One day **Breana**, a fifty-year-old female, came to me for treatment of depression and chronic abdominal pains, which she had suffered off and on for several years. Her physical examination, laboratory tests, and gastroscopy were all normal. She wanted to try hypnotherapy to see what was causing her abdominal pain.

Under hypnosis, when I asked her to go back to the source of her abdominal pain, she found herself in another time and another life. When patients find themselves in another life, I usually ask for identifying information, such as the name, age, sex, what year it is, and what country they are in. When I asked Breana these questions she said, "I am a fifty-five-year-old white male, I live in Pittsburgh, and this is 1974."

I realized that this information could not be correct because Breana was fifty years old and was born before 1974. So it could not be her past life. I asked Breana to check again and see what was going on. She became emotional and said, "This is my father John. He died in 1974 of stomach cancer. His spirit is here with me and I can see him clearly." I was very surprised. While reading different literature on past life regression therapy, I had noticed Irene Hickman, D.O., mention in her book, *Mind Probe Hypno-*

sis, about the spirits of deceased people possessing her patient, but till now I had never come across one.

I was curious about why and how he came into Breana. So I asked him the following questions.

> **Dr. Modi:** "John, why are you here?"
>
> **John:** "I love my daughter. After my death, she was having problems so I came in to help her."
>
> **Dr. Modi:** "How have you helped her?"
>
> **John:** "Not much; she does not even know I am here. She is suffering with my stomach pain because I died of stomach cancer, but she thinks it is her pain."
>
> **Dr. Modi:** "Tell me, exactly how did you come in?"
>
> **John:** "After my body died, she was sad. I just came in to comfort her but then I couldn't leave her. I got stuck here."
>
> **Dr. Modi:** "Since you are here, look inside her, and tell me who else is there."
>
> **John:** "There are many people here inside her, but I do not know who they are."

Breana could not recognize them either. They were strangers. I wondered what to do with these spirits of different people in her. During past life regression therapy, my patients had often reported seeing angels and their departed loved ones in the bright white Light coming to help them after the death of their physical bodies. So I asked John to look up and tell me what he saw.

> **John** [surprised]: "I see a bright white Light filling the entire room and my deceased mother in it wearing a white flowing gown. She does not look sick or old as she was when she died. She is smiling and asking me to come with her. There are also many beautiful angels in the Light."

John and the spirits of other people who were inside Breana were sent into the Light with John's mother and angels, after saying goodbye to Breana. After the session, Breana and I were both surprised. Breana was very emotional about seeing her father and grandmother. On one hand, she was sad, but on the other hand she felt happy and at peace, knowing that they were really not dead and that they both were in heaven. Breana had no doubts whatsoever about what she saw during the session. She did not think that she was making it up.

During the next session, Breana reported that she was free of her longstanding depression and stomach problems. She recalled that her father had cancer of the stomach and he had been very depressed after he learned of it.

I was surprised to find that spirits of deceased people can come on board in patients and affect them physically and emotionally. Many questions ran through my mind. Breana's father and the other people in her: were they real or was she fantasizing about him because she missed him? Maybe this was her way of grieving and letting go of her father? But why the strangers? And if it was all her fantasy, then how was it that her longstanding depression and stomachache were completely relieved after that session?

If the spirits were real then why was it that none of my patients ever reported them before? Could it be there were spirits in other patients too, but we had not recognized them? I did not know. All I knew was that my patient was free of her longstanding symptoms in just one session, and that was good enough for me.

After that session, many of my patients, under hypnosis, reported having spirits of deceased people inside them. Some they knew and some they did not. Releasing the spirits released their emotional, mental, and physical symptoms in just a few sessions. Sometimes in just one or two hypnotherapy sessions patients' long standing psychological and physical symptoms started to disappear.

About one and one-half years after I began to work with these earthbound spirits, a psychologist, Edith Fiore, published a book, *The Unquiet Dead*, which had information and techniques similar to those given by my hypnotized patients.

I do not know whether these spirits are real or not, or if my patients' subconscious minds made up these fantastic stories. It really does not matter to me. All I know is that releasing these so-called spirits relieved my patients of their symptoms. As a psychiatrist working with patients who are suffering with their psychological and physical symptoms, results are more important than the proof.

My Accidental Discovery of the Demon Spirit (Entity)

A few months later, I was surprised and shocked when a patient under hypnosis told me that he had a demon inside his head. It would perhaps be logical for a person raised in the American culture to describe his problem as being demon-caused because of cultural and religious beliefs; but I was at a loss. How do you deal with a demon? The only exposure I had was through the movie *The Exorcist* and my patient was not acting and behaving like the character portrayed in that movie.

This patient, **Nick**, a thirty-five-year-old man, had a history of frequent migraine headaches since he was a teenager. He also described suffering from depression and chronic fatigue for several years. I explained to Nick about hypnotherapy and the different reasons my patients in the past have given for their physical and emotional problems, including the problems caused by the current and past life traumas and the earthbound spirits. Nick was willing to try it.

As we began the session, Nick started to experience severe headaches. I asked him to look inside his head and tell me what he saw. As Nick looked inside his head he said he saw nothing except darkness. As he continued to focus on the darkness inside his head, he said that it was kind of moving around and it looked like a black blob. I thought there might be an earthbound spirit in his head trying to hide, as I had found this phenomenon many times in the past with other patients. So I tried to communicate with the one who was moving in his head. The following is the transcript of what happened.

27

Entity in Nick's head: "I am a foul one. Why do you want to bother with me?"

Dr. Modi [in an effort to establish a dialogue with the entity]: "Tell me, are you a male or a female?"

Entity [arrogantly]: "Why would I want to be a human?"

Dr. Modi [surprised]: "What do you mean? If you are not human, then who are you?"

Entity [laughing arrogantly]: "I am a demon. I am a disciple of Satan. He is my master and he sent me to torture this person."

I was shocked and surprised. The only change I saw in Nick was a change in the tone of his voice and angry expressions and arrogance on his face. Nick normally spoke softly and was gentle and polite. At this point the only logical step, it seemed to me, was to continue the dialogue to find out more about this so-called demon.

Dr. Modi: "How old was Nick when you joined him?"

Entity: "Fifteen, when this dumb kid was using drugs. This opened him up and I came in."

Dr. Modi: "You said you are here to torture Nick. How did you torture him?"

Entity [laughing]: "Now lady, why do you think he is having the headaches? I am doing it. I also siphon his energy so he feels tired and drained all the time. I can create any type of problem for him. It is fun."

As this so-called demon talked more, Nick's headaches became worse. Nick stated that the whole room was filled with brilliant white Light and many angelic beings were there. He saw the angelic beings surrounding this black being, the so-called demon in his head, with the Light. The being was reacting very violently to the Light and screaming, "Take this Light away from me. It will destroy me; it will kill me."

Nick described the dark being like a fish in a net of Light struggling to get out. At this point Nick was holding his head because of the severe splitting headache he was experiencing.

Totally amazed at what was going on, I continued.

Dr. Modi: "What is happening?"

Entity [upset]: "This Light, it is burning me and now it will kill me. We are told by Satan never to go close to the Light because it is death. If Light does not kill me, Satan sure will, because I failed. [He sounded very scared and angry.] I do not want to fail. I do not want to be punished by Satan again."

Dr. Modi: "What do you mean by, 'you failed'?"

Entity: "We are not supposed to fail in our jobs. If we fail, then Satan punishes us by torturing us in a worse way."

Dr. Modi: "How did you fail?"

Entity: "You located me, which is considered failure by Satan, and now this Light!"

Nick described that the angels were pressing and squeezing the black entity with the Light and they were asking the entity to look inside itself. The entity, still struggling with the Light and squirming around in a helpless way, started to look inside itself and screamed, "What is it?"

Dr. Modi [not knowing what the entity was talking about]: "I don't know. You tell me what is happening."

Entity: "I see this star, this diamond of Light in me. How is it possible? I am a black, ugly thing. [scared] And now it is growing and consuming me. My darkness is disappearing. What is happening to me? Am I going to die? [silence] I look like them, the angels. I am all Light, but do not feel dead. [surprised and excited] I feel different. I feel good. I do not remember feeling this way before."

Nick watched in amazement and confirmed what was happening. As the entity looked inside itself and found the spark of Light, even Nick could see the Light in the black demon and said that as the Light grew, the darkness started to dissipate almost like magic until the entity totally changed into the Light. According to Nick, the entity looked like a being of pure Light, like an angel, after its transformation.

Not only the entity but Nick and I also were shocked and surprised while trying to absorb all that happened. Nick was even more surprised to realize that his splitting headache had vanished completely after the entity was transformed into the Light.

The Transformed demon described experiencing feelings of peace and joy that it never felt before. The being mentioned how Satan deceived and lied to it and all the other demons about the Light. It expressed sadness that it had caused damage to Nick and to humanity from the beginning of the time.

At this point, Nick said angels were saying that this transformed entity was a being of the Light and it needed to go back to the Light (heaven). Nick described how loving and accepting these angels were toward that transformed being. There was no judgment or condemnation from them. Before leaving, that transformed being apologized to Nick for causing all the problems and thanked me for helping it. Then Nick said that the angels took that being into the Light through a large gate which he believed was heaven.

He also saw angels cleansing, healing, and filling with the Light the space in his head where the demon was. The next week, Nick reported being free of depression and headaches and was feeling more energetic.

I did not know what to make of that session except that Nick was free of his headaches, chronic fatigue, and depression. Traditional psychotherapy and medication had not given this type of miraculous result before.

My mind was filled with many questions. Was that demon, which Nick described in his head, real or a figment of his imagination? Maybe his subconscious mind made up this fantastic story so he would not have to be responsible for his problems. But if it was just his fantasy or a figment of his imagination, how could this session totally cure his longstanding crippling headaches and depression? But then I realized that it did not matter. What really mattered was that Nick was free of his problems.

Later, I was even more surprised to find that other therapists discovered similar information and techniques with their patients and had similar results. It proved to be an extremely effective method in curing patients' psychological and physical problems.

My patients, under hypnosis, also reported that with the physical and emotional traumas, their souls fragmented into many pieces, causing the weakness of their souls and thus of their bodies, leading to different symptoms. These soul parts can remain in the body as an inner child or leave the body and go to different people and places. Locating and integrating these soul parts caused a great deal of improvement in their conditions.

Over the years, I have come to realize that the formal induction of hypnosis is not necessary for locating and releasing spirits. Some patients can just look inside and see, while with others, somatic and affect bridge techniques can help to locate an entity inside. Just by looking in and focusing on the entity or their feelings, patients slip into a self-induced state of hypnosis.

Over the years, different sources and reasons for patients' emotional and physical problems unfolded before me. I developed further insights into their treatment and prevention. I realized that neither the patient nor the therapist has to believe in past lives or spirits for the treatment to work. I found that we the psychiatrists and other mental health professionals have a limited understanding about the true nature and causes of mental illness. I learned to keep my mind open and continue to ask questions and stay away from providing my interpretations. I understand that the patient's subconscious mind not only has the knowledge of the reasons for his problems but can also provide solutions and even the healing.

After many years of receiving similar information over and over from a cross-section of my hypnotized patients, I felt compelled to write about this mind-bending knowledge. What you are about to read is by no means offered as proof of anything. You may believe or disbelieve what you read in this book—except for one thing: this approach to therapy works.

In this book, the words *possession* and *attachment* are used synonymously. Similarly, *spirit*, *entity*, and *soul* are used synonymously.

The word *Light* is used synonymously for *God*, for *heaven*, and for the *emanation of Light coming from heaven.*

The contents of this book make some startling revelations and may upset some readers. You may experience some physical and emotional reactions, anger, and difficulty in concentration while reading this book. In my experience, these are often the signs of having one or more spirits inside a person. My aim is not to cause any fear or to discourage you from reading this book. On the contrary, my aim is to educate you about these earthbound and demon spirits and explain to you that having them with you is not the end of your world. Releasing them is not difficult and can free people from their longstanding physical and psychological symptoms, sometimes in only a few sessions.

These symptoms are usually the problems of the possessing or attached spirits, which they experienced while they were living in their physical bodies; usually due to their death experiences. These problems are transferred over to their host, who in turn may begin to experience them.

According to my experience and my research, most of the acute psychological and psychosomatic symptoms for which patients are seeking help are due to these possessing spirits within them. These are not the patients' symptoms to begin with and no medication, psychotherapy, and medical treatment can permanently cure them. As long as these spirits remain within them, they will continue to suffer with their symptoms. Only by releasing these unwanted guest spirits can people be free of their debilitating symptoms. By reading this book, you can gain more knowledge about these spirits, how to free yourself from them, and how to remain free of them.

The subject of "demon spirits" is perhaps the most delicate in the book and potentially the most misunderstood. How many times have we said or heard the following phrases? "The Devil made me do it." "He is wrestling with his demons." "She acts like she's possessed." "He's behaving like a devil." What we view as mere figures of speech, my patients tell me, have a real basis in fact. There are truly dark forces, they say, which influence our emotions and our behavior, which we innocently assume as our own feelings and behavior. We all wrestle with demons quite often all our lives. According to my hypnotized patients, the things that are wrong with us mentally and physically, in our society, and in the world, are often caused by these dark spirits.

Releasing demon spirits is not a religious exercise. It does not require adherence to any specific religious belief or practice. It is not the traditional exorcism as it is practiced by the Roman Catholic Church.

Exorcism is a religious ritual marked by the forceful expulsion of a demon entity. It is confrontive, wrenching, and physically and emotionally exhausting to the exorcist and the subject. It directs judgment upon the entity itself, damning it and casting it out of the subject. It can be grabbed by Satan and punished brutally, it can go to another host, or it can return to the person from whom it was cast out.

Releasement, on the other hand, is practiced with compassion for the entity. The demon entity is treated as a secondary patient. My hypnotized patients report that demons are fallen angels, tricked and trapped by Satan, and are in intense pain. Releasement is practiced with care for that pain. While the therapist must sometimes take a firm stand in getting the entity to talk, to identify itself, at no time does the therapist make negative statements to the entity. There is no judgment by the therapist, by the patient, or ultimately by the beings of Light (heaven) to whom the demon returns after it is transformed into the Light.

The terms *Satan* and *demons* may offend or upset some readers. I personally like to call these beings "dark spirits," "dark beings," or "negative energies," because of their dark appearance and negative actions. But, because this book deals with the information given by my hypnotized patients as accurately as possible, it would be false and misleading to refer to these dark beings by my own labels. Instead, I address them as they are named by my patients consistently as "Satan" and "demons." None of the information written in this book is based on any religion or spirituality. It is based only on the information reported by my hypnotized patients.

It is important to clarify that having earthbound or demon spirits does not mean that a person is evil. Because of our human frailty, every one of us is open for possession and indeed may have been possessed at some point in our lives.

This book, when viewed with an open mind, can provide lay readers and professionals alike with an explanation of psychological and physical problems and human behavior. It will also give a profoundly expanded understanding of life in its broadest sense, which will impact the rest of your life. What you will read will dispel any fear of death, knowing that we really do not die with the death of the physical body. It can provide hope to those who are sick and in despair. It can change lives, rearrange priorities, and put "the details" of living in their proper perspective.

The material in the pages that follow is offered on two levels: as an exciting and inspirational piece of reading for the general public, and as a guide for other professionals to use in applying these techniques to their patients. Please read with an open mind.

Because the weight of this book rests upon the information my patients and I discovered together, I have used numerous case histories. I have taken extreme pains to protect the identity of my patients without changing the essence of their information.

I claim no ownership of any of this information. It is quite simply a condensation of information given to me through my hypnotized patients.

I have provided a glossary near the end of the book. Please read it first, so you can properly understand the information given in this book.

A forewarning: This book is not a technique manual. The techniques you are going to read about are simple but should not be treated lightly and are not to be used by lay people. Only trained health professionals should attempt to use them.

History of Mental Illness

Over the course of the recorded history of humanity, people have puzzled over the mysteries of mental illness. What accounts for diseases of the mind? What makes a seemingly "normal" person suddenly behave in strange ways?

The history of psychiatry reflects a backward movement. Primitive practitioners, shamans, and medicine men had a better concept of what really causes mental illness. Over the years psychiatrists have wandered down countless blind alleys, looking for other more "worldly" answers, mostly as a result of societal pressures and beliefs.

The purpose of this book is to examine that history briefly and then to present evidence that, just in recent years, psychiatrists and other mental health professionals have begun to come full circle, back to the understandings of their early counterparts.

In early times, during the pre-Christian era, people believed that mental illness was caused by one of three phenomena: (1) acting against one's nature, (2) possession by evil spirits, or (3) divine madness, imposed by the gods as either a punishment or a protection. Later, some practitioners recognized that physical disease might account for mental disorders to some extent. Senile dementia and character disorders were isolated as causes of aberrant behavior.

A look at some specific beliefs and practices will show how psychiatry developed, got sidetracked, and finally found its way back to the idea that the psyche is spiritual and that restoring mental health is largely a matter of healing the spirit within.

Acting against One's Nature

In earlier times, people believed that they were created directly from God. As pieces of God, people believed, they were given good and loving souls. What went against basic human nature was doing things that were not good and loving. In this context, Plato, in *The Republic* (c. 400 B.C.), described "madness" as a state in which the wanting soul loses the thinking soul. When this happens, people act against their rational nature.[1]

35

In the second century A.D., Galen determined that the health of the soul depended on the harmony of the rational, irrational, and lustful parts of the human soul. Wrongful acts committed for personal gain cause in one's nature an imbalance that is hard to correct and eventually leads to mental illness.[2]

In the fifteenth century, Henry Kramer and James Sprenger, Dominican monks, designated witchcraft as "unnatural" behavior and considered it to be the most dangerous kind of mental illness. They advocated keeping "witches" away from others, and recommended killing those most feared.[3]

During the late 1700s, psychiatry became recognized as a field of medicine. The German physician George Stahl first identified the function of the soul in maintaining health. He divided mental illness into those types with a physical and organic basis and those that are caused by inhibiting the soul's functioning. This latter category, animism, which accounts for most mental illness, became widely accepted in the eighteenth century.

At about this time, psychiatry took a turn—not, however, for the better. Those suffering from mental illness were all classified as "morally unfit, physically intemperate, and greedy." As a result, mental illness then became a punishable crime.

Possession by Evil Spirits

The earliest evidence of the need to deal with spirits is the work of the shamans, primitive medicine men. The function of the shaman was to conduct a cleansing séance for mentally disturbed people. This involved inducing a trance state within the shaman through the use of music, smoke, and certain herbs and drinks. Then the patient would confess sins or request that certain problems be removed, and the shaman would free those afflicted by removing evil spirits. Through the shamans, spirits spoke. Shamans were especially vulnerable to possession by the spirits who spoke through them. Individuals who became shamans possessed what we refer to today as psychic ability. They practiced healing by spirit releasement and reclaiming the lost soul parts.[4]

Later, the medicine man emerged as the community mental health agent. Like the shaman of primitive times, the medicine man used prayers, herbs, drinks, and music to induce the spiritual awareness that was necessary to ward off evil spirits and heal. The emphasis was on communication between the medicine man and spirits who invaded people.

The earliest beliefs in primitive cultures were based in the influence of the spirits of ancestors. The standard treatment for mental illness was trepanation, or drilling holes in the skull so the evil spirits could escape.[5] Greek and Roman cultures believed that mania was the result of possession by evil spirits who represented the "cult of the dead."[6]

Witchcraft, born innocently enough in the early Middle Ages when women met by night to worship the goddess Diana, was denounced in 1147 by the Church of England. The Church felt that these were meetings of "deranged minds" who worshiped the Devil.[7] During the time of the Spanish Inquisition, people who were delusional or hallucinating were feared, imprisoned, viewed as vixen intent on destroying men, and ultimately put to death. While witches were feared and punished throughout the Middle Ages and into the time of the Inquisition, they were also regarded as capable of spiritual healing. They were identified as people with special psychic wisdom and power. They used potions and elixirs made from animal parts, herbs, and barks. These were given as a part of a special ceremony to a suffering person. Throughout this time, people could not deny the spiritual awareness and power of these misunderstood practitioners. Aside from ancient cultures, Thomas Sydenham, in the seventeenth century, was the earliest to actually attribute mental illness to spirit possession. He held that hysteria was caused by "disturbed animal spirits." Thomas Willis followed him by adding that female hysteria was also caused by disturbed animal spirits, instead of a "wandering uterus" as had been previously thought.[8]

Divine Madness—Blessing or Burden?

Plato was the earliest to describe divine, or poetic, madness. This was not meant to be a punishment by the gods, but a gift with an attached purpose, mainly to enhance creativity. Beyond this, however, many others defined madness as a natural consequence of angering the gods. As far back as the book of Deuteronomy in the Old Testament, we read that "God will punish those who violate his commands with madness, blindness, and astonishment of the heart," which translates to mania, dementia, and stupor.[9]

The Greeks and Romans believed that dementia was caused by supernatural phenomena at the hands of gods and goddesses. They also believed that the gods caused dreams in order to communicate with the dreamer. The Arabs, on the other hand, felt that the insane were loved by God and sent to tell the truth. In that culture, they were worshiped as saints.[10]

Throughout the ages people have believed that the human psyche is eternally linked by its soul to its creator. Understanding and seeing the relationship between that soul and its creator holds the key to mental health, mental illness, and the continuum of emotions between. People have recognized the fact that the human body is powered by the spirit. When the spirit is threatened, the individual responds in fearful and unnatural ways. It seemed, in those earlier times, spiritual healing was the logical answer.

But let's see what happened . . .

Current Theories of Mental Illness

At the dawn of the nineteenth century, psychiatry turned its attention toward the physical and social aspects of mental illness. Inevitably, psychiatry moved outside the person to look for causes. A social illness? A community epidemic? A public scourge? Care of the "insane" became a cause, focused on "caretaking" rather than treatment. Moral issues became a concern. Care of the mentally ill became a moral cause worldwide.[11]

In asylums everywhere, the focus on treatment of mental disease rested in physical measures. In America in the eighteenth and nineteenth centuries, purgatives, emetics, and bloodletting were believed to rid the patient's body of poisonous humors that affected mental functioning.[12] Tranquilizers soon became popular as they quieted restlessness and agitation, masking patient symptoms and creating the illusion of "wellness."

In the late nineteenth century, psychiatrists began to ascribe mental illness to mental degeneration. The French psychiatrist Morel stated that this degeneration became worse as it passed through generations. Building on this concept, another French practitioner, Magnan, explained that alcoholism, obsessive-compulsive behavior, and delusions were also results of degeneration.

But it was the work of Sigmund Freud—his studies of childhood development and resulting sexual behaviors—that set the stage for the development of psychiatry and psychoanalysis in the twentieth century. Using the unconscious to investigate and treat mental illness, Freud widened the gap between psychological and organic approaches to mental illness. Freud's interpretation of dreams, his later studies of the elements of the conscious personality—the ego, id, and superego—and his studies of defense mechanisms and of life and death instincts have made him the most influential psychiatrist in the history of psychiatry to date.

The 1930s saw the introduction of electroshock therapy. Both insulin shock therapy and electroshock therapy were introduced in Europe for treatment of schizophrenic and manic-depressive patients. Along with these therapies came a host of psychotherapeutic drugs designed to alleviate or mask the symptoms of a variety of mental illnesses.

Thus began an era of chemical therapy. For many years now the primary treatment of psychiatric illness has been based on medication. This approach creates a problem: masking the symptoms does not get at the source of the problem, and it gives the patient a false sense of wellness.

Prefrontal lobotomy, a type of psychosurgery, became a widely used technique for actively psychotic patients who did not respond positively to shock therapy. While it proved an effective measure for some patients, in others it produced irreversible brain deterioration.

Community psychiatry as defined by Adolf Meyer in 1957 described mental illness as the result of a person's maladaptation to the environment. His beliefs, based upon Kurt Lewin's concept of the person interacting with the environment, stated that when behavior was "out of synch" with the social structure, mental illness was the result.

Current theories hold that social and physical factors contribute to one's predisposition to mental illness, as well as the onset and persistence of the disease. One's inability to deal effectively with environmental stress has been attributed to social factors. A holistic or total approach to traditional psychiatry includes these psychological and social factors.

Psychosomatic illness is considered to be a major contributor to a variety of mental illnesses. Even though these symptoms manifest themselves in a variety of gastrointestinal, cardiovascular, respiratory, musculoskeletal, and skin disorders, the underlying causes are more subtle. Stress, anxiety, depression, and obsessive-compulsive behaviors are some of the more common causes of psychosomatic illness. The extensive study of general paresis, a disease marked by psychological and physical deterioration, further strengthened the notion that mental illness has a clear organic base.

Biochemistry has emerged as a partial explanation for certain mental illnesses. The identity of several neurohumors, or chemicals that affect the brain, have become associated with schizo-phrenia and certain types of depression. Treatment with medi-cations believed to restore balance to the brain is focused on hopefully restoring the brain to "normal."

Brain imaging permits a detailed analysis of brain tissues that may be associated with certain disorders. New microscopic and x-ray techniques are currently popular in evaluating brain function. Trans-lating brain function into visual images or numerical printouts, brain imaging permits the clinical investigator to study the whole brain, looking at the total function rather than at isolated parts.[13]

Purely structural brain imaging is done by CT screening. Other brain imaging detects some aspects of structure and func-tion. Magnetic resonance imaging (MRI) is the most commonly known of these techniques.[14]

The primary use of brain imaging in psychiatry is to rule out organic brain disorders (tumors, blood vessels) in the diagnostic phase of treatment. Research has, however, shown through CT scan studies of schizophrenic patients that there is conclusive organic cause in that disease.[15] The importance of these tech-niques is that they can provide detailed evidence of brain func-tion/dysfunction, which in time may permit researchers to establish links between certain mental illnesses and the brain. To date, little basis for mental illness has been found in organic research for most mental illness. Psychiatrists still grope for answers to effective treatment.

Through time, practitioners have tried everything in an at-tempt to heal their patients. Psychiatrists have gone through a range of vain attempts, from ancient times to modern, to find answers in psychiatric treatment. They have drilled holes in skulls, performed surgery to literally destroy frontal brain tissue, used shock therapy, insulin therapy, nutrition therapy, and chemical therapy. In all these attempts, psychiatrists have met with little true success. At best, they have masked symptoms, giving patients a false sense of well-being that goes away with the therapy.

Where do we mental health professionals stand in our quest for a cure for mental illness? Where we stand is back at the door of those early practitioners, those "medicine men," and those "shamans" who possessed a measure of understanding, which today's mental health professionals are just beginning to reclaim. The human psyche is not a physical entity; it is a spiritual manifestation of our soul's connection to "the source." Whether we refer to that source as God, Allah, Buddha, Shiva, Mohammed, Jesus Christ, Messiah, or Jehovah is not the issue. The issue is simple: we are all souls (spirits), pieces of our creator, on a journey through eternity.

And what is the goal? Consistently, my patients affirm one thing: our destiny is with Our Creator and our longing is to return to Him. Understanding this, we can understand how treating mental illness—feelings of loneliness, despair, isolation—must be a spiritual, soul-restoring process. The early shamans and medicine men understood this. Humans are spiritual beings; we can operate on them and remove their stomachs, their hearts, their kidneys. We cannot, however, remove their spirit. Organs cease to function; bodies die; but the spirit, the soul, lives on. It is eternal, and it is linked to its creator.

In recent years, some psychiatrists, psychologists, and other mental health professionals have "happened upon" evidence that tells them it is time to return to the age-old practice of dealing with the spiritual essence of patients. And they are finding, through regression of patients, that our psychological problems are based in the "history of our souls," both in this life and in past lives. In dealing with this spiritual side of patients, psychiatrists, psychologists, and psychotherapists are finding not only lasting cures for mental and physical illness, but so much more.

That is the subject of this book. Please read with an open mind. The time has come for people to face themselves spiritually, a task that through time has met with fear and mistrust. What you will find in the pages that follow will not only calm your fears and erase your mistrust, but bring you a wellspring of hope and understanding that can change the course of your life.

A New Theory of Mental Illness

Consistent experiences with my hypnotized patients have fostered my understanding that mental illness can be attributed to several sources that include:

- Current life traumas including prenatal and birth traumas
- Past life traumas
- Possession or attachment by earthbound spirits
- Possession or attachment by demon spirits
- Soul fragmentation and soul loss

The theory of mental illness that I present here is not derived from any existing psychiatric theory nor from any of my personally held beliefs. These new insights are based solely on what my patients have told me consistently under hypnosis. The approach is unique because the hypnotized patients tell what is wrong and also provide the reasons for their problems, which range from current life traumas, including the prenatal and birth traumas, and problems carried over from past lives to possession by earthbound and demon spirits and soul fragmentation and soul loss.

Current Life Traumas Including Prenatal and Birth Traumas

In psychiatry, current life traumas from early childhood are well recognized as a source of mental illness. As a result, this cause will not be covered in this book, permitting me to discuss other causes of mental illness in detail.

During the sessions with my hypnotized patients, I have found that another source of mental illness finds its roots in prenatal and birth traumas. The experiences of the fetus are far more dynamic and penetrating than we ever suspected. The scars the fetus sustains in the prenatal months and during birth carry over later in life.

The fetus in the womb tunes in to its mother's emotional, mental, and physical feelings and accepts them as its own. It listens to its mother's interactions with others, and even if it does not understand her language, it still picks up on the emotional content of the exchange. The physical shock and trauma of the birth process can also create multiple physical, emotional, and personality problems later in life. The baby, upon its birth, feels rejected and cast out into a cold world from the warmth and security of the womb.

I find problems and feelings of separation anxiety, rejection, inferiority, inadequacy, anger, remorse, loneliness, depression, fear, panic attacks, paranoia, claustrophobia, headaches, asthma, and sinus problems can stem from prenatal and birth traumas.

To heal the patients of these problems, we need to help them in recalling, releasing, understanding, and resolving these prenatal and birth traumas.

Past Life Traumas

It would seem that one must believe in the theory of reincarnation to accept past life trauma as a cause for mental illness. Interestingly, it does not require that the patient or the therapist believe in reincarnation or past lives for this therapy to be effective. The only requirement is that the patient be willing to go through the experiences provided by the subconscious mind to resolve the symptoms and problems.

During therapy, when directed to focus on a symptom to find its source, the patient frequently is led to another life, in another body at an earlier time. The patient spontaneously regresses to an event that appears to be the cause of that symptom. When that past life problem is treated and resolved, usually the symptom is much improved or completely relieved.

Symptoms that have been traced to past life origins are many and varied. Sometimes the cause is found in more than one lifetime. Usually psychosomatic conditions, autoimmune disorders, and deep-seated personality disorders have their origins in one or more past lives. Typical symptoms that come from past lives are as follows:

Depression and anxiety disorders	Head and neck pain
Fears and phobias	Back pain
Premenstrual symptoms (PMS)	Arthritis
Sexual disorders	Fibromyositis
Eating disorders	Other aches and pains
Personality disorders	Skin conditions
Perfectionism	Sinus problems
Passive-aggressive personality	Asthma
Obsessive-compulsive personality	Allergies, etc.

Attachment or Possession by Earthbound Spirits

I was greatly surprised when a past life of a patient during regression turned out to be the life of the spirit of a deceased person who was the patient's father. Since that first occasion, several patients have reported finding inside them another spirit, a human soul separate and distinct from their own soul. This soul is reported by the patients to be a visitor or, as we say, an attached or possessing earthbound spirit who did not make its transition to the Light (heaven) after the death of its physical body and has remained on the earth plane.

The hypnotized patients report that the visiting or possessing spirits are influencing them and causing them problems, either intentionally or unintentionally. Before there can be any resolution of the patients' symptoms and problems, all possessing earthbound spirits must be treated and released from the patients.

This approach is not in keeping with the psychiatric tradition and definitely is not part of my training. This information also is not based on my beliefs or personal experiences, but solely on the experiences reported by my patients while under hypnosis.

The guest entities found within my patients can usually be conversed with. They speak through the patient with the patient's permission. Many of the visiting spirits report being attracted to my patients and admit that they joined the patients while they were physically or mentally debilitated after an accident, during a surgery, after a loss, or while they were under the influence of drugs and alcohol.

Several patients reported that a spirit was with them for more than one lifetime, while others said that the earthbound spirit had been originally with another family member before it joined them. Sometimes my patients reported that their possessing human spirit has other human and demon spirits inside it who came on board with it.

Frequently, the spirits' experiences are seen by the patients as part of their own current or past experiences. The experiences of the possessing spirits frequently cause physical and emotional problems for the patients. Usually it is a possessing spirit's death experience and its cause that contribute to the patient's problem. Possessing spirits' thoughts, experiences, and voices can be very distressing to patients, who think they are insane because they hear and react to these thoughts and voices.

Possession or Attachment by Demon Spirits

My hypnotized patients not only report having possessing human spirits inside their bodies, but also report finding black, gray, or red entities that they say are demons. These demon spirits can also be conversed with through the patients' vocal cords, with the patients' permission and cooperation.

My patients vividly describe the power of Satan and his demons to inflict misery upon the human race. Based on the results of my treatments, it seems that these demon entities are frequently the cause of many emotional, mental, and physical problems. According to my patients, these possessing demon spirits are the single leading cause of psychiatric problems, especially depression and its associated cluster of problems. Demon spirits have a greater influence in patients' lives than any of the previously mentioned causes.

Many people have a preconception of what demon possession is like, based upon their religious beliefs and their experiences with the entertainment media. Many of my patients find it hard to believe that they are being influenced by demon beings even though they themselves report such influence.

These possessing demon spirits, speaking through the patients, provide reasons for their presence and tell how they have affected the patients. Frequently they reveal facts about patients' lives and plans. Some possessing demon spirits claim to have been with the patients since birth, before birth, or even from previous lives. Some patients also report that their possessing human spirits are also possessed by demon spirits and other human spirits.

Some patients have revealed that their possessing demon spirits have a part of their soul or another human soul trapped inside of them. Patients have reported possession by as few as one and as many as hundreds of demon spirits.

Patients consistently claim that these demon spirits have great powers, but with the help of God and his angels the patients are more powerful than Satan and his demons, and are capable of controlling them. Patients often report that Satan and his demons have only as much power as we give them and that Satan and his demons operate within limitations. This concept is in contrast to what most people believe.

None of this information is based on any religion. During the treatment, only what my patients report under hypnosis is taken as evidence. No spiritual claims or suppositions are made. Their information is usually dealt with in a very straightforward, down-to-earth manner with no religious or spiritual implication or association.

Soul Fragmentation and Soul Loss

My hypnotized patients consistently report seeing their souls in their chest, neck, or head. They describe *soul* as an immortal energy essence, a part of God, which resides in each of us. It empowers the body, which cannot live without it. At the time of death, the body dies, but the soul continues to survive.

During the therapy, sometimes patients were resistant to spirit releasement and past life regression therapies. As we searched for reasons for their resistance, they reported that their souls were fragmented due to some trauma. The soul fragments can stay inside the patient and appear as the patient at a younger age when the trauma occurred that caused the fragmentation or they can go outside the body.

My patients describe the soul fragments as similar to what we call sub-personality, alter personality, or an inner child in traditional psychiatry. However, there is a difference. The patients report that this fragment is not just symbolic or their imagination. They report literally seeing their child parts or personalities clearly inside them, including their age, clothing, and hair styles. Each fragmented soul part is still suffering from the memories and emotions of the trauma that caused its fragmentation and separation from the main body of the soul. Some patients report that the fragmented soul part or inner child is being controlled by the possessing earthbound or demon spirits. This relationship creates problems during the treatment.

Patients also report that portions of their souls are in the possession of other people. Husbands, wives, parents, children, and other relatives and friends are the most frequent possessors of the missing soul parts. Sometimes patients report their soul parts were in possession of people who abused them physically, emotionally, or sexually, causing them continued fear and emotional turmoil. In these cases, patients are influenced by the abusers' experiences, behavior, and problems.

Sometimes patients claim that some portions of their souls are in possession of Satan and his demons, who are outside and continue to reinforce their influence and manipulate patients' thinking, attitudes, behavior, and emotional and physical problems through these captive soul parts.

Patients frequently report they have possession of other living people's soul parts. These soul parts of living people act in the same way as a possessing spirit of a deceased human being and influence patients physically, emotionally, and mentally.

Treatment is usually stalemate and is less effective until these soul parts are returned, cleansed, healed, and integrated with their rightful owners. This is particularly true in the cases where Satan or his demons are the possessors of patients' soul parts.

By recognizing all these possibilities, we can clearly understand that any emotional, mental, or physical disease is in fact the disease of the soul. To heal the mind and the body, we need to heal the soul by removing all the possessing earthbound and demon spirits and soul parts of the living people. Then we need to heal the traumas from the current and past lives by recalling, reliving, releasing, and resolving them and reclaiming all the lost soul parts from the current and past lives and integrating them with the main body of the soul. By healing the soul we can heal the physical body from its emotional, mental, and physical problems.

None of this theory is based on any religion or spirituality. It is based on the information given by patients, under hypnosis. If the patient has a basis in religion and spirituality, that basis may of course influence what the patient's subconscious is telling us. No claims are made for the accuracy of the religious or spiritual information provided by the patients.

Whether or not these patient accounts are "true" is not the issue. You may view them as the patients' creative subconscious being extraordinarily inventive in creating explanations for their problems, you may consider them as incredibly vivid and realistic psychodramas tailored to the patients' specific needs, or you may think, if you choose, in terms of patients being accurate reporters giving literal accounts of the events of their lives.

It does not matter what explanation you believe. What does matter is simple: these therapies work. Patients are freed from their crippling symptoms. As a physician and a psychiatrist, I am satisfied with the dramatic results regardless of the explanation. I have sometimes seen a 100% improvement, a complete cure, of both physical and emotional problems in a single hypnotherapy session: a success rate that is far beyond the usual standard for psychiatry.

Protection Prayer

All You Have To Do Is Ask

And the angels watched me their aspect all concern
For others had fallen to the delusion

And they danced about me, singing
"Fear not. We are always near

"All you have to do is call for us,
Only ask, and we are yours."

—Jane

As I began to recognize, locate, and release human and demon spirits from my patients, I realized that just by being human we are all open for spirit attachment. I began to wonder about how we can protect ourselves. During a session of releasing spirits, a patient, **Mona,** saw the whole room filled with bright white Light and a large angel with wings and loving eyes in it.

According to Mona, the angel said that his name was Gabriel and he could answer our questions. In the past, while working with different patients under hypnosis, I realized it was also possible to converse with the angels and other Light beings through the patients with the patients' permission. Since many of my patients reported seeing angels who helped us while we were releasing spirits, I asked angel Gabriel who he was and about angels and who they are.

> **Gabriel**: "I am an archangel. We angels are spiritual beings of the Light and we have never been human. Our job is to defend the earth and protect and guard human beings. We are as real in the invisible world as you are in the visible world."

Wondering about Satan and his demons, which many of my patients reported, I asked angel Gabriel whether they are real or not and who they are.

> **Gabriel**: "Yes, they are real. They are also spiritual beings like us, but they are of very negative energy. They have been lost in the soul of the earth. They are the lost souls, as you have been told, and as your work is leading you, you will detect more and more.
>
> "You need to treat them as patients and you need to help them to see the Light within them, as opposed to perhaps allowing your patient in the chair to be frightened or to remain powerless. These demons can cause different types of physical, mental, emotional, and other problems for humans. All psychiatrists and other physicians, therapists, and other health professionals should pray for protection and guidance regularly every day because they do not know what they are dealing with."

I then asked how we can protect ourselves from human and demon spirits and their influences.

> **Gabriel**: "Protection techniques are partly a matter of faith, partly a matter of belief, and partly a matter of will. Protection can be invoked in many ways. The first and the most important and basic of the protection techniques is prayer. Pray to God to cleanse, heal, shield, protect, illuminate, guide, enlighten, balance, transform, and bless you. Turning the mind to God and the Light provides the first layer of defense and shielding against the demonic attacks. The mind that is turned to God and the Light will eliminate half of the possible demonic attacks." He continued, "The next important form of protection is to form an intent not to be possessed and influenced by Satan and his demons and to reject all their works and everything that

is evil and dark. Also, to form an intent to accept the work of God and achieve God's purposes, by dedicating your life to God.

"When you dedicate your life to God and God's purposes, it establishes a strong connection and constant communication back and forth between you and God. That means you will always be in the Light.

"Now it will not mean that every action will be a correct action or every thought a correct thought. But it will establish that what is good or done well literally serves as an act of worship to God and gains benefit for the person.

"You should also pray for your family members, friends, coworkers, and other people you care for and even for people with whom you have problems. When everybody around you is free of negative influences and is protected, you can live in peace and harmony with each other. Also remember to pray for protection for your surroundings, such as your homes, workplaces, and cars."

Based on what different Light beings have suggested about how to pray for protection, I have prepared the following protection prayer, which my patients and I found very effective in protecting us from the negative entities, energies, and influences. It should be used every night before sleeping and in the morning upon waking.

Protection Prayer

"I pray to God to please cleanse, heal, shield, illuminate, and protect me, all my family members, friends, coworkers, and all our surroundings such as our homes, workplaces, cars, and everything in them and miles and miles around them, from Satan and all of his demons, all human beings under Satan's influence, and all the negative energies and entities. Please fill, shield, and illuminate all of us and our surroundings with your Light and Love. Keep all of us and all our surroundings under your protection as long as our souls shall exist and balance us, transform us, enlighten us, bless us, and guide us in the right direction. Please keep us loving, giving, caring, forgiving, and humble all the time.

"I form an intent not to be possessed and influenced by any spirits and reject all the work of Satan and his demons. I also form an intent to accept the work of God and achieve God's purposes by dedicating my life to God and achieve my goals and purposes which I planned in heaven for this life."

These protection prayers and techniques will be explained in more detail in the later chapters.

Different Therapeutic Techniques

The following techniques are used to locate and treat different sources of emotional, mental, and physical problems, whether they are current life traumas including prenatal and birth traumas, past life traumas, possession by earthbound or demon spirits, or soul fragmentation and soul loss.

- Hypnosis
- Bridge techniques
  - Affect bridge technique
  - Somatic bridge technique
  - Linguistic bridge technique
  - Visual bridge technique
- Spontaneous recall
- Dreams

Hypnosis

History of Medical Hypnosis

If we look at the history of hypnosis, we find that since the time of the ancient Egyptians, there is a recurring theme: persecution of the practitioners. Although the use of hypnosis for healing has been successful through the centuries, people continue to fear what they do not fully understand. Despite the fact that when we cure through hypnosis, introducing nothing into the body, and the healing occurs, the persecution persists. Hypnosis has always endured and continues to endure a bad reputation, and those of us who use it pay a dear price in its defense.

The earliest users of hypnosis were the ancient Egyptians, who used it as "sleep therapy" to promote healing. It has also been practiced worldwide over countless years by shamans and medicine men of various tribes using drums, chants, and herbs to induce a trance state to heal people. Hypnosis in those days was disparaged as "voodoo art" and was appreciated only in the realm of the occult.

In the eighteenth century, however, physicians attempted to employ hypnosis as a viable treatment for illnesses that did not respond to more traditional approaches. One by one, they were ridiculed by their colleagues, stripped of their professional status, and thoroughly humiliated in spite of their success.

The earliest of these was Franz Anton Mesmer, an Austrian physician who practiced in Vienna in the eighteenth century. He achieved a great deal of success in practicing what he called "mesmerism" or "animal magnetism." He was investigated by a commission of the Royal Academy of Science and the Faculty of Medicine in Vienna and, in spite of his great success, was expelled from the medical society.

He moved to Paris in the late eighteenth century and again became very successful, using his methods to heal people by stroking the patients with his fingers to induce a trance state. Once again he was investigated by the Royal Commission of Science. They denounced his methods in spite of his success, claiming that his findings were only a product of his imagination.

Some years later, in the 1840s in England, John Elliotson, a surgeon who first introduced the use of the stethoscope, became interested in hypnosis or mesmerism, as it was called. He performed surgeries using hypnosis as the sole anesthetic. He was ridiculed by his colleagues in spite of his success.

Around the same time, James Esdaile, another Scottish surgeon, was working in India in a prison hospital. He successfully performed several hundred surgeries using only hypnosis for anesthesia. He was also professionally humiliated.

Dr. Parker and Dr. Ward were other physicians who also performed surgeries under hypno-anesthesia around the same time. They were also ridiculed by other doctors.

Dr. James Braid was a British physician who coined the terms *hypnosis* and *hypnotism* from the Greek word *hypnos*, meaning *sleep*. He used eye fixation and verbal suggestion. In spite of his success, his colleagues ridiculed him and called his work "Braidism's Artificial Insanity."

Once again the interest in hypnosis declined. Then Dr. Jean Martin Charcot of France authorized the use of hypnosis with hysterical patients in 1879. He classified hypnosis in three stages: lethargy, caused by muscle relaxation; catalepsy, when the limbs can be placed and will remain in any position; and somnambulism, the deepest level of hypnosis.

In about 1880 two French physicians, Bernheim and Liebault, revived the practice of hypnosis, using induction through verbal suggestions after the example of James Braid. Their collective successes caught the attention of a young Austrian physician, Sigmund Freud, who came to study their methods along with many others.

For a brief period, hypnosis enjoyed a measure of respect in Europe and America. But by the turn of the century, interest again diminished largely because Freud, who by that time was very famous, had abandoned its use. He was reportedly not a good hypnotist and had realized little success using the technique. He effectively criticized it for another twenty years.

After both world wars, psychologists and psychiatrists turned to hypnosis to treat battle fatigue since it proved to be a useful shortcut in dealing with this postcombat syndrome. Still, it was not applied in any other illnesses. It was saved by a few physicians who managed to keep very quiet about its use.

A breakthrough came in 1955, when the British Medical Association issued a report stating that hypnosis was a valuable medical tool. The association endorsed and encouraged medical schools to instruct students in its uses and techniques. The British Medical Association was followed by the American Medical Association, which officially sanctioned the use of hypnosis by physicians in 1958, and by the American Psychiatric Association in 1962.

Despite the fact that the official stamp of approval has been put on hypnosis by the governing medical societies, it continues to struggle for its rightful place among respected treatments for illnesses. People continue to fear what they cannot accept as a thoroughly scientific method.

Although hypnosis works time after time, resistance to its use, the failure of insurance providers to acknowledge its legitimacy, and a pervasive negative attitude toward it continue to hamper its use. As a result, many health professionals and their patients are being deprived of a technique that could succeed where others have failed.

It is time to lay the myths aside. It is time to recognize that the power to heal lies largely within that untapped portion of the human mind that is our subconscious mind.

Venture with me into that unexplored territory. Follow me into the case histories of my patients who, in their respective journeys into that region, have recovered and brought back treasures of knowledge and understanding.

Looking beneath the Surface: The Subconscious Mind

To understand hypnosis and how it works, we need to understand our conscious and subconscious minds. The conscious mind is the thinking, reasoning, and problem-solving part of our mind, which is also known as our left brain. It is the part of our mind that deals with our day-to-day functioning. It is the normal state of our awareness.

The subconscious mind functions at a deeper level than our conscious mind. Everything that has ever happened to us is recorded in our subconscious mind—from this life and all the other lives, from the beginning of time. No matter how important or unimportant, exciting or boring, traumatic or nontraumatic, happy or sad, nothing is erased. The unresolved traumatic memories from the current life and also from past lives can surface from our subconscious to our conscious mind in bits and pieces and can create emotional and physical problems because of their severity.

The subconscious mind is also the storehouse for the inner wisdom into which we all can tap. It is not restricted by time and space. According to my hypnotized patients, the subconscious mind in reality is our soul, which contains all the memories from the beginning of time.

Normally, our conscious mind or left brain is booked with our day-to-day thoughts and problems. It is busy, cluttered, and also constantly aware of everything that is happening around us. In this state we cannot bypass the conscious mind and get in touch with our subconscious mind, to give suggestions or retrieve information.

The goal of hypnosis is to relax and set aside our constantly chattering conscious mind and selectively block the peripheral awareness, by guiding patients to focus on their breathing and to relax different parts of their bodies. When the conscious mind is calm and quiet and not preoccupied by unnecessary thoughts, it is easy to bypass the conscious mind and get in touch with the subconscious mind. Here the conscious mind is not asleep or unconscious. It acts as a passive observer. It is always aware of what is happening during a session but does not interfere with its doubts, constant analysis, and interpretations. We achieve a similar state of focused concentration daily, normally and naturally, when we are absorbed in reading a book, watching a movie, listening to music, or daydreaming, as described later.

With this understanding, we can also see why traditional talk therapy works only as a Band-Aid approach and is slow and less effective. During talk therapy, we are dealing only with our conscious mind and knowledge, which is often superficial and based on intellectual interpretations, but it is really the subconscious mind that holds the understanding and knowledge about the real reasons for our current problems. By recalling, reliving, releasing, and resolving the problems under hypnosis, patients can be completely cured in a very short period.

In therapy, hypnosis can be used in two different ways:

Directive Approach: Here, after calming and setting aside the chattering conscious mind, the therapist bypasses the conscious mind and gives directly to the subconscious mind positive suggestions, which are effectively accepted by it. It is important to know that even at the deepest level of hypnosis a person will not accept any suggestions that are against his or her morals and ethics. Patients are free to accept or reject any suggestion they choose. This approach can be used for insomnia, anxiety states, fears, phobias, eating disorders and addictions, to produce analgesia and anesthesia, and to treat a variety of other conditions.

I usually make relaxation tapes for my patients with positive suggestions to suit their needs, which they can listen to every day at home so they require less or no medication. Usually these tapes work well and people feel better, but they are just a symptomatic treatment. What a tranquilizer, a sleeping pill, or a pain pill can do, a relaxation tape with positive suggestions can achieve in a motivated patient. But, just as these pills do not cure a problem, the relaxation techniques and tape relieve a problem temporarily but do not cure it.

Nondirective Approach: In this approach, instead of suggestions being given under hypnosis, the reasons for the problems are explored by asking the patients questions. Under hypnosis, I usually ask patients to go to the source of the problems. By getting in touch with their subconscious mind under hypnosis, patients can find not only the reasons for their problems, but also the solutions and even the healing. After recalling, reliving, and resolving the emotional, mental, and physical residue of the traumatic events, patients can be free of their problems. Hypnosis can bypass the conscious mind and tap and access information from the subconscious mind, which is the storehouse of all the memories, emotions, and knowledge.

Misconceptions about Hypnosis

The general public has many misconceptions and fears about hypnosis based upon what they understand from television, movies, and stage hypnosis. In order for people to benefit from the treatment, we need to dispel a number of these misconceptions. It is important for people to understand exactly what hypnosis is and what it is not. This understanding is important so they may enter into the experience free from fear and with the appropriate expectations. Let us look at some of these misconceptions.

In hypnosis people are asleep or unconscious: This is not true. All of us enter this state of focused concentration, or hypnosis, several times a day. For example, when we are so absorbed while watching a movie, listening to music, or reading a book that we lose track of time or awareness of our surroundings, we are in a hypnotic state. Students who study for several hours continuously and sometimes lose track of time are in fact utilizing this state of focused concentration or hypnosis.

Highway hypnosis is another example known to many of us. While driving we sometimes lose track of time and we wonder how we got to our destination, even when we were wide awake all the time. Similarly, while daydreaming we are focusing on a person, place, or an event. We are not concerned about our surroundings nor are we distracted by the events near us.

In all of these cases our concentration is focused on whatever we are doing and we are not asleep or unconscious. Other examples of hypnosis that we experience every day include the time just before we fall asleep and the beginning stage of waking up from a natural sleep in the morning.

Hypnosis occurs only when induced by a hypnotist: This statement is not true either. Every hypnosis is a self-hypnosis, just like the different examples of the daily hypnosis described above. We go in and out of the state of hypnosis several times a day without any formal induction. In therapy, a therapist is acting only as a guide in assisting the patient. It is the patient who controls the level of the trance and what happens during it.

A hypnotherapist has special powers: Not true. Hypnotherapists are ordinary individuals who are trained in using the tool of hypnosis in the therapeutic situation. They do not have any special powers.

Under hypnosis the subject reveals all: Another concern people have is that they will be totally under the control of the hypnotist and will end up revealing secrets they do not wish to reveal. This is not true. First of all, nobody can be hypnotized against their will. During hypnosis, the patients are in control of what happens and what is said and revealed during hypnosis. Nobody can make them say or do anything they do not want to. They cannot act against their ethical and moral codes. They can accept or reject the suggestions as they choose, and can come out of the hypnosis any time they desire.

Hypnosis is dangerous: As I have explained, it is a normal and natural focused state of mind, which we use several times a day. With a trained therapist, hypnosis can be used very effectively in treatment to find the source of problems, resolve them, and heal the patient.

Deep trance is necessary in therapy: Therapy can be done at any level of hypnosis, from light to medium or deep trance, with good results. I personally do not prefer to work in deep trance because people tend to have amnesia for the session. Although healing is achieved effectively, patients are not able to remember what happened during the session and therefore cannot integrate the knowledge and understand the reasons for their problem.

Hypnosis itself is the treatment: Hypnosis is only a tool that can be used in therapy. It allows us to uncover the source of the problems and heal them. Just the act of hypnosis can relax a person, but in itself it is not a therapy.

There are a variety of induction methods to achieve a state of hypnosis that differ from therapist to therapist and are a matter of individual preference.

Bridge Techniques

Here an intense emotion, physical sensation, words, phrases, or a vision can instantly bridge a present life conflict to a conflict in the past, from the current or a past life. While focusing on them, patients automatically shift into an altered state of consciousness and there is no need for a formal hypnotic induction. There are several types of bridge techniques:

- Affect bridge technique
- Somatic bridge technique
- Linguistic bridge technique
- Visual bridge technique

Affect Bridge Technique: An affect is a person's emotional feeling tone. During a session, if the patients are experiencing intense and sometimes exaggerated and inappropriate emotions, such as anger, fear, anxiety, sadness, etc., they are asked to focus on them and allow those emotions to take them back to another time, when they felt the same way. The emotions from present conflict can bridge to a past conflict in this life or in a past life. Here two different events are linked by a specific emotion. This is an emotional residue of an unresolved present or past life trauma that is carried over to the present time.

Brandy, a twenty-five-year-old female, was in treatment off and on for different symptoms. During one session, as she sat in the chair, she started to cry. She was sobbing so much that she could tell me only that her boyfriend was leaving and going back to California. I was surprised at the intensity of her feelings because she had told me before they were not getting along well and had decided to go their separate ways.

Since she was not able to speak much because of her crying and sobbing, I decided to use her intense emotions to find why she was having such a strong reaction to his leaving. I asked her to close her eyes and focus on her feelings about her boyfriend leaving and let those feelings take her back to another time when she felt the same way.

She instantly regressed to another life in Israel, when she and her boyfriend were husband and wife. He had suddenly drowned and died. She lived the rest of her life sad and lonely, missing her husband. When she came out of the trance she understood why she had such an intense sadness about her boyfriend leaving. Her crying and sobbing stopped right away and she felt calm and peaceful.

Somatic Bridge Technique: During a session, while describing the problem, if a patient is experiencing a physical sensation such as a pain, a numbness, a tightness, palpitations, or difficulty in breathing, the patient is asked to focus on those physical feelings and sensations and let those feelings lead to the source of the problem, to another time when the patient felt the same way. Those current physical feelings often link to the similar feelings in a present life or a past life trauma. It is a physical residue of an unresolved current life or a past life trauma, carried over into the present time.

William, a forty-year-old male, complained about tightness in his jaw and often found himself biting down. So I asked him to close his eyes and focus on those feelings and let the feelings in his jaws take him to the source of the problem.

William instantly regressed to a life as a twenty-two-year-old soldier in 1863, in the Civil War. His name was Benjamin and he was in a military hospital awaiting the amputation of his leg. The leg had been shattered by a cannonball. He was in pain and was feeling despairing, sad, and lonely. Two attendants took him to the operating table and put him on it. An attendant shoved a wooden object in his mouth and instructed him to bite down hard!

The purpose was to distract his attention from the pain in case ether did not work. Next, an ether-laden rag was placed on his nose and mouth area. Ben faded in and out of consciousness during the operation, once even seeing his spirit leave his body only to return immediately. Later he died at the age of thirty-five of an unrelated injury, feeling bitter and angry. William's symptoms were relieved after that session.

Linguistic Bridge Technique: As the patients describe their problems, certain words or phrases might be used over and over to describe emotional, physical, and other problems. In these cases, patients are asked to repeat them several times and allow those words and phrases to take them back to another time when they felt the same way. This process will often elicit a conflict or trauma from the current life or a past life that is carried over to the present time.

These phrases usually contain words such as "always," "never," "forever," etc. These are the mental residues, the unresolved decisions, conclusions, and promises made during a conflict, a trauma, or in death and dying in an earlier lifetime. The following are examples of this kind of phrasing:

"I will never be hungry again."
"I will never take this much responsibility ever again."
"I will always love you."
"I will always be there to take care of you."
"I will never make the same mistake again."
"I will never let anybody hurt me like that again."
"I will never tell people what they do not want to hear."
"I will never write again because it got me killed."
"I will never be poor again."

Blanche, a thirty-year-old female, came to me for multiple problems, including marital difficulties. During one session, she was very upset with her husband and while expressing her feelings she kept repeating the following phrases:

"He makes me feel like a kid."
"I am not good enough."
"I cannot do anything right."
"I want to run away from him."

I asked her to close her eyes and repeat those phrases and let them take her to another time when she felt the same way. She instantly regressed to a life in England, where she was a sixteen-year-old girl living with her aunt who was very mean and strict and did not show much affection. Blanche in that life had to do a great number of household chores and no matter how well she did things, her aunt was not pleased with her. As a result, she was planning to run away from home. Later, when she went to heaven after the death of her body at the age of forty, she recognized her aunt in that life as her husband now.

Visual Bridge Technique: Sometimes patients describe having vivid visions or flashbacks from current or a past life. Usually it is a traumatic event and the patient is made aware of it by his or her subconscious mind in an effort to resolve it.

In therapy, I usually ask patients to focus on the vision, expand their awareness, and recall the whole story. Patients are often able to recall the whole story from the beginning to the end.

Nora had a history of headaches and neck pain. She also described having a vision as follows: "I was having one of my migraine headaches. It was in the middle of the day. I lay down on the couch with my arm over my eyes to protect them from the light. As I was lying there, I was asking myself 'why. Why do I always get these headaches?' As I asked myself this, I saw a battlefield with knights in armor fighting. They had swords. Some of the knights were on the ground, some still on horseback. I saw all of this in great detail as if watching a movie. As I watched, I focused in on a man in armor. I knew this was me. I was fighting another in armor on the ground. I saw my opponent draw his sword back and cut off my head. I saw the head fly and I saw the neck where the head had been and I saw the arteries still trying to pump blood, but I did not see any blood."

During a session, I asked her to focus on that vision she had and expand her awareness to recall the whole story. As Nora focused on her vision, she recalled that she was a knight fighting with invaders in England. His name was John Castleberry. He had armor on his head and chest.

John recalled being beheaded by the sword of another knight. After the death of his physical body, he recalled his spirit out of the body looking at his dead body. He saw the neck where his head had been. The blood vessels were still pulsating and squirting the blood out, just the way Nora saw in her vision.

After the death of his physical body, when John went to the Light (heaven), he saw soul parts from his head still lying in the battlefield; they were cleansed, healed, and integrated with Nora with the help of the angels. She also clearly saw and understood that that lifetime was one of the sources of her migraine headaches and neck pain, which were then relieved.

When patients come to me, they are already feeling intense emotional or physical feelings or sensations associated with the conflict, or they may be using certain words or phrases to describe their problems. Any of the bridge techniques, individually or all together, can elicit the source of the problem.

In these cases, the problem is very close to the conscious mind. It is not completely out in the conscious mind but is ready to surface into it. It makes no sense to relax the patient with a formal hypnotic induction and push the problem back to the subconscious and then ask the patient to recall it by bringing it out into the conscious mind again.

Andy, a thirty-five-year-old man, became anxious every time he went to the doctor's office, and his anxiety caused his blood pressure to rise. During a session, I asked him to recall and focus on his thoughts and feelings when he went to the doctor's office. He used the following phrases repeatedly to describe his emotional and physical problems:

"I am afraid."
"I feel very tense and taut."
"My heart is beating fast."
"I can feel my blood vessels constricting."

After a few repetitions he regressed to a life when he was a thirteen-year-old female. Her name was Frances White. Her abusive, unloving parents left her in a park and never came back. She was taken to a state institutional home. There she felt despair and fear and was anxious because of the unkind and unloving staff. She heard stories about a sinister doctor who performed sterilization on the girls who lived there.

At the age of fifteen she was taken to that doctor. She felt powerless, helpless, and hopeless as the attendants wrestled her to the operating table and the doctor performed the sterilization against her will. He said that he wanted to make sure that no more of her kind could be born. She died after the operation due to an infection, feeling helpless, anxious, and unloved. After recalling, reliving, and releasing that life, Andy's fears and anxiety about going to the doctor's office were relieved.

Hypnosis and bridge techniques are also used to locate the possessing earthbound, demon, and other spirits.

Spontaneous Recall

Some of my patients describe having spontaneous memories from their past lives. Usually they recall vivid scenes and realize that they are viewing their past lives. These past life memories often are fragmented and may contain traumatic events. As a result, they can be confusing and frightening. These memories can be initiated by a person or place, an event, emotional feelings, or physical pain or sensations. Sometimes they can be triggered by sight, sound, smell, taste, or touch. Some of my patients reported having spontaneous past life recall while they were using hallucinogenic drugs. Other patients have reported having spontaneous past life memories while they were meditating.

Young children can sometimes spontaneously recall events from past lives, but are often discouraged by the family from talking about the experience and gradually they learn to block those memories.

When I have patients with spontaneous recall, I use that memory to access the past lives. I ask the patients to close their eyes and focus on that memory. They are then requested to expand their awareness and recall the rest of the story. The whole past life can be accessed this way.

Allen, a ten-year-old boy, was brought to me by his parents because he was having multiple physical and behavioral problems. He had head shakes, facial tics, and twitches and jerking of his whole body. According to his mother, in school they told him that he had a learning disability and yet he had knowledge of things he was never taught. During the first session, while I was taking his history, Allen told me that he had knowledge about different things, but he was afraid to talk about it. He was afraid that he would be locked in a mental institution.

When I promised him that I would not put him in a mental institution, he told me he could go into his past or his future any time at will, but sometimes he did not have any control over it. He simply rolls his eyes and he is there. He told me he remembered many of his past lives that he had lived in different places.

He had a fascination with airplanes. Sometimes in school, he drifted away with any noise and found himself in an airplane. He felt he knew all the buttons and switches in the plane and knew how to fly it. His teachers thought he was daydreaming and his grades suffered.

During the next session, his mother told me that just after the first interview there was a dramatic change in Allen's attitude. She felt as if she were taking a different child home. Allen was less anxious and hyper because I was willing to listen to him and did not think he was crazy.

During the following session, I asked Allen to close his eyes and focus on that airplane and expand his awareness and tell me what else he was aware of. He recalled that he was a twenty-six-year-old man, a fighter pilot, and his plane was attacked by an enemy, injuring his face, head, and his whole body and he died.

He also recalled many other lives. Just after one hypnotherapy session, most of his symptoms, such as his head jerks, facial twitches, and behavioral problems, were relieved.

Dreams

When taking their history, I always ask patients about any recurring dreams or nightmares. They can be due to an unresolved conflict from the current life or a prior lifetime. They may be the subconscious mind's way of resolving an unresolved trauma or a conflict.

During the session, I usually ask the patient to close his or her eyes and recall and focus on the dream, expand the awareness beyond the dream, and complete the story. This focus will often uncover a current life or a past life trauma. After processing and resolving the trauma the dream usually stops.

Wilbur, a forty-year-old man, had a repetitive dream about being on a boat in a storm. He often awakened feeling panicky. He also had a fear of water and could not swim.

During a session, I asked him to close his eyes, remember and focus on his dream and expand his awareness and recall the whole story from the beginning to the end. As he began to focus on his dream, he remembered being a twenty-year-old female in a past life. She was on a boat with her baby. Suddenly a severe storm came up and the boat tilted and everybody was drowning. Somebody pulled her out of the water but her baby drowned. She felt extremely sad about the loss of her child. After that regression, Wilbur's fear of water was relieved and he did not have that dream any more.

Betty came to me because of severe depression she had had for about one year. She had many dreams and nightmares daily. During a session, she told me about eight different dreams she had repeatedly. Later, as we proceeded in the therapy, each dream turned out to be a memory from a different past life. I regressed her through those dreams, resolving the traumas and conflicts from those lives, leading to a great deal of improvement with her emotional and physical conditions.

In any of these techniques, closing the eyes helps to focus better, but doing so is not necessary. I had a few patients who could regress and recall past events and lives without closing their eyes. They were able to focus and block their peripheral awareness, even with their eyes open.

If we really think, all these techniques are a state of focused concentration—focusing on emotions, physical sensations, words, phrases, memories, visions, and dreams; thus, they are in fact states of hypnosis. But there is no need for a formal induction. Most of the time these are the techniques I use in therapy, and I have referred to them as hypnosis throughout this book.

Different emotional and physical feelings, spontaneous re-calls, visions, and dreams can also be due to a possessing earth-bound entity that needs to be treated and released.

Short Cases

It is very gratifying when miracles occur, when patients are cured dramatically of their debilitating emotional and physical symptoms after only one or two hypnotherapy sessions. I have seen these miracles many times, but it never ceases to amaze me. Following are some of the examples of such dramatic cures. In all these cases, most of the symptoms were primarily caused by earthbound and demon spirits; releasing them from the patients relieved most of their crippling acute and chronic symptoms.

Trinity

Trinity, a forty-two-year-old married female, had had claustrophobia since the third grade. As a child, she was afraid of water and while washing her hair couldn't breathe with the water falling on her face. She couldn't stand to have water above her neck and as a result could not swim. Since the age of sixteen she was not able to ride elevators or ride in cars or buses with the windows up and was uncomfortable driving through tunnels. She also was afraid of traveling at night. Everywhere she went she had to leave before dark. She had a fear of dead people and was afraid of being in the casket; as a result, she wanted to be cremated.

When she was in any of these circumstances she had severe panic attacks. During these attacks she had tightness in the chest, palpitations, and shortness of breath, and she became very nervous, shaky, and dizzy and felt as though she was going to pass out. Before she came for the treatment, while approaching a tunnel one day, she became very anxious and panicky. She stopped the car before entering the tunnel and jumped out of the car. Her uncle, who was also in the car, drove home. At this point she realized she had to get some help. She admitted having mild depression from these problems and was taking Imipramine 25 mg., at bedtime.

She had repetitive dreams that she had to go to the bathroom but the toilets were dirty. On two occasions she dreamed that she was being locked in prison in a small cell and was climbing the wall but could not get out. She had a flashback of the same dream when she was experimenting with marijuana.

My office was located on the fifth floor and she refused to use the elevator because she was too frightened to ride in it. For the first two visits she walked up the steps.

During the second session, I made a relaxation tape for Trinity and explained about hypnosis and hypnotherapy. During the third session, we proceeded to use hypnotherapy, after an explanation of earthbound spirits, demon spirits, and past life traumas that my patients had reported as being the source of their problems. Under hypnosis, she found the following earthbound spirits inside her.

Peter was a dark-looking, tall, white man in a blue suit who claimed to have raped and killed a five-year-old girl named Jane in a park. He went to jail for the crime. Peter could not stand to be locked up in a small cell room because he had claustrophobia. So he climbed out of his cell into a path like a tunnel, and fell into a river and choked to death in the muddy water. Trinity's dreams about being locked in a prison cell with a dirty toilet and climbing the walls to escape were due to Peter. Peter also had a red demon spirit in his penis who bragged that it made Peter rape Jane. His feeling of claustrophobia was transferred to Trinity, who began to experience them after he came on board with her.

Jane was a five-year-old girl who claimed that she was raped and killed by Peter.

Mary was a twelve-year-old who claimed to have drowned in a swimming pool. Her feelings of suffocation while drowning were transferred over to Trinity after she came in with her.

Ann was a little girl who was raped by her father. He put his hand over her mouth so she could not scream and she was smothered to death.

Grandmother, who died in a hospital where she had been put in a room that was very small and had no windows and door knobs (like an elevator).

All these entities were released into the Light (heaven) after some therapy with them. Trinity clearly saw that they were separate and different from her. While she was still under hypnosis, I asked her to visualize going up and down in an elevator, and as she did so she had no anxiety attacks. Then, after the session, I told her to go up and down in the elevator in the office building and come back and tell me how she felt. She came back after a few minutes and was extremely euphoric. She was able to ride the elevator several times without any panic attacks. A phobia she had for many years was totally cured after just one hypnotherapy session and without any insight psychotherapy or medication.

During her next session, Trinity reported she was no longer afraid of riding in elevators, driving after dark, and driving through tunnels. She was not afraid of dead people and was able to ride in the back seat of the car with the windows up.

Eight years after her treatment, Trinity wrote that she still is doing well and none of her symptoms have returned. She described how that one session changed her life:

> It was truly the beginning of the rest of my life. I was able to get a job and ride the elevator every day to get from floor to floor. I can ride in the cars and buses with the windows up, drive through tunnels, and drive during the night without becoming panicky. I cannot thank God enough for letting Dr. Modi help me.

Hope

Hope, a forty-two-year-old female, described her condition:

> I feel like I am a walking dead person. I am as low as a person could get. I feel there is somebody else inside me, controlling me and making me do things which I do not remember later. I feel like I am being possessed. I want to take a gun and end it all.

Hope appeared very depressed and withdrawn. According to her, she had been depressed, irritable, agitated, withdrawn, and upset off and on for fifteen years, but more so in the past three years before she came to me. She described feeling tired and drained, with poor concentration and memory. She was not able to function and felt totally hopeless, helpless, and like a failure. She often had crying spells. She had a hard time falling asleep and slept only four to five hours and would wake up early in the morning.

Hope was admitted twice to a hospital for depression. She had counseling until a year before she saw me. She had suicidal preoccupation. She was thinking of ending her misery by taking an overdose of pills or shooting herself. As a result, her husband hid the guns and was afraid to leave her alone.

On two occasions she had violent outbursts of which she had no memory. According to her husband, the first time she seemed to be fine and then all of a sudden she threw a glass and started to scream and curse. The second time, for no reason, she started to throw things, kick, and curse, and became very violent. Normally, Hope never cursed. Both times her husband had to hold her down until she recovered from those outbursts, which lasted just a few minutes.

She also had severe panic attacks during which she felt extremely shaky, had chest pains, difficulty in breathing, and palpitations and felt she was going to have a heart attack. She felt as if everything were closing in on her and she had to get out. She also had a fear of losing her mind. These attacks occurred two or three times a day, each lasting five to ten minutes.

Hope also had severe migraine headaches daily for about five months. She had injured her back and had severe back pain ever since and it was getting progressively worse. She had a difficult time moving, sitting, and lying down. As a result, she had a hard time in doing her daily work.

She was also having sexual problems. She was raised in a very strict environment. She was told by her dad not to talk about sex and not to look at her body below the neck while taking a shower. Recently while having sex with her husband, she heard her dad's voice saying, "Hope, what are you doing?" Her dad had died of pneumonia seven years before. He was very violent, abusive, and paranoid and also attempted suicide once.

One time while wide awake she saw her dad standing at the foot of her bed. She had recurring dreams about her dad since his death. She also had constant conversations going on in her head. She felt as if she was possessed by an evil spirit and she was "Damian" as in the movie. She felt that there were many people inside her, including another Hope. She often had flashbacks from her childhood when her father was violent and physically abusive toward her and others. She had a fear of snakes and had nightmares about snakes chasing her.

Hope suffered from many physical problems besides headaches and back pain. She had arthritis, asthma, sinus problems, and laryngitis. When she had laryngitis, she sometimes lost her voice completely for months. She was allergic to dust, mold, grass, trees, animals, smoke, and dampness. She had to take allergy shots on a regular basis. She also had PMS symptoms, during which her nervousness, depression, and irritability became worse. She was taking the antidepressant Pamelor, the tranquilizer Tranxene, and pain pills for about three years.

During the next session, I made a relaxation tape for Hope with positive suggestions that she could listen to at home daily. It helped her sleep better and feel calmer. I also explained to her about hypnotherapy and about earthbound and demon spirits, and past life traumas that my patients found as the source of their emotional and physical problems. Hope was willing to try. So we scheduled a three-hour session.

First Hypnotherapy Session

Under hypnosis, as Hope scanned her body, she saw two large black blobs. One was in her head and one in her heart. Each claimed to be a demon working for Satan.

Black demon blob in the head: It claimed to join Hope when she was five years old. It bragged about making Hope afraid of getting in trouble. It also claimed to cause her depression, anger, and headaches. This black blob had trapped soul parts of Hope and the earthbound spirits inside it as follows:

Hope's father: He was eighty years old. He joined Hope after the death of his body seven years before she came for treatment.

Hope's father claimed he had severe arthritis, fear of snakes, depression, suicidal thoughts, and a violent temper, which Hope started to experience after he came in.

Soul part of Hope's father when living: He fragmented when he was forty-three years old and joined Hope when she was five years old. He claimed he came in Hope to make sure she behaved and made her afraid and ashamed of sex.

The dark entity was transformed into the Light and was helped into heaven. Both parts of her father were integrated and then he was sent to heaven after some therapy. Hope saw many dark blobs falling out of him as he entered into the Light.

Five-year-old Hope: A subpersonality, a fragmented soul part of Hope, which appeared to the older Hope as when she was five. She fragmented when her father was angry with her. Her trauma was processed and resolved. She was cleansed, healed, and filled with the Light and then integrated with older Hope, with the help of the angels.

Gray demon blob in her heart: It claimed to join Hope when she was young and was in a car accident. It bragged about causing Hope depression, anger, fear, and panic attacks. This gray blob was transformed into the Light and was released into heaven.

Fragmented soul part of her mother: She was living at the time of the treatment and was eighty years old. Hope saw a soul part of her mother, who looked forty-five years old. Her mother said that she came in to help Hope. This soul part of the mother was cleansed and healed and was taken back and integrated with her mother's soul in her body by the angels of the Light, who, according to Hope, were helping us during the whole session. As the angels took the part of her mother back to her body, Hope saw her mother in an aqua-green flowered dress, sitting in a chair, quilting. Later, her mother confirmed that she was wearing the same dress Hope saw and was quilting at that time.

Hope's soul part with her husband: As Hope was looking for any other fragmented parts, she saw a silver thread coming out of her soul. She traced the cord going to her husband, where it was connected to a part of her that was with her husband. The angels, at our request, brought that part back, cleansed, healed, and then integrated it with her soul.

Second Hypnotherapy Session

During the next session, Hope reported that after the last session there was a miraculous change in her. She did not have any sexual problems or inhibition. She just kept saying, "I am free, I am free." Her headaches, arthritis, nervousness, anger outbursts, depression, suicidal thoughts, fear of going crazy, and panic attacks were all relieved. She did not have any crying spells and felt very energetic and alive. She slept well all night. Most of those symptoms were due to her father and the demon entities. She reported she was still suffering from back pain. As Hope scanned her body under hypnosis, she found many dark demon entities in her back, hips, and throat.

Black demon blobs in the back and hips: They claimed to have joined Hope when she hurt her back. They all said they caused her back pain and kept her from doing things.

Gray demon blob in the vocal cords: It claimed to have joined Hope when she was a baby. It said that it caused her throat infections and pain, and sometimes took away her voice.

Melinda, a forty-year-old earthbound spirit who had a cough, throat infection, difficulty in breathing, chest pain, and fever and died after one and a half weeks of sickness. After she died she did not go to the Light and joined Hope when she was a little girl and caused her asthma, throat infections, and laryngitis.

Soul part: After releasing all the demon and earthbound spirits to heaven, I asked Hope to check for any fragmented parts of her soul. She saw a cord going to her sister. With the help of the angels, this part was brought back and was cleansed, healed, filled with the Light, and integrated with Hope's soul.

Hope also saw another silver thread or cord coming out of her soul. She traced it going into heaven, to Jesus and then to God. Jesus told her that things will be all right for her now. He also told her that her daughter, who had had two miscarriages, would have a child. Hope saw two rosebuds, at each foot of Jesus. She recognized them as her daughter's two miscarried babies.

After just two sessions, after releasing all the attached earth-bound spirits and demon spirits and locating and integrating all her soul parts, Hope was completely free of all her primary and secondary symptoms. She gradually reduced her pain pills and Tranxene and within three weeks she stopped all the medications. She was sleeping and functioning well without any pills. After her first hypnotherapy session, Hope wrote telling how she was feeling:

> *I felt like I had been asleep since 1989 and just woke up. I feel like I missed so much and now I want to do everything. I feel like I am all bubbly inside and just want to tell everyone how great I feel. Everyone is noticing a change in me. I just cannot thank you enough for what you have done for me so far. Thank you for giving me back my life. I cannot wait for our next appointment.*

After five years, she is still doing well. None of her symptoms have returned. She had gone through many personal and family crises during the past five years. Her husband was laid off and there were financial problems and serious sicknesses and deaths in the family, but she handled them well without falling apart. Also, within a month after her therapy, she found out that her daughter was pregnant, and after nine months had a child just as Hope was told by Jesus.

Grace

Grace, a thirty-five-year-old married female, came to me with symptoms of severe depression, insomnia, poor concentration and memory, and had no energy or motivation to do anything. She was not able to function at home or at work, and as a result was on sick leave. She was nervous, irritable, and agitated and was contemplating suicide. She had lost her appetite and was losing weight.

She had severe panic attacks, during which she felt nervous, shaky, dizzy, cold, and sweaty and had palpitations, dry mouth, and a fear of the unknown. These attacks lasted anywhere from a few minutes to one hour. She also had recurrent nightmares in which everything was chaotic. She had crying spells for no obvious reasons.

She complained of severe headaches, burning in her eyes, back pain, severe gastritis, and stomach pain. She also had PMS, during which she became depressed, moody, and irritable. She described herself as a perfectionist all her life. According to Grace, "I maintained a totally capable exterior while the interior battle was getting worse all the time."

A year before she came to me, she had severe depression, insomnia, loss of appetite, and was suicidal. She had to take off from work for five months because she was not able to function, in spite of the fact that she liked her work. She was treated by her physician for depression with antidepressant medications, which helped some, but not much. She had counseling with a psychologist for four to five months with some improvement, and she pushed herself to go back to work. All those symptoms came back in full force again two months before she came to me for help.

During the next session, I made a relaxation tape for her with positive suggestions. I explained to Grace about different ways I could try to help her. I told her we could try some antidepressant medications and talk therapy, which would help, but there was a good chance the symptoms may come back again as before, or we could try hypnotherapy to find the source of her crippling problems and work with them. She did not want to use medication, and traditional talk therapy did not work for her before. She wanted to get to the root of her problems, so she decided to try hypnotherapy.

I explained to her about different possible reasons for her problems, which were found by my other patients, such as traumatic events from her younger age, from prenatal and birth traumas, and traumas from past lives. I also explained that some patients reported their problems being caused by earthbound and demon spirits. Grace was willing to try and was enthusiastic about it.

First Hypnotherapy Session

During the next session, under hypnosis, Grace saw a gray entity surrounding her body and many small and large gray and black blobs in her head, eyes, throat, heart, and female organs. They claimed to be demons and said Satan was their master. They said they were assigned to Grace by Satan to cause her emotional and physical problems and to retard Grace's spiritual progress. They told how old Grace was when they came in, what opened her up for them to come in, and what type of problems they caused for her.

Dark demon blob around Grace: It joined Grace when she was three years old and was having an out-of-body experience.

Effect: It claimed to cause Grace the fear of men, low self-esteem, depression, and suicidal thoughts.

Dark demon blob in the head: This entity joined Grace when she was twenty-four, at a time when she was afraid and therefore opened up.

Effect: It said that it caused Grace confusion, insomnia, depression, suicidal thoughts, headaches, and the desire to drink alcohol.

Dark demon blob in the eyes: It joined her when she was drinking at the age of thirty.

Effect: It claimed to cause her bad eyesight and burning in her eyes, make her not able to see the truth, and make her think she was not good.

Dark demon blob in the heart: It joined Grace when she was eight and was afraid.

Effect: It claimed to cause her panic attacks, depression, fatigue, and inability to feel anything.

Dark demon blob in the uterus: It joined Grace when she was fifteen.

Effect: It made her irritable and depressed and caused cramps during her menstrual periods.

All the dark entities were transformed into the Light and released to heaven after counseling with them.

Fragmented soul parts: Grace also saw many fragmented soul parts of her or little Graces inside her, ages two, six, eight, eleven, and fifteen. They all looked to Grace as she looked and felt at those ages. Each was encouraged to speak individually and, after their issues and traumas were resolved, they all were integrated with Grace. Grace described the experience of integration as feeling whole, strong, and all together. She saw angels of the Light cleansing, healing, and filling her with the Light.

Second Hypnotherapy Session

During the next session, Grace reported that since the last session her panic attacks, depression, suicidal thoughts, burning in her eyes, and stomach pain were all relieved. She was sleeping and eating well and had more energy. She still had some headaches and back pain.

Again, under hypnosis, she saw gray blobs in her head and back. They both said that they were hiding during the last session.

> **Dark demon blob in back**: It joined Grace when she was ten and was having an out-of-body experience.
> **Effect**: It claimed to cause her backaches, depression, and confusion.

> **Dark demon blob in the head**: It joined Grace when she was five and was sad.
> **Effect**: It caused her headaches and pain and burning in her eyes.

All the dark entities were transformed into the Light and released to heaven after counseling with them.

During the next session, Grace reported that every one of her symptoms was completely relieved. She didn't have any earthbound entities. Only the demon entities were responsible for her symptoms. She took no medication and no other therapy was done.

Six years later, she is still completely free of all her problems and doing well. She wrote about how she felt about her therapy.

> *Experiences during those two sessions made such major changes in my life that I still find it hard to believe. The world still has its problems, but I deal with them in a much better manner. I no longer have to fight with the "others" within, and I am free to be me.*

Adrian

Adrian, a thirteen-year-old male, was referred to me by his family physician because he had been having fainting spells for about six weeks. During those spells he sometimes passed out and fell to the floor. After these fainting spells he felt weak and dizzy, had headaches, and had no memory of the events. He had been depressed after his grandfather died of cancer one year before, on Adrian's birthday. Since then Adrian had repetitive dreams and nightmares about his grandfather chasing him. He was afraid and was convinced that on his birthday, which was coming up in two weeks, he would die.

For two months before Adrian came to me for treatment, his depression had been getting progressively worse. He was having crying spells and poor appetite, was feeling tired and drained, and had difficulty sleeping. He started to see his grandfather standing at the bedroom door asking Adrian to come to him. He did not tell his parents or anybody about the vision because he was afraid they would think he was crazy. After a while he could not cope with it and told his parents about it. Since he could not sleep in his room because of his fears, he started to sleep in his parents' room. He also had been having intermittent panic attacks for about one year. During these attacks he felt out of control, weak, dizzy, and hot and had palpitations and ringing in his ears. He also started to have aches and pains all over his body. He was becoming nervous and moody. He had been an A and B student, but he started to get D's.

His physical examination, blood and urine tests, blood sugar, EKG, EEG, and other tests were all within normal limits. He was also examined and tested by a neurologist, who did not find anything physically wrong with him.

During the second session, I made a relaxation tape for Adrian. I mentioned to him and his parents the possibility of exploring his problems under hypnosis. I explained to them that sometimes my patients had found spirits of their deceased loved ones and other spirits with them, and how they experienced those spirits' physical and emotional problems. I also explained that releasing those spirits from the patients freed them from their crippling physical and emotional problems. They agreed to try it.

During the next visit, Adrian reported that during the whole week his nightmares about his grandfather chasing him and all his symptoms had become worse.

Under hypnosis, Adrian found his grandfather's spirit with him. The grandfather expressed a desire to be with his grandson because he loved him. I explained to him that his grandson was suffering from the physical and emotional problems that he had had before he died and that were transferred to Adrian after he joined him. After he realized how his presence was affecting his grandson negatively, he was more than willing to leave and was released to the Light (heaven). It was a very emotional session for Adrian and his parents.

During the next session, Adrian and his parents reported a great improvement in Adrian. He did not see his grandfather and was able to sleep soundly in his own room without any nightmares. He didn't have any fainting spells, panic attacks, headaches, ringing in his ears, dizziness, and aches and pains. He had no depression or crying spells and was feeling more energetic. Seven years later, Adrian told me that he is still doing well and none of those symptoms have returned. He described his experience:

> Looking back on my therapy, I realize now that I had to go through this experience in order to go on with my life. With the

love and support of my family and Dr. Modi's treatment and guidance, the process I went through was a positive experience with miraculous results and has given me a new understanding of life and death. Thank you, Dr. Modi. You are a miracle worker.

Just one hypnotherapy session totally relieved all of Adrian's crippling emotional and physical problems.

Sources

1. Harold I. Kaplan, M.D.; Benjamin J. Sadock, M.D.; and Jack A. Grebb, M.D. *Synopsis of Psychiatry*, 7th ed. (Baltimore: The Williams and Wilkins Co., 1994) 836.

2. Alfred M. Freedman, M.D., and Harold I. Kaplan, M.D., ed. *Comprehensive Textbook of Psychiatry* (Baltimore: The Williams and Wilkins Co., 1967) 10.

3. Kaplan and Sadock, *Synopsis*, 837.

4. Freedman and Kaplan, *Comprehensive*, 4.

5. Ibid, 3.

6. Ibid, 6.

7. Ibid, 12.

8. Kaplan and Sadock, *Synopsis*, 838.

9. Freedman and Kaplan, *Comprehensive*, 5.

10. Ibid, 12.

11. Ibid, 23.

12. Ibid, 25.

13. Kaplan and Sadock, *Synopsis*, 112.

14. Ibid, 113.

15. Ibid, 115.

Chapter II

Prenatal and Birth Traumas

Cast Out of the Womb

Pushed and tugged and tossed about
First I'm pulled in, then I'm cast out
I try to remember, but try in vain
Why it is I feel such pain.

Sometimes I think I almost see
The "why" of what's become of me
But then I lose it, for once again
I'm pulled, and pushed, and shoved, and then
I'm blinded by a burst of light—
What happened to eternal night?
The warmth and comfort of that place
I'd come to love, but now I face . . .

The world again. Have I been here?
It feels so strange, and yet I fear
I know it well, but why, and when?
Well, here I go—around again.

Why do they always cast me out—
Am I the one they don't care about?
Have I been bad, or just not good
To go back home . . . I wish I could—

But maybe if I do this right
They'll take me back into that Light
That's softer, sweeter, brighter than day
And if I'm lucky . . . This time I'll stay!!

— Jane

Prenatal and Birth Traumas

Prenatal and Birth Traumas

My hypnotized patients have recalled in detail the memories of their prenatal life in the womb and of birth as they try to locate the source of their physical or emotional problems. Contrary to popular belief, the fetus has memories and feelings while in the womb and during birth.

According to the reports of my hypnotized patients, from conception the fetus feels and records all the mother's thoughts, feelings, and experiences, including depression, anxiety, anger, guilt, rejection, and also the physical discomfort and pain, and accepts and absorbs them as its own. It is also aware of the words spoken by the father, doctors, nurses, and others, through the mother.

The fetus, however, has not developed a separate identity or ego and has little ability to differentiate its mother's experiences and feelings from its own. The information is uncensored and accepted by the fetus without any discrimination.

David B. Cheek, M.D., an obstetrician, did an interesting clinical experiment several years ago in Chico, California. He kept detailed birth notes of a few babies, especially about how their head and shoulders were positioned at birth and how they were delivered. Positioning was selected as a measure of reliability of birth memories because information like this rarely finds its way beyond the obstetrician's delivery notes. Dr. Cheek locked up these delivery notes for more than two decades.

Later, under hypnosis, Doctor Cheek regressed these young men and women to their birth. They all accurately described how his or her head had been turned and shoulders angled at birth, and also the way he or she was delivered. The information was exactly the same as he had written in their files. (*The Secret Life of the Unborn Child* by Thomas Verny, M.D.)

The reason the fetus can recall events even before the development of the body and brain is because the memories and events in fact are recorded in the soul (the subconscious mind), which might be partly or completely in the fetus. Part of the soul consciousness of the fetus is connected with it from the time of conception even though the rest of the soul may be outside watching and enters the body just before or after birth.

The experiences in the womb and during birth become deeply embedded and continue to affect the person after birth, in childhood, and in adult life. Many physical and emotional problems can be traced to the traumas in the womb and during birth. The feelings of the mother and father when they learn of the pregnancy, or their reaction to the sex of the baby, has lasting effects on the fetus and can imprint the personality patterns of the person later in life.

All the traumatic events involving the mother while the fetus is in the womb have profound effects on it. If the baby was unwanted and the mother unsuccessfully tried to abort the fetus, this usually has devastating effects on the fetus, creating feelings of rejection, anger, violence, inferiority, worthlessness, rebelliousness, and relationship problems later in life.

Problems Caused by Prenatal and Birth Traumas

My patients tell me that birth is one of the most painful experiences of their lives. The following birth situations can be the origins of problems:

Process of being pushed and coming out: In some it can cause: fear of change; feelings of rejection, alienation, insecurity, inferiority, separation anxiety; paranoia (nobody likes me or cares for me); etc.

Difficult birth: It can cause panic, terror, feelings of being stuck in different situations in life, claustrophobia, anger, and frustration.

Cord around the neck: It can cause headaches, hypertension, asthma, feelings of choking, seizure disorders, etc.

Mucus in the throat: Can cause feelings of choking and suffocation.

Traumas in the womb and during birth can stimulate memories of similar past life traumas that the patient needs to resolve in the current life. It can also reactivate the feelings and memories of the first birth, when the soul was first created in God.

Under hypnosis, my patients have recalled four different types of births:

The First Birth: Cast out from God.
The Second Birth: Cast out from Godhead, into Paradise/ Garden.
The Third Birth: Cast out from the womb.
The Rebirths: Experience of being reborn again and again.

The First Birth: Cast Out from God

Amazingly, many of my patients were even able to recall the creation of their soul under hypnosis. They describe the process of creation of their individual soul similar to birth. They describe it as being something intense going around them, being shaken and squeezed. Finally, the intensity becomes great and all of a sudden they find themselves being thrust out as a separate soul from the core of God (the mother), but still connected to God with a silver cord (like a cosmic umbilical cord).

During this process of creation and separation they describe feeling anxious, confused, scared, angry, apprehensive, sad, rejected, alienated, and being cast out. Others feel joy, excitement, and feelings of adventure. Most of our feelings of inferiority, inadequacy, imperfection, fear, depression, rejection, and separation anxiety have their roots when we were first created by God (the first birth).

Following are some examples of the memories of patients under hypnosis, when they were first created and separated from God.

Ann

"*Something is happening here. I feel intense vibrations and buzzing around me, which builds up and builds up. Everything is tremulous. I feel confused, excited, and scared. I never felt these feelings before. Then all of a sudden the shaking and buzzing stops and I am out there.*

"*I hear the most beautiful music [patient looks shocked]. It just stops me dead. Music comes from God and I am supposed to make people understand that fact in the future. I am supposed to write it, play it, and translate it. I know it as I am separated and I feel humbled.*

"*I feel excited and adventurous. But at the same time there is this feeling of reaching back. It is like a child who is leaving his mother for the first time and wants to reach back and grab hold of her. I feel like I want to hold on. I am scared and sad because I am not 'Home' any more. Part of me wants to go back 'Home,' but honestly the biggest part of me wants to go out there and feels adventurous.*"

Sheila

"*I feel shaky, I feel like I am being tossed around. I am being shaken like in an earthquake. It is confusing and frightening. Then the shaking stops and I feel being thrust out. I realize that I am outside the core of God but still connected.*

"*I feel like, what am I doing out here? I need to be there where I belong. Why are you bumping me around? I feel angry, sad, and alone. I feel I ought to have stayed there with God. I feel I am being rejected and pushed out.*

"*I am seeing through times of what is going to happen. I can see how we are going to evolve. I can see life and death, birth and rebirths, worlds and universes and how all will eventually evolve and come back to God. I have this ability to see through times and have foreknowledge.*

"*I see my purpose and I feel overwhelmed. I am supposed to bring this knowledge to people and help them to know their purpose and understand their place in this whole scheme. I am supposed to teach and heal and bring hope for people.*

"*I feel overwhelmed with this foreknowledge. Why me? Why do I have to do it? It is such a big job. In a short time I accept it and feel O.K. If this is what I am supposed to do then I will do it. I am not afraid. I am strong. I feel more positive. First, I was looking backward feeling angry, rejected, alone, overwhelmed, sad, and resigned. Then quickly I became more positive and excited like it can be adventurous and became charged with it.*"

Aaron

"*I feel excited. All this activity around me is stimulating. What is happening? Something big must be about to happen. And I feel a burst and I am out here.*

"*I feel confused. I feel being cast out. I cannot get oriented. What is happening? It takes me some time to figure out that I am separate. I do not want to feel it so I feel numb for a while. I am not mad, sad, or unhappy. I do not register emotions for a long time. Then I feel resigned. It takes a long time for me to adjust to it.*

"*It takes a long time to realize that I have a purpose and what it is. Then I get excited but in a serious way, almost task oriented. It is like I have a job to do and I am going to do it right.*"

My hypnotized patients report that God is surrounded by the Godheads. Each soul emerges from the core of God and after a time, when ready, it enters one of the Godheads. For a time after its separation from God, each soul waits in the Godhead. Feelings of nervousness, anticipation, and abandonment surround the soul as it waits. Some feelings of excitement or anticipation (waiting in the wings) create an ambivalence within the waiting soul. This mixture of good and bad feelings results in a profound feeling of nervous confusion. Patients describe this waiting in the Godhead like waiting in a cosmic womb. After a time however, the soul adjusts to being part of the Godhead, only to be cast out again at the point of incarnation.

The Second Birth:
Cast Out from the Godhead, into Paradise/Garden

Under hypnosis, some of my patients have even recalled when God first created human life and several souls were infused into adolescent human bodies and placed in strategic places throughout the universe to generate human life. These original couples can be identified as the "Adam and Eve" concept. That is, they were the first humans on earth, placed there to create more like themselves.

At the point of infusion, the soul once again suffers grief, separation anxiety, loneliness, and the feelings of rejection and anger that it felt when it was emitted from God. After a period of adjustment, however, the Garden or Paradise looked very much like heaven, and the soul began to feel once again at home in this place of warmth, beauty, purity, and light. Paradise was lovely; it was free of all adversity, pain, and trouble.

Just at the point of infusion of the soul into the body for the first time, patients often have memories from before, for a split second, and then the memories are wiped out. Then they begin to wonder where am I, why am I here, and finally they conclude this place is pretty. Following are some examples of such memories.

Ann

"I feel real strange and alien at first. I feel alone. I had somebody. Where is he? I am scared. Then almost instantly I forget everything. Then I begin to wonder where I am and how I got here. I feel a mixture of awe, fear, and loneliness. Not so much rejection.

"It is a beautiful place. Music is still here. It has changed some. Right now it is the music of nature. It is the music of water, birds, and animals."

Sheila

"Why do I have to go through this? Why couldn't I just stay there? Why do I have such a big job to do? Was I bad? Am I being punished? And then quickly these thoughts are wiped out. I look around and feel maybe this is not so bad after all. This is kind of exciting. I do not know where I am, but I guess it is O.K."

Aaron

> *"Where am I? I feel confused. What happened? Why am I not where I was? Where is everybody? I feel alone and rejected. I do not know why I am here. I want to go back. Then I instantly forget everything. I look around. It is kind of beautiful. Maybe this is not so bad after all. This is kind of exciting."*

At the point when temptation overcame the so-called Adams and Eves and they ate of the fruit, innocence was lost. Paradise was no longer pure, shining, and a perfect Light. Once again the soul suffered the loss of perfection, the experience of rejection, inadequacy, and being cast out. For the first time, the soul felt guilt, accompanied by remorse, sadness, and extreme loneliness.

The Third Birth: Cast Out from the Womb

According to my hypnotized patients, when the soul is first incarnated it feels alienation as never before. Moving from God into the Godhead, accompanied by all the feelings of rejection, inferiority, and ejection is a profound shock to the soul; now, in addition, it has been ejected from the Godhead into paradise, feeling confused, hurt, and rejected again.

Now, abandoned and rejected, the souls experience another ejection: physical birth, born of human physical love, facing an imperfect world. Being incarnated not only evokes all those painful memories and feelings of the first and second birth, but includes the experience of being in a totally strange place. The womb is dark, wet, and confining, not light and airy. The soul, feeling trapped and frightened, once again mourns the loss of its "Home." But, as in the Godhead, time passes and the soul begins to adjust and even feels comfortable in the womb. It begins to forget its grief and once again experiences the feeling of "waiting in the wings."

Then comes the birth experience. Feeling pulled and squeezed and tugged and torn, the soul experiences a different type of shock. At the point of birth, the soul is cast out from the womb into a cold, foreign place. It feels angry, upset, confused, frightened, and ultimately abandoned. At this point of birth the soul loses all its memories of its prior experiences and of its rightful "Home."

The Rebirths

Subsequent incarnations or reincarnations carry no less pain, but in fact pile pain upon pain. Feelings of inadequacy run high. "I must have really been bad . . . done wrong . . . done a poor job . . . not been good enough . . . because I have to do this again."

The experience of rebirth carries all the memories of ejection from God, from the Godhead, from Paradise, and from the womb in prior births. In addition, rebirth carries a karmic burden: in each life, we plan certain experiences in order to resolve problems from past lives. Many times we plan painful, unpleasant circumstances so that in resolution our souls can grow.

Once again, the soul waits in the wings, for things it knows and for things about which it has no idea. Once again the soul endures ejection from the womb, feelings of rejection and abandonment by God and Light, feelings of fear, inadequacy, and grief. Once again, at the point of birth, past memories are erased and replaced by confusion, uncertainty, and insecurity. Once again the soul begins a journey into a cold, alien world.

Memories of Past Life Traumas

The memories of different traumas from past lives are reactivated during pregnancy and birth by the thoughts, emotions, and experiences of the fetus, the mother, and others around and by different types of traumas during labor and birth as follows:

Pregnancy: It can stimulate the memories of rejection, loneliness, depression, anxiety, anticipation, relationship problems, being thrown in a dungeon, and being buried alive from different past lives.

Labor: It can evoke memories of rejection, violence, reluctance, abandonment, anger, and anxiety from the first birth and subsequent rebirths in past lives. Contractions and compression of labor pain can stimulate the memories of being crushed or tortured and other violent past life events.

Difficult labor: It can evoke memories of violence, torture, being stuck, being buried alive, and dying slowly in past lives.

Limbs being pulled: It can trigger memories of being drawn and quartered, being mutilated, and different types of tortures from past lives.

Forceps delivery: It can evoke memories of decapitation, hanging, head being crushed, and other types of traumas to the head from past lives.

Cesarean-section births: It can trigger memories of being cut with knives or swords, war memories, and being aborted in past lives.

Mucus in the throat: It can evoke memories of being choked and suffocated in past lives.

Cord around the neck: It can trigger memories of being hanged, choked, suffocated, or decapitated and other tortures to the neck area in past lives.

Use of anesthesia during delivery: It can dull the consciousness of the mother and the fetus, triggering the memories of being knocked unconscious, dying slowly, bleeding, and passing out in past lives.

Bright lights at birth: It can trigger memories of dying due to lightning or burning in fire.

Techniques to Access Prenatal and Birth Memories

The prenatal and birth memories can be accessed in the following ways:

1. They can be accessed by regression therapy moving from the present backward to birth and prenatal states.

2. During a past life regression, when the patients make their transition to the Light (heaven), after the death of their physical bodies, they are directed to move to their planning stage in heaven for the current life. Then from heaven, they are progressed forward when they come down to the earth to be born.

3. Prenatal and birth memories can also be accessed through one of the bridge techniques.

Example of a Prenatal and Birth Regression

During one session, when Ann (one of the long cases in Chapter VIII) was in the Light (heaven) going through planning for her life, I asked her to move ahead in time when she comes down to the earth to be born as Ann. Following is the transcript of the session.

Ann: "I planned to come down just before the conception or at the point of conception."

Dr. Modi: "Describe to me how you go down."

Ann: "My guardian angels come with me as far as they can. They are very reassuring. I come down through my cord and stay in the cord and hover around my parents. The cord is my protection and it is very, very strong and cannot be influenced by darkness. At the end it is almost like a crust. I stay in the cord around my parents until I am ready to be infused in the fetus.

"I send a part of my soul to the embryo at conception. It goes like a laser beam from me to the embryo. I can see outside through the cord. It is translucent. I just hover around my parents and watch till it is time to enter the fetus."

Dr. Modi: "How do you feel?"

Ann: "I feel nervous. I really do not want to do this, but I know I have to."

Dr. Modi: "At this point do you have all the memories from the Light (heaven)?"

Ann: "Yes. I forget them at the point I enter the body."

Dr. Modi: "What do you feel as you wait outside?"

Ann: "I get the feeling like you get before jumping off the high diving board. It is like I know I am going to do this and I know I am going to be all right, but God I do not want to do this because it is going to be rough. I feel reluctant."

Dr. Modi: "Now I want you to tune into the soul part, which went into the embryo at the conception. What are you aware of? What are you feeling?"

Ann: "I have to go in and protect this baby."

Dr. Modi: "Do you go during or after conception?"

Ann: "Just after conception."

Dr. Modi: "What are you aware of?"

Ann: "I am aware of a swishing sound. It is my mother's heartbeat. I am aware of all kinds of sounds like her body sounds and sounds outside her body. It is dark in here. But it is kind of comfortable. I sleep a lot. It is restful."

Dr. Modi: "How old are you?"

Ann: "Just days."

Dr. Modi: "Describe as you grow day by day in the womb. What happens?"

Ann: "Not a lot. Just the same."

Dr. Modi: "Move ahead to the time when your mother finds out that she is pregnant. What is her reaction?"

Ann: "I am two and a half months old. She is excited but scared because she lost babies before. She does not want to lose another one. She is very careful. It is like she is walking on eggshells. She is sick a lot. She does not feel well."

Dr. Modi: "Do you feel sick with her?"

Ann: "It is kind of unsettling but I do not feel sick like her."

Dr. Modi: "Move ahead in time when your father finds out that your mother is pregnant."

Ann: "She does not tell him for a while. She does not want to tell him. When she tells him he does not say anything.

He does not want any kids. I feel confused, puzzled, and angry. But not surprised. I feel rejected and unwanted."

Dr. Modi: "Move ahead when you are three months old in the womb. What do you look like? What do you feel?"

Ann: "I do not look like much at all. I feel fine. I am comfortable most of the time except when she is sick. I worry about her."

Dr. Modi: "Look at your body. Do you have hands and feet?"

Ann: "Sort of funny looking. My hands do not have much configuration. But there is separation. I just look like a sea horse or something funny."

Dr. Modi: "Move ahead when you are five months old in the womb. What are you aware of?"

Ann: "Something is wrong. She is bleeding."

Dr. Modi: "How does that affect you?"

Ann: "I cannot get enough food. I am losing my nutrients. I get really scared. I do not get enough food. I do not get enough oxygen. I am hungry. We are very quiet now."

Dr. Modi: "Who is quiet?"

Ann: "My mother and I. She lies down a lot. They make her lie down. They are going to put her in the hospital if it does not get better. I am so scared. I feel hungry. I am afraid I will die. I remember my lives when I died of starvation. Especially the life in a concentration camp when I was starving."

Dr. Modi: "Look at your body. How does it look?"

Ann: "I look pretty good. I have some definition now. I just float. I sleep a lot. I lost something when she bled. Like energy or something. I am not as active as I was before. I think I am feeling my mother's feelings of being tired and drained because she lost blood. She sleeps a lot and I sleep a lot. Like we are one and the same."

Dr. Modi: "Move ahead when you are six months old. How do you feel?"

Ann: "We are still very quiet. She stopped bleeding."

Dr. Modi: "Move ahead when you are seven months old. What is happening?"

Ann: "Same. We stay quiet."

Dr. Modi: "Move ahead when you were eight months old. What are you aware of?"

Ann: "It is getting awfully crowded. I will be glad to get out of here. My mom is O.K. now, so I feel O.K."

Dr. Modi: "Move ahead to the time when your mother begins to have labor pains. How do you feel?"

Ann: "It feels a lot like the first time."

Dr. Modi: "What do you mean by the first time?"

Ann: "First time when I was created by God. I began to remember when the things began to move around me and squeeze me."

Dr. Modi: "How?"

Ann: "Everything around me starts to move and vibrate and squeezes just like the first time. Our heartbeats are faster. I feel being pressed, squeezed, and pushed. I feel like I am about to be cast out."

Dr. Modi: "How does that make you feel?"

Ann: "Scared and anxious. I am not ready to do this again."

Dr. Modi: "Move ahead. What happens next?"

Ann: "They grab me on the head with this thing, a clamp. It squeezes my head to pull me out because I cannot get out."

Dr. Modi: "How do you feel?

Ann: "I cannot breathe. I feel stuck. My head is going to explode. My head hurts. I feel like my head is going to burst. I remember feeling this way before in another life. I do not like it.

"I just want it to be over so I can get out of here and get some air. I just cannot get any air. I feel like I am suffocating. My head is going to blow up.

"Here comes one big push and that clamp tightens over my head and the doctor pulls and I am out. [Breathes deeply.]

Dr. Modi: "What is the doctor saying?"

Ann: "It is a girl."

Dr. Modi: "How does your mom feel?"

Ann: "My mom is talking nonsense. They gave her some kind of gas. She is just babbling."

Dr. Modi: "How did you feel when they gave your mother gas when you were in the womb?"

Ann: "Tired. I was half aware. It was a creepy feeling. I did not like it. I felt like I was going to die if I did not get out of there. I knew things were happening around me but I could not do anything. I felt drugged.

"Now, I do not know where I am and yet I feel I have been here before. This does not feel like a new experience to me. The lights are too bright, too invasive. I do not like it. I feel lost. There is nothing holding me. I am scared. I am cold and tired."

Dr. Modi: "When are you taken to your mother and father?"

Ann: "The next day. My father says I have a red face. My mother says I am ugly. She is teasing. My doctor thinks I am pretty."

Dr. Modi: "Do you have any memories of the Light at this point?"

Ann: "Some. Not much."

Dr. Modi: "When did the rest of your soul enter the body?"

Ann: "When the doctor put the clamp on my head."

Dr. Modi: "What did that feel like when your main body of the soul entered the body?"

Ann: "I felt I had more strength. It almost came in to save me. I was all worn out."

As we look at Ann's prenatal and birth memories and experiences, we can clearly understand how her experiences in the womb and at birth stimulated the memories of past life traumas and the trauma of her first birth when her soul was created by God as follows:

- At two and a half to three months in the womb, when she found out that her father did not want her, it stimulated the memories of past lives when she felt rejected and unwanted.
- At five months in the womb, when her mother began to have bleeding, Ann felt hungry and weak, triggering the memories of a past life in a concentration camp when she was starving.
- The labor pains of her mother and process of birth while being squeezed and pushed brought the memories of her first birth, when her soul was first created by God.
- When her mother was given gas during the delivery, Ann, in the womb, felt drugged and not quite aware of what was going on. This feeling triggered memories from the past lives of being helpless and that she was going to die. It also created a feeling of chronic fatigue and feelings of the dragging that Ann experienced during most of her life.
- The experience of her head not easily coming out triggered her memories of being stuck, not being able to breathe and of suffocating, from past lives.
- When the doctors applied the forceps to the head to enhance the birth, she felt like her head hurt and was going to explode. This stimulated the memories from past lives when she felt the same way.

Most of these physical and emotional feelings from her prenatal and birth traumas stimulated the memories of her past life traumas, i.e., hunger and weight problems, headaches and feelings that her head is going to explode, chronic fatigue and feelings of dragging all the time, feelings of suffocation, and feelings of rejection. These problems continued during most of her current life. They were treated and resolved through past life regression therapy during the treatment. (Read case of Ann in chapter 8.)

Summary

According to the reports of my hypnotized patients, many of our personality traits and physical and emotional problems can be traced to experiences in the womb and during birth. From conception until birth, the fetus feels and records all the experiences, thoughts, and feelings of the mother as its own. The information is uncensored and accepted by the fetus as its own without any discrimination.

The fetus can recall the events even before the development of the body and the brain because they are recorded in the soul consciousness (the subconscious mind). According to my patients' reports, the soul may enter the fetus any time from conception till birth. Most commonly, the soul enters the body just before or after birth. In any case, a part of the soul consciousness (soul fragment) is attached to the fetus from conception, recording all the experiences of the fetus in the womb.

The memories, experiences, and traumas from conception on, until birth, can also trigger memories of different traumas in past lives. These are often the problems that patients need to resolve in this life.

Many emotional and physical problems, such as feelings of loss, alienation, rejection, loneliness, grief, relationship problems, separation anxiety, panic attacks, depression, claustrophobia, paranoia, asthma, headaches, and sinus problems, can be traced back to the traumas surrounding birth—not just the birth in this life but any number of preceding births, going all the way back to the beginning of the creation of the individual soul when it first became separated from God.

In treatment, with regression therapy, we can help the patient recall, relive, release, and resolve the source of his or her emotional, physical, and personality problems that were rooted in prenatal and birth experiences and traumas.

This knowledge that the fetus in the womb feels and records all the feelings, thoughts, and experiences of the mother as its own, can have tremendous impact on parenting. Mothers and fathers can communicate with their unborn babies and let them know that they are welcomed and loved. They can pray for protection and healing for their unborn babies and for themselves. Thus they can provide the spiritual education while their babies are in the womb and also can continue to educate the babies about the spiritual reality, even after the birth as they grow into adulthood. This way, some of their problems will not manifest because from the beginning they are already aware that God is always present in their lives.

I usually make a relaxation tape for expectant mothers with protection prayers and positive suggestions for their day-to-day functioning. By listening to this tape, not only mothers but even the unborn babies can feel better and also be protected and healed. Parents can use this knowledge and actively contribute to the well-being of their babies, and can help to shape the personality of their unborn children.

A couple planning to have a child can also go through regression to their own prenatal life and birth, giving themselves firsthand understanding of what a fetus goes through in the womb and at birth and resolving their own personal issues as well. In this way, they can be better prepared to love and nurture their unborn children.

This understanding can also help the doctors and nurses in the delivery room to pay attention to the lights, sounds, and temperature in the room, and how newborn babies are treated at birth and after.

Chapter III

Past Life Traumas

Key to Yesterday

Glimpses of a movie that I have never seen,
Memories of someplace else that I have never been,
Shadows of another day flash across my mind,
Places, people, pictures of things I left behind.

So many things I seem to know, I don't remember learning;
It's like I had them long ago, and now they are returning.
And how long have I known you, a thousand years or so?
Or maybe even more than that. Impossible—although—

How is it we communicate, when not a word is spoken,
The deepest secrets of our hearts, in dialogue unbroken?
Why has my heart this wistful ache when nothing can explain
Why I am drawn to things unknown, time and time again?

Sometimes I feel I'm someone else; that I've been here before,
I take the key to yesterday and open up the door—
I'm shuttled back through history, I watch with bated breath,
The panorama of my soul through birth and life and death.

I see the golden beacon that leads me to its core,
Where I am bathed, and healed, and charged to do it all once more.
And so I see the answers, I know what I must do;
Love, and trust, and persevere—and so, my friend, must you.

— Jane

Past Life Traumas

Search for Literature

I was very impressed and excited when my patient Martha spontaneously regressed back to a past life and, after recalling, reliving, and releasing her emotional, mental, and physical feelings, experienced relief in just one session from her longstanding, crippling claustrophobia and panic attacks. As I began to do research on the subject, I was surprised to find that there were many books written on the subject of past lives and past life regression therapy, by professional and lay people. Some of the books that impressed me were as follows:

Ian Stevenson, M.D., professor in the Department of Psychiatry at the University of Virginia, has researched and documented more than 2,000 case histories. He studied very young children who seemed to consciously and vividly remember their past lives without any hypnosis. Some of these children recognized their former homes and neighborhoods as well as relatives and friends from their former lives who were still living. These kids sometimes had birthmarks that corresponded to the wounds they had during their previous deaths.

Many of these children exhibited xenoglossy, the ability to speak a foreign language to which they had not been exposed in this life. About half of these children came from Western countries where people had no belief in reincarnation.

Dr. Stevenson wrote several books on the subject, including *Twenty Cases Suggestive of Reincarnation*, *Cases of the Reincarnation Type* (four volumes), *Xenoglossy*, and *Telepathic Impressions—A Review and Report of Thirty-Five New Cases*.

Frederick Lenz, Ph.D., wrote the book, *Lifetimes: True Accounts of Reincarnation*, which gives accounts of 127 people who had spontaneous memories of one or more of their past lives. These people came from many different walks of life, religions, and ethnic and geographic backgrounds. One hundred nineteen of these people had no belief in reincarnation prior to their past life remembrances.

Helen Wambach, Ph.D., a psychologist, wrote two books based on her research: *Reliving Past Lives: The Evidence Under Hypnosis* and *Life Before Life*. In the first book, she tells of regressing more than 1,000 people to their past lives to specific time periods under hypnosis in small groups in different parts of the country.

In *Life Before Life*, she documented accounts of regressions of 750 people under hypnosis in small groups and explored the fascinating answers to the questions about life before birth. Some of the conclusions from her two years of research were as follows:

- Her subjects divide 49.4% into past lives lived as women and 50.6% as men.
- 90% of the people definitely flashed on images from a past life.
- 81% of her subjects said that they themselves chose to be born.
- 59% of her subjects mentioned more than one counselor in the Light before birth who helped them in the planning of another lifetime.
- 10% of her subjects reported people in their current lifetime—mother, father or relative—counseling them before birth.
- 68% of her subjects felt reluctant, anxious, or resigned to the prospect of living another lifetime.
- Only 26% of her subjects looked forward to the coming lifetime. Many of these subjects reported that they had planned carefully and felt that there would be help from the other dimension in achieving their goals in this life. It

was a hope of achievement and not pleasure that made life worth living for them.

- Death was experienced as pleasant by 90% of these subjects but being born and living another lifetime was unhappy and frightening.
- 87% of her subjects reported being aware that they had known important people in their current life from past lives. They all said that we often come back with the same souls, but in different relationships. We live again not only with those we love, but with those we hate and fear. Only when we feel compassion and affection are we freed from the need to live over and over with the same souls.
- 86% of all subjects said that they became aware of the feelings, emotions, and even thoughts of their mothers before they were born.
- Birth and living another life is perceived as a duty and not a pleasure.
- A soul can elect to leave the fetus's or the infant's body and return to the Light. Perhaps the sudden death syndrome in infants may be the result of a soul's decision not to go ahead with the life plan.
- Most of her subjects, no matter how enthusiastically they chose to enter the world, found the actual experience one of loneliness and alienation from the "land of Light" that they lost when they once more entered the physical world.

Life between Life, by Joel L. Whitton, M.D., and Joe Fisher, includes descriptions by Dr. Whitton's hypnotized patients about the mysteries of the between-life state in the Light and what we do there.

Mind Probe Hypnosis, by Irene Hickman, D.O., described cases in which her patients under hypnosis regressed to past lives to find the reasons for their fears, allergies, sexual problems, and aches and pains, which were completely alleviated after the sessions. She also described a case of possession by a human earthbound spirit.

Edgar Cayce, one of the best-known psychics of the twentieth century, was one of the first to explore the inner dimensions of health. From 1925 through 1944, he conducted some 2500 readings, in a hypnotic trance state, describing the past lives of individuals as casually as if everybody understood that reincarnation was a reality. Mr. Cayce was brought up in a fundamentalist Christian family and initially had a hard time accepting what he was saying during these trance states. Later, as he came to trust in the accuracy of the readings, he gradually understood the basis of reincarnation and karma and how they help us comprehend the seemingly incomprehensible aspects of human life. (*Scars of the Soul*)

Subjects, such as deep-seated fears, physical ailments, mental blocks, vocational talents, innate urges and abilities, marriage difficulties, child training, etc., were examined in the light of what Cayce called the "karmic patterns" resulting from previous lives of the individual's soul on the earth plane. (*Born Again and Again*)

The Search for Bridey Murphy, published in 1956, was the first heavily publicized case of a past life regression through hypnosis. It gained a lot of attention when a Pueblo, Colorado, housewife, Ruth Simmons, was regressed by an amateur hypnotist by the name of Morey Bernstein. Mrs. Simmons recalled in detail the life of an Irish girl named Bridey Murphy, who lived in Cork in the early 1800s. Because of the controversy surrounding it, some people tried to prove that her experience was valid, but most tried to prove that it was not.

There were other numerous accounts of past life regressions and of the attempts to prove or disprove their validity. Some people seemed to be very concerned whether the information was coming through past sources or present knowledge. Others wanted to prove or disprove the existence of reincarnation.

As far as I am concerned, these are immaterial concerns. What is important to me as a psychiatrist is that these regressions are capable of healing patients' emotional, mental, and physical problems. I make no judgment. I do not attempt to prove the accuracy or reality of these past life recollections. It is enough for me to know that this is a good and effective way to help and heal the patients.

During my research for literature, I also learned about the Association for Pastlife Research and Therapies, founded in 1980. Its purposes include the progressive development of the use of past life therapy, the advancement of research in this field, the improvement of standards of practice, the development of criteria for training past life therapists, and the provision of vehicles for the exchange of information and experiences.

The objectives of APRT are to improve human welfare, to provide meetings and seminars, and to inform the public about the field of past life therapy and research.

My literature search showed that I was merely one independent discoverer of a phenomenon already known to many others. Many other books have been published on past life regression therapy since my work took this direction.

Process of Past Life Regression Therapy

Utilizing past life regression therapy for about eleven years, I have developed certain steps of evaluation and therapy with my patients as follows:

Identifying the problems: The first step is to get a good psychiatric history and identify different emotional, mental, and physical symptoms and other core issues. If a patient is going through a crisis, it should be resolved first. The presenting crisis might be related to drugs or alcohol, a marriage or family problem, suicidal or homicidal preoccupation, or any other crisis in which the patient's life may be in danger.

Once the patient is stabilized, an inventory of emotional, mental, physical, and relationship problems helps to decide which symptom should be addressed first, depending on which symptom is most debilitating. For example, if a patient has severe panic attacks, fear of heights, chronic headaches, and chronic arthritis, it would be wise to work on the panic attacks first, then headaches. Chronic arthritis and the fear of height should be treated last, unless the patient has to fly often or has a job that requires climbing poles or being in other high places.

Deciding which technique is best for a particular patient: Most often, when patients come to seek psychiatric help they are suffering from acute emotional, mental, or physical problems, indicating that the problems are surfacing from the subconscious mind close to the conscious mind but not completely in the conscious mind. As a result, they are feeling the symptoms but are not aware of the real reasons for the symptoms.

When the problems are close to the surface, there is no need to relax the patient with progressive relaxation technique. Using that technique simply pushes the problems back into the subconscious mind, after which we again ask the patient to get in touch with the source of the problem and bring it into the conscious awareness. This is not necessary.

For example, let us say a patient is having a panic attack, experiencing difficulty in breathing, palpitations, and a fear of dying. I can use hypnosis with progressive relaxation, calming the patient and getting rid of the panic attacks by pushing them back into the subconscious mind. I can then ask the patient to find the source of the panic attacks and the patient may experience the symptoms again with the memory of the trauma. This is an unnecessary waste of time, and it really makes no sense. Instead, I ask the patient to focus on the symptoms and allow those symptoms to take him or her back to the source of the problems. The patient usually slips into a self-induced trance automatically.

I usually use one or more bridge techniques individually or together and they almost always elicit the traumatic event that is responsible for the problem.

Similarly, if a patient has a repetitive dream, a vision, or a spontaneous memory that may be connected to a past life or related to the patient's problems, I ask the patient to close his or her eyes and focus on that dream, vision, or memory and expand the awareness. As the patient begins to focus, the whole event unfolds from the beginning to the end.

If a patient does not have any acute emotional or physical symptoms during a session, then I utilize traditional hypnosis, using progressive relaxation to contact the subconscious mind and access the memories.

Steps of Past Life Regression Therapy

During past life regression therapy, I usually employ the following sequence. Any of the regression techniques can be used effectively.

Grounding and identification: When patients find themselves in past lives they are asked to look at their feet and describe what they are wearing on their feet, what type of clothing they are wearing, whether they are male or female, the color of their skin, their name, age, name of the town and country they live in, and the year. These questions help them to become aware of their identity in that life and focus on it. Questions are asked in the present tense and the name of the past life personality is used because that past life is the current life for the patient who is being regressed.

Processing the traumatic event: The patients are guided through the traumatic event. They are encouraged to recall, relive, and release the trauma completely. Often the event will lead to the death of the body in that life. Patients are encouraged to stay in the body and experience it completely.

They are directed to pay attention to their emotional, mental, and physical feelings and release them completely as they pass through different traumas and their death. Patients are also asked to pay attention to their last thoughts, decisions, and promises they made to themselves. These are the unresolved emotional, mental, and physical residues that are brought to the current life with their souls and are creating the problems. The patients are encouraged to release them completely.

If needed, the patients are asked to return to the beginning of the traumatic event and are encouraged to reexperience it fully. They must be kept in the experience while moving to the end of the event, which is usually the death. If the event does not end in death, patients are guided to their death in that life.

If the death occurs suddenly, the patients are asked to look at the event when their spirit is out of the body. They are directed and encouraged to describe their emotions, physical feelings, last thoughts, promises, and decisions, which are brought to completion, allowing the healing of the residue. If these are not resolved, problems in the current life will persist.

Process of death: Patients are consistent in their descriptions of the process of death. They describe that their body is sinking while their spirit is lifting up out of the body. There is no loss of consciousness or of continuity. There is an immediate freedom from any pain and discomfort they were experiencing before death. They can see their dead bodies below. Their memories, personalities, and attitudes continue. They feel as alive as they felt when they were in their physical bodies.

Transition to heaven: Most of the time, after the death of their physical bodies in past lives, patients describe seeing a bright white Light and find themselves drawn into it. Often they see their departed loved ones or angels or other beings of the Light coming from heaven to escort them.

Sometimes, after the death of the physical body, the spirit is so confused that it does not know what to do and where to go. Patients report that they try desperately to talk to others but nobody sees or hears them. They go to their funeral and try to comfort their loved ones without much success.

Sometimes they describe staying on the earth plane for many years, till they can find their way to heaven. Other times they describe going into some other person's body and staying there till that person dies. They then find their way to the Light with the one they possessed, or they go to somebody else and possess them.

Experiences in the Light (Heaven)

Greeting: The patients describe being lifted up and drawn toward the bright white Light. They describe feeling loved and free of the concerns they felt before and just after the death of their body. Patients often describe being greeted by the Light beings, who can be angels, a religious figure, a guide, or anyone they believe in. At times they see their departed loved ones in the Light, who look younger and in perfect health, compared with how they looked during the death of their physical bodies. Patients usually describe them as beings of Light with loving eyes, wearing white robes and totally surrounded by the white Light.

As they move into the Light, the patients find themselves also looking like a being of Light. They still have the same form and identity they just left, but they have no solid body or earthly clothing.

Ventilation: This step is not consistent with all patients. It is only if the life that they just lived was extremely traumatic and they are still feeling confused, angry, or guilty; then they are taken to a room where there are some Light beings waiting for them. Here the patients are allowed to ventilate their feelings about what happened. The Light beings, just by being good listeners, help the patients by allowing them to ventilate their feelings.

Cleansing: According to my patients, everybody goes through the stage of cleansing before they enter the main part of heaven. Patients describe different representations or symbolism for this stage. Some mention the similarity to taking a shower, where a burst of Light cleanses them; a sauna; a process of dry cleaning; bathing in the river; or walking through a river of Light. Some report standing under a waterfall and being cleansed from all impurities. Others describe a mechanical spinning process where the negative stuff is thrown off, or a vacuum cleaner sucking out all the impurities. Patients' reports differ in details, but the basic idea of cleansing before entering the main section of heaven is the same in every case.

Patients state that this process removes from their being anything negative, such as negative energies, devices, and any possessing human and demon spirits that came along with them. Negative emotions and attitudes are also removed, but not the memories of them.

Review phase: Patients describe going to another room after cleansing, where there are one to five or even more beings waiting for them. Patients say that if they are at a very high level spiritually, in the Light, then there are usually a master and other very high beings. If the patients are less developed spiritually, there may be angels or other wise beings of heaven. These beings serve as counselors who help in reviewing the life. They usually have a broader perspective and clear understanding of the nature of the Light and the universe.

Patients describe reviewing their whole life with the help of these counselors. Together they review their purpose for that life and the lessons they learned or failed to learn. They also evaluate their spiritual achievements.

According to patients, the function of the Light beings who help them review their life is not to judge or condemn them. Their function is to help them get the information out in such a way that the patients can see and understand it clearly. Patients usually say this is the most difficult stage, because it is they who judge themselves. There is no judgment or punishment by God or the Light beings who are helping them. Patients are their own harshest judge and jury.

Patients often describe this as a process of self-analysis and evaluation of the life they just lived. They alone interpret their success or failure in meeting the goals they set in the Light (heaven) for that life. Their feelings of disappointment and bitterness over lost opportunities and wrong actions cannot be adequately described. Their feelings of success and triumph about goals they achieved and good acts are just as remarkable and hard to convey. This is the stage in which patients come to grips with the harm they did to themselves and others by suicide, murder, and other negative actions.

During the review, patients not only assess every good and bad thing they did, but also experience other people's feelings. In heaven, patients describe themselves as nonphysical spirits. There are no barriers of time and space. Patients can return to any movement in the lifetime they just departed and observe the events from different points of view. In heaven, patients also have access to their other past and future lives.

Recognizing people: In past life regression therapy, at this stage in heaven I ask the patients to look back and see if they recognize any people who were there in the life they just recalled who may be here in the current life. Patients tell me that the people in this current life frequently show up in past lives in different relationships. This recognition helps the patients understand their interpersonal problems and feelings toward different people. They are helped in exploring, understanding, and resolving their conflicts with different people in the present life. Sometimes this improves their relationships instantly. This form of therapy not only changes the patients' attitude toward those people but, according to my patients, there is even a sudden and dramatic change within these other significant people in their lives.

Recognizing the problems and connections between the past life and the current life: I ask patients to recognize and understand different problems and issues coming from the past life they just recalled and relived. This step gives patients a better understanding about themselves and their current emotional, physical, and relationship problems. They can understand the unresolved issues that are carried over from that past life into the current life and resolve them.

Forgiveness: The next and most important step in past life regression therapy is forgiveness. I usually ask the patients at this stage if they choose to forgive the people who hurt them in that past life. Sometimes the patients are willing to forgive them without any problem. Other times they have a hard time forgiving. Their typical response is, "How can I forgive that person? He killed me . . . He raped me . . . He tortured me."

I ask the patients to look back in that life, into the event where those people are raping, killing, or hurting them and tell me how those people look to them. Patients often describe these people as totally dark and being demon-possessed, or surrounded by the demons who are encouraging them to commit the evil acts.

All of a sudden the patients have a better understanding about these people and their reasons for hurting or killing the patients in that life. They are able to understand that although these people are partly responsible for their actions, they were influenced and motivated by demon entities and were like puppets in the hands of the demons. With this understanding, almost always the patients are willing to forgive people who hurt them in that life.

I then ask the patients to locate and collect all the people who hurt them in any way, and fill them with the white Light. They are asked to tell the abusers who hurt them whatever they need to tell them, individually or in the group, to forgive them. As the patients fill these people with the white Light, all the darkness from them dissolves and disappears, along with their anger, hate, jealousy, guilt, and all the other negative emotions. The patients often see the abusers smiling. In this process, even those people who harmed the patients are also healed. The patients later describe a definite change in these people if they are here in the current life.

The next important step in the therapy is asking the patients if they need to ask for forgiveness from people whom they hurt. Usually they are willing to do so because in heaven they know they did hurt those people without making excuses for their actions or rationalizing them. In heaven they have an awareness of the truth.

Lastly—and the most difficult step in forgiveness—I ask the patients if they choose to forgive themselves for hurting others.

They find this most difficult. So I ask the patients to look back in that lifetime when they were hurting somebody. Almost always they see demon entities in and around them telling them and pushing them to do the wrong things. This realization gives them a better understanding about their behavior and actions. The patients can see that, although basically the problem was theirs, they were infested and influenced by the demon entities who pushed them into negative actions and behavior. Understanding this, the patients are willing and able to forgive themselves.

Locating, retrieving, and integrating the fragmented soul parts: From heaven, patients often describe losing many soul parts throughout that past life, especially during mental, emotional, and physical traumas. At this point, I request the angels to locate and bring back all the fragmented soul parts that the patients lost during that lifetime, from different people and places, including the ones that are in darkness in the possession of Satan and his demons, and cleanse, heal, and integrate them with the patients. It is important for the patients to watch and see where those parts are coming from and how they were used to create problems for them, especially when they are in the possession of Satan and his demons in hell. It is extremely important to retrieve and integrate those fragmented soul parts, otherwise the healing will not be complete. These lost, fragmented soul parts are the ones that create holes and weakness in patients' souls or beings, creating problems, and need to be brought back, cleansed, healed, and integrated with them to avoid any future problems.

Integrating the past life personality with the patient: The patients are asked to visualize that past life personality in front of them, fill it with the Light, and tell it whatever they want to tell. Then patients are asked to give that past life personality a hug and allow it to integrate and become one with them.

At this point I ask the patients to take a deep breath and check and tell me if any emotional, mental, or physical residue is left from that past life. If they say yes, then they are asked to locate it and go back in that life to the event that is responsible for the problem and resolve it. The process is repeated until all the problems coming from that lifetime are resolved. This concludes the regression therapy with that past life.

Sometimes, from heaven, the patients can see the same problem coming from more than one past lives, which are worked on in future sessions.

Resting phase: After the review stage, patients describe going to a place where they rest. Occasionally, if they led a very traumatic life, they are sent for resting right after the cleansing phase and review the life after resting.

Different patients give different representations of this place in heaven. The more common representation is of a beautiful garden, an open field with a meadow with trees and flowers, or a house with a bed. Some patients describe it like sleeping on the clouds, or sitting on the cloud with angels and playing a harp. The patients' needs govern how they see that representation. The purpose is the same: resting, healing, and allowing the experience to integrate.

The hallmark of the resting phase that the patients describe is limited activity. Whatever activity is there is very contained in nature and it is not vigorous. It is the concept of rest, sleep, recuperation, and preparation for continuation.

My patients state that the length of the resting phase depends on what is needed for individual beings. More spiritually advanced people tend to need a longer resting phase, because there is more work done and more to integrate. Also, if the life was hard and traumatic, the resting phase is longer.

Here patients report that they let go of the past life personality. They do not destroy it, but incorporate it into themselves, making "themselves" much greater than the individual personality they just lived. That life is no longer their way of functioning; they get their real spiritual self on the surface.

After resting, patients see paths that go to different gates and then into the inner part of heaven. Up to the resting phase, everything is on the outer level of heaven, where everything is in human terms: the table, the chairs, the garden, and human forms. Everything looks more like the things on the earth.

Patients say that after they go through the path into the inner gate, they are into the inner area of heaven and are no longer in a human form. This is where my patients describe that they shed the representation of the body and the body's weaknesses and limitations. Here they describe themselves as a complete and total spirit, a spark or a ball of Light. For the first time after several years they are free from the body's influences. They are able to act with their full spiritual capacity. Here the integration of knowing and taking the knowledge into their own being takes place.

Patients describe heaven as a sphere, which has two sections. The outer section is like the porch of a house or an inset into the building where cleansing, reviewing, and resting take place. Here everything is in an earthly form. Then, depending on their spiritual development, they go down one of the pathways into the gate to the inner section of heaven, where everything is in spiritual form.

Learning and planning stage: In the inner part of heaven, patients state that they learn, have discussions with others, and plan for the next life. Some people who are at the higher level say that they go and teach the beings at the lower levels, while they learn from the beings who are at the higher levels, including the masters. Some patients describe working in groups toward divine goals and purposes. Their planning includes personal goals and group goals.

The patients describe choosing their parents, spouses, children, and other significant people, usually because they need to make up for some negative problems between them, from one or more past lives.

They also claim to plan not only all the positive events of their lives but also the negative and traumatic events. They say that they learn and grow by facing and dealing with those negative and traumatic events. According to my patients, when the bad things happen in our lives it is not really God punishing us, but it is we who have planned those tragic events to grow and evolve spiritually, and it is we who are seeking to understand and evolve by resolving our negative actions from our past lives.

In therapy, I make a point to regress the patients to their planning stage in heaven for their current lives. This stage helps them understand their problems and purposes.

At the end of the session, after the regression, I spend some time discussing with the patients their understanding about the session and how it sheds light into their current life situations and problems. This step allows the patients to integrate the experiences, insights, and information from that past life into the present life.

An Example of a Past Life Regression

Sophia, a thirty-nine-year-old female, had trouble with her joints for many years. As a child she was extremely flexible and many times would hyperextend her joints, particularly her shoulders and knees. As she got older the pain in her joints became more chronic and hyperextension of the joints became constant. Her joints, after the age of twenty-eight, became sensitive to cold and dampness. Exercise and inactivity both seemed to hurt her joints, particularly her knees. The backs of her knees also had cysts, which swelled to the size of baseballs and were very painful when she had fluid retention. She had to take ibuprofen, an anti-inflammatory medication, to control pain.

During the session, as we were planning to explore the reasons for her joint pain, a vision came to her mind. She saw that in a past life she was being drawn and quartered by a horse, tied to each of her extremities, pulling her apart.

I asked her to close her eyes and focus on that vision, expand her awareness and tell me what was happening. The following is the transcript of that regression.

Sophia: "My name is Ravene. I am a thirty-four-year-old man. I am scared. I sense I am in a courtyard and I am going to be persecuted for my beliefs."

Dr. Modi: "Tell me more about yourself."

Ravene/Sophia: "I am kind of a hermit, a beggar. I talk to people about God. I tell everybody who will listen to me that God has nothing to do with fear."

Dr. Modi: "Fear of what?"

Ravene/Sophia: "Fear of retribution, fear of punishment, fear of burning in hell. My belief is that God is all-loving and forgiving and he does not punish anybody."

Dr. Modi: "What year is this?"

Ravene/Sophia: "1043. I am in a small town ruled by a king."

Dr. Modi: "Why are they persecuting you?"

Ravene/Sophia: "I always hang out in the courtyard. I am speaking to people about what I believe. Somehow the young princess was passing through and she heard me speaking and began to ask me questions. She liked what I was saying. Later she innocently told the king about me, who in turn talked to his bishop. They decided that I am a heretic and for that reason I must be publicly punished to discourage anyone else from speaking against the church."

Dr. Modi: "What happens then?"

Ravene/Sophia: "The whole town is there to watch. I am terrified. I am praying like crazy. I ask God to be merciful. To take me out of this as fast as possible. To take my soul straight to heaven."

Dr. Modi: "Uh-huh."

Ravene/Sophia [crying]: "If it is to affect all those who are watching, let it be in a good way. They lay me on the ground. The guards stand on my ankles and my wrists."

Dr. Modi: "Why?"

Ravene/Sophia: "So I can't pull free; and now they put the chains around me. Then they bring four horses.

They are big Belgians; they are huge. They tie one horse to one leg, the second horse to another leg, the third horse to an arm and the fourth horse to the other arm, all pointed in different directions."

Dr. Modi: "As they are doing this, what are your last thoughts?"

Ravene/Sophia: "Please God, help me. Please God make this quick."

Dr. Modi: "What other thoughts?"

Ravene/Sophia: "I know what I was saying was true. I believe in heaven. I know I am going to a better place. It is just this death is so horrible, so hard."

Dr. Modi: "Yes."

Ravene/Sophia [crying]: "They are whipping the horses. Oh, the pain is so excruciating. All my joints first rip free of their sockets and then the meat begins to tear off my bones. The pain gets so great that I pass out, thankfully, before I am split into four pieces. Then I'm above it all; so it was nice that God was good to me. It does not hurt anymore."

Dr. Modi: "Tell me what are you seeing from above."

Ravene/Sophia: "I see four hunks of meat beings . . . and that is all, it is really four hunks of meat beings, dragged across the courtyard in four different directions. It is horrifying and everybody who sees it is horrified. Even the horses are having a hard time with it. I screamed very loud because of the pain. I do not want to look anymore. It is disgusting. Man's inhumanity to man, and this was done in the name of the Church. I know deep down, I was right."

Dr. Modi: "What happens then?"

Ravene/Sophia: "I see a bright white Light coming down, and there are many beautiful angels in it. They pick me up and take me to heaven. They put me in a protective capsule of golden Light. It is almost like they sew me back together and put me in a bandage of golden Light all around me so I can heal. I feel like I am suspended vertically in this liquid Light, because I do not want to lie down and rest in the horizontal position after that lifetime. I rest for a long, long time."

Dr. Modi: "Move ahead in time after you are all rested and healed."

Ravene/Sophia: "Angels come and take me to another place. There are four beings in white robes. They look wise. They are very loving and kind. They do not judge or criticize. They want me to look back in that life. It is like a movie. I can see every little detail."

Dr. Modi: "Tell me what you see and understand."

Ravene/Sophia: "These counselors are telling me in a loving and nonjudgmental way that, although I was right in my beliefs, I really did not have to martyr myself for my beliefs. Everyone comes into their awareness of God and the truth in their own time. Although I believed in it, I did not have to be such a crusader. It was good that I offered people hope, but it was not good that I did myself in. I was as valuable in God's eyes as the people I was offering hope to.

"This was not really necessary. I could have carried this message much longer and influenced a lot more people if I would have been more diplomatic about it. When one is extreme in life, it is going to be counterbalanced by those who are just as extreme in another direction. I should have more regard for my personal safety and should be more careful in future lives. Although I did not feel like I was forcing anybody, I was too intense. I kind of invaded other people's psychic space. Everybody has to make those decisions for themselves."

Dr. Modi: "What are the connections between Ravene's life and Sophia's life? How has that life affected Sophia's life?"

Sophia: "My joint pain, including my shoulders and neck pain, back pain, knee pain, ankle pain, cysts in the back of knees, and pain in all the other joints came from Ravene's life. Also, hypermobility of my joints and weakness of my muscles because each joint was made loose and pulled apart.

"Thanks to Ravene I have learned not to be extreme in this life. I guide my kids gently and give them plenty of room to make their own decisions.

"In this life, I guard my spiritual knowledge and am careful about whom I talk to and how I talk about it. I also kind of distrust organized religions."

Dr. Modi: "Now look back in Ravene's life and see if you recognize anyone who was there who may be here in this life."

Sophia: "Yes, the bishop in Ravene's life is a lady I know in this life. I am afraid of her in this life, too, and I cannot trust her. The princess is a good friend in this life who also has pain in all her joints."

Dr. Modi: "Okay, now look back in Ravene's life and see if he lost any soul parts during the trauma or at any other time."

Sophia: "Oh, yes. Many, many."

Dr. Modi: "Okay. I request the angels of the Light to locate and bring back all the fragmented soul parts of Ravene from wherever they may be. Cleanse them, heal them, fill them with the Light, and integrate them with him, please. Sophia, you watch and tell me where those soul parts are coming from and how they have affected you."

Sophia: "I see many of Ravene's soul parts with the bishop as if through his religious authority or power he took those soul parts from him. He really enjoyed seeing Ravene being pulled apart. Oh, I see. There are many black cords from the bishop going down into hell, to a large dark being. I think it is Satan. Now I understand why he thought that I should be killed for my beliefs. They were different than his. He was under the control of Satan and his demons and he did not even know it.

"I also see angels bringing many of Ravene's soul parts that fragmented when his body was being pulled apart. These are soul parts that belonged to all his joints, muscles, eyes, etc.

"It is interesting that the princess felt so guilty that even she felt the empathetic pain in her joints and body as she was watching Ravene being torn apart, and she too lost many soul parts from her joints, which Satan and his demons grabbed and which are still with them. I am asking the angels to bring the princess's soul parts back and integrate them with her after cleansing and healing."

Dr. Modi: "Look down and see how Satan and his demons used those soul parts to affect you."

Sophia: "Oh, I can see it. What they are doing is through the cords that connect those soul parts with the main body of my soul, they are infusing a black, murky-looking fluid into my joints and also putting my soul parts in hell's fire. It produced inflamed, swollen, hot joints."

Dr. Modi: "Now do you choose to forgive all those people who hurt you in that life?"

Sophia: "Oh, that is so hard. They were so cruel to me."

Dr. Modi: "Look back in that life as the bishop and the king were making the decision that you should be persecuted. How do they look to you?"

Sophia: "I can see. They are filled with black demon entities. They are all dark and also many dark demons are lurking around them. Also, Satan is controlling them through their soul parts by whispering negative thoughts to them."

Dr. Modi: "Now do you understand why they took such cruel action toward you? Now do you choose to forgive them?"

Sophia: "Oh yes. They were possessed and controlled by evil and did not even know it."

Dr. Modi: "First ask the angels to fill them with the Light and heal them and then tell them whatever you want to tell them to forgive them."

Sophia: "I am asking the angels to fill everybody with the Light and heal them, including the king, the bishop, and the people who were involved in it including the princess, although she did not mean any harm to me. She was just an innocent child. I can see the darkness just falling apart and they are all smiling.

"I forgive all of you for your cruel and inhuman actions. You were totally controlled by the darkness and you did not even know it. May God bless you and heal you."

Dr. Modi: "Do you need to ask anybody to forgive you?"

Sophia: "Yes, I ask the princess to forgive me for getting her into trouble."

Dr. Modi: "Does she?"

Sophia: "Oh yes. I think I need to forgive Satan and his demons so they do not have any hold on me."

Dr. Modi: "Okay. See them in front of you and tell them whatever you need to tell them to forgive them."

Sophia: "Satan and all the demons, I forgive you all for influencing all those people in torturing me. You are the real source of all the inhuman acts on earth. I forgive you all and I will pray to God for your salvation. [looks surprised and smiles] Oh, Dr. Modi, you should see this. They cannot stand it. They squirm and literally seem to shrink and run away as I forgive them."

Dr. Modi: "Yes, isn't that interesting? Now look at Ravene, your past life personality standing in front of you. Fill him with the Light and tell him what you need to tell him."

Sophia: "Ravene, I am sorry for the pain you went through. You were very brave. In the future we need to be careful about who we talk to and what we talk about."

Dr. Modi: "Now give him a hug and watch him integrate with you. [She does so.] Now take a deep breath and let go. Tell me if anything is left with you from Ravene's life physically, emotionally, mentally, and spiritually that you need to release, understand, or look at."

Sophia: "Nothing."

Dr. Modi: "Good. Now feel God cleansing you, healing you, and filling you with the Light and love."

Sophia: "I feel free. I feel good."

After Sophia came out of the trance, we discussed what happened during the session and how it was connected with her arthritis.

During the next session, Sophia told me that her severe arthritis was almost gone. Not only that, the arthritis of the friend who was the princess in that life also improved through forgiveness and by having her soul parts brought back and integrated with her, without going through her own regression.

Experience of Past Life Regression

Over the years, I have realized that patients' experiences during their past life regressions vary widely. For some, it is a firsthand, in-the-body experience. For others there remains a degree of detachment, almost as if they were viewing a rerun on TV. Following are the different types of past life experiences my patients have reported.

1. Sometimes patients see and hear nothing. The knowledge simply flows into them that they are now a different person, in a different place and the meaning of the words that are spoken comes to them. They are aware of the feelings and the situations, but they really see or hear nothing. This is the most elemental way of perceiving.

2. Some patients report experiencing their past life as watching a movie, where they observe a life on the screen. In this case they do not hear a voice but simply observe the action and receive the feelings and the knowledge from within, as in the first category.

3. In some cases patients see the scenes being played out on a movie screen. They hear the voices, conduct the action, and receive the feelings and the knowledge from within.

The most important part in all the above examples is the fact that the patients receive the feelings and the emotional turmoil while perceiving the conflict going on.

4. In most advanced cases, patients report they actually entered the life and it is as if they are actually reliving it with the real people around them. They describe receiving the feelings directly, not just having the knowledge of the feelings. However, they also receive knowledge of the situation in the most elemental way, as in the first category. They also have the perception of what is going on with other people rather than just the interpretation they have of that life. They have more knowledge in reliving and looking back than when they lived that life the first time.

All of these experiences are therapeutic and promise success in releasing symptoms. As patients move up the scale in experiencing, the success of therapy increases.

During a past life regression, patients often have parallel awareness of both the past life and the current life. At other times they forget about the person they are now and go completely back into the former life as in the most advanced case. Patients still can respond to my questions. They say that they are aware of me but have forgotten they have a self in the present.

Some patients relive every moment emotionally, physically, and mentally, screaming, crying, and sobbing in agony while reliving a traumatic movement. Others remain calm and unemotional while reliving the traumas. Either way, the experience can be therapeutic and can release the symptoms. However, it is much more effective when the patients relive and release the events emotionally, physically, and mentally by staying in that past life body rather than watching from outside the body.

Reasons Why Some People Cannot Access Their Past Life Memories

Sometimes patients are unable to recall their past lives. They report the following reasons for the inability.

Fear of not coming back from the past life or death experience: Sometimes people are afraid that if they recall a past life and go through the death in that life they may really die and may not come out of the trance. This is not true. Recalling past life events and experiences is the same as recalling current life experiences.

Fear of finding negative lives: Another reason some people cannot recall their past lives is that they are afraid they will not be able to deal with lives in which they were guilty of some negative actions. If somebody has past lives in which they have done wrong things, those unresolved issues are already creating a problem in the current life, regardless of whether the person realizes it or not. By recalling, reliving, releasing, and resolving those unresolved issues and understanding them, an individual can be completely free of the problems that are carried over from other lives.

Possession by demon entities: This is one of the most common reasons some people cannot be regressed, especially if demons are in the person's eyes, ears, or brain. The demons prevent patients from seeing, hearing, and receiving. For this reason, it is extremely important to completely remove all the entities from a person and shield that person completely before attempting a past life regression.

Direct influence of Satan and his demons from outside: According to my patients' reports, Satan and his demons can create a block by putting a device like a black curtain, or standing between them and the Light. They can also insert false memories through different soul parts.

Missing soul parts: Sometimes patients cannot do past life regression because their soul parts are missing from their eyes, brains, and ears. These parts are usually in possession of Satan and his demons. The demons use those soul parts to block patients' visions, memories, and hearing by clamping the connecting cord between patients' souls and lost soul parts. They also send entities, devices, energy absorbers, or negative thoughts through the soul parts and their connecting cords to the patients' eyes, ears, and brains, causing interference.

After removing the negative entities, energies, and devices, and locating and retrieving the lost soul parts and integrating them after cleansing and healing, patients' vision can be restored and they can recall and see past lives vividly.

Satan and his demons planting the idea that it is all hocus-pocus: Another common reason, according to my patients, is that Satan and his demons have planted an idea or an attitude in them that this is all hocus-pocus and foolishness and that there is no such thing as past lives. Patients have a difficult time getting over that attitude.

Rejection of the idea of God and of the soul and its Continuation: Another reason some people cannot do past life regression is their rejection of the idea of God, soul and its continuation, and the cycle of reincarnation. As a result, they cannot access a past life.

Doubts and guilt about trying past life regression because of their religious beliefs: Although belief in reincarnation is not at all necessary for the treatment to work, sometimes patients' reluctance and guilt in trying past life regression, due to their religious and intellectual beliefs, block them from receiving the information from within. This guilt also opens them up for possession and influence by outside entities. As a result, they cannot recall a past life or may get confusing information.

Holly came to me for past life regression for allergies. She was a good subject and was able to release spirits from herself but, because of her religious beliefs, she felt guilty about wanting to try this therapy. As a result, she was not able to access the life responsible for her problems. I asked her, under hypnosis, to look inside the Light and see if there was somebody from heaven who could give her some answers to her questions. As she looked up she described seeing Jesus in the Light with kind and loving eyes. She asked Him about Satan and his demons, if they are real, and if we live more than one life. According to Holly, Jesus explained to her in the following way:

> "Yes, Satan and his demons are as real as you and I, creating constant problems and confusion for humanity. Nothing makes Satan more happy than to make everybody think that he and his demons do not exist.
>
> "Satan uses religion to create disbelief in people. Every religion on earth is a gift from God, but God is not the only spiritual being working on this earth. It also has input from Satan. He has taken the truth and twisted it to keep the knowledge and the truth from humanity by working through the corrupt human beings who are influenced by demons. It allowed people from different religions, and within the same religion, to fight with each other over what is the truth. The belief that 'Our religion is the only possible correct religion,' is another example of Satan's influence. Human and animal sacrifice also came through perversion of Satan.
>
> "Satan has implanted the idea in religions that the souls do not continue and we live only one life. The truth is that people live many lives to learn and grow. How they live this life affects their next life or lives further down the line. People need to make up for their negative actions from past lives; otherwise they will follow them in the current or future lives."

After that, Holly felt comfortable about the therapy and was able to recall the past life trauma that was responsible for her allergies and was relieved of them.

Blocked on purpose from the Light: Some patients, under hypnosis, say they are blocked on purpose due to the decision they made in heaven for some special divine purpose. That is why they cannot recall their past lives.

A new soul: In extremely rare cases, the person may be a new soul coming to earth who does not have any or has only a few past lives.

Confounding Factors that Complicate and Interfere with a Past Life Regression

Occasionally in some patients a peculiar similarity and repetition appears, so that many patients recall the same past life. Suppose seven people make claim to the same past life; it is possible that all seven lived that life, but it is highly unlikely. It is clear that either all of these individuals are suffering from a common delusion or there are reasons for what they recall. As I worked with different patients, it became evident that not every reported past life actually belonged to those patients who are reporting it.

In this situation, an analysis of the patients' reports is necessary. Are there other factors that interfere with and confuse a past life regression? Are the patients tuning into someone else's past life? Or do these patients give other reasons for their psychiatric difficulties that may impinge upon past life regression therapy?

Different patients have provided the following reasons for these problems:

- Cross talk
  - Complete cross talk
  - Incomplete cross talk
  - Internal cross talk

- Memories of a possessing earthbound entity
- Possessing earthbound entity's cross talk
- Falsely planted past lives

Cross Talk

Occasionally, while doing a past life regression, patients recall a past life that they later describe as not their own. They say that they were tapping into somebody else's past life.

Patients explain the reasons for this cross talk in this way. They say that from God come seven or more beings called masters, Godheads, or oversouls. We all descend from one of these Godheads. Each person is connected to one of these Godheads by a silver cord. Each Godhead has many silver cords coming from different people who descend from that Godhead.

According to my patients, these connections or cords act as tunnels or pathways through which memories, emotions, feelings, and information of past lives travel. Each individual's life is transported to his or her Godhead through the connecting cords, which can be tapped into by others through their connections with the same Godhead. To each it may seem like his or her own life.

The Godhead is the main expression of our being in the Light (heaven). Each Godhead lives many lives through many people at the same time. The lives that are picked up by other people through their Godhead are either positive or negative lives with very intense emotions and feelings that resonate strongly in the Godhead.

This explains why sometimes people find themselves recalling the same important or famous, well-known life even though it is not their own. According to my patients, a life that was very ordinary does not produce much vibration and does not resonate in the Godhead. Therefore, it is not picked up by others.

The patients' therapy is effective only when they recall their own past lives. Recalling somebody else's past life cannot help the patient, unless it is creating problems for them, too.

CROSS TALK
(Drawing by a patient)

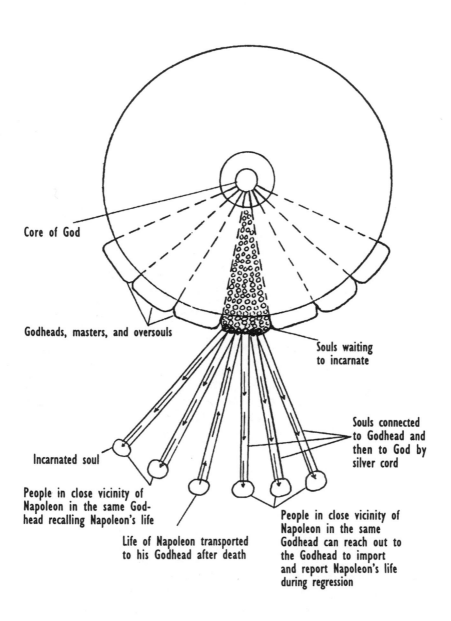

Core of God

Godheads, masters, and oversouls

Souls waiting
to incarnate

Souls connected
to Godhead and
then to God by
silver cord

Incarnated soul

People in close vicinity of
Napoleon in the same God-
head recalling Napoleon's life

Life of Napoleon transported
to his Godhead after death

People in close vicinity of
Napoleon in the same
Godhead can reach out to
the Godhead to import
and report Napoleon's life
during regression

Lifetimes that are picked up through cross talk can be complete or incomplete.

Complete Cross Talk

Patients can reach back in the Light (heaven) to the Godhead and pick up a whole past life of somebody else, import it, and report it as their own past life. Sometimes patients become aware that the life is not their own only after they make their transition to heaven and look back and review the life.

Emma had severe feelings of guilt and failure all her life with no good reason. During one session, under hypnosis, as I asked her to go to the source of her guilt feelings, she recalled a life of Eve with Adam; Eve died with intense feelings of guilt and of failure.

As she went into heaven, I told her to go to her planning stage for Emma's life. There she saw Eve as one of the counselors who was helping her plan her life as Emma. She saw Eve as a separate entity from her and she realized that she was simply tapping into Eve's life and it was not her past life. In the Light (heaven) she saw herself in close proximity to Eve in the same Godhead and thus she was able to tap into Eve's life and even feel her feelings. After that session, her feelings of guilt and failure were relieved.

Incomplete Cross Talk

Sometimes, while patients are recalling and reliving their past life, they get partially polluted by a fragment of somebody else's past life. Here a name, a place, or an incident from somebody's past life can be picked up and fed into what is the patient's own past life.

Internal Cross Talk

Sometimes patients recall memories from many of their own past lives in one session as the memory of one life. Patients describe the recalled events as true, but some of the details are mixed up. These are usually similar lifetimes. The same issues keep coming up in different lifetimes and have not been successfully worked through. So the patients keep trying different lives with the same sort of events, trying to get it right, and trying to learn and integrate the lessons that have to be learned.

The patients come back with the same basic story in another time and another place to work through the issues. In these cases, events are similar but the details such as names, dates, and places are different. As long as they are the patient's past lives, therapy will be effective.

Jacob, a forty-year-old male, had problems with his wife and felt trapped. He wanted to leave her but couldn't. He also had trouble recovering from a lung infection. During one regression, he began to get confusing information in which different names and places kept popping up in his mind. I told him to focus on one name, place, and story at a time. He recalled three different lifetimes when he tried to resolve the same conflicts and learn the same lessons. In these lives the basic theme and events were the same but the names, places, and dates were different.

First life: He recalled a life as a thirty-year-old female in 1800. Her name was Jane Carmon. She recalled being in a log cabin sick with pneumonia and unable to take care of her family. She died of pneumonia, feeling angry with God. Her last thoughts were "I have no control. I wish somebody would help me." She promised herself "I will never leave my husband again." From the Light (heaven) Jacob recognized Jane's husband in that life as his wife in the current life.

Second life: He recalled another life as a thirty-five-year-old female in 1843 in Indiana. Her name was Rachel Pierce. She had four children. The youngest child was two months old and was very small. Rachel was sick with bronchitis with a constant cough and was unable to take care of the family and died of pneumonia, feeling helpless and useless and feeling that she was abandoning her baby. Her last thoughts were "I am abandoning my baby. I am angry at God for taking me away." She promised herself "I will never abandon him. I will always be there to watch over him."

From heaven, Jacob recognized the little baby, whom he promised never to abandon, as his wife in the current life.

Third life: Jacob recalled a third life as a forty-year-old female in 1898. Her name was Amy Smith and she lived in Wyoming with her husband and three children. The youngest child had brain damage. At the age of forty-three, Amy died of pneumonia. Her last thoughts were "Who is going to take care of my baby? I am angry at God." She promised the baby that she would always be with him and would never abandon him. From heaven, Jacob recognized the baby in that life as his wife in the current life.

Jacob understood that in all these lives, including the current life, he was facing similar problems of feeling trapped, having no control, and being angry at God for not helping him. He could not leave his wife in the current life because of the old promises in his past lives of never to abandon her and to always take care of her. The lung infection in this life brought back memories of the conflicts from those past lives. He needed to learn the lessons of being more accepting of the situations and not to blame himself or God for situations over which he had no control.

Memories of a Possessing Earthbound Spirit (Entity)

Sometimes during a past life regression, what initially seems to be the patient's past life turns out to be the life or a past life of a possessing earthbound spirit. Here the past life events were usually related to the patient's symptoms, but it was not his or her past life. These were the events in the possessing spirit's life that created symptoms for that spirit, and in turn for the patient it was inhabiting.

For this reason, again, it is very important to locate and release all the possessing entities from the patient before attempting a past life regression.

Dawn was a forty-year-old female who came to me for severe depression, suicidal preoccupation, and anxiety attacks. She always felt trapped and wanted to run away from everything. During one of the sessions, she was very upset and was crying. During the conversation she repeated the following phrases several times.

"I am worthless. I feel like I am trapped. I do not want to be by myself."

I asked her to close her eyes and repeat these phrases, with feelings, and let them take her back to another time when she felt the same way. After repeating those phrases a few times with emotion, she found herself in another life as a man in jail. His name was John. At the age of forty-five he robbed a woman and killed her by cutting her throat. In jail he felt alone and trapped and did not want to live like that so he committed suicide by cutting himself with a piece of metal.

After death, he saw the Light and found himself floating up into the Light, where there were angels and other Light beings. He felt unworthy of the warm reception, so he turned away from the Light. He wandered around until he joined Dawn, who in turn began to feel his symptoms. After some psychotherapy with John, he was released to the Light.

After that session, Dawn's depression, suicidal thoughts, anxiety attacks, and the intense feelings of being trapped, being unworthy, and being alone were improved a great deal. They were caused by the earthbound entity's life and were not the patient's past life.

Possessing Earthbound Spirit's Cross Talk

A possessing earthbound entity can also draw information from its past lives or from somebody else's past life, through its connections with its Godhead. The possessing earthbound entity's cross talk can also intrude upon its host, the patient.

Falsely Planted Past Lives

Based on my patients' reports, sometimes false past life stories can be planted by Satan and his demons. Usually these lives, as patients describe them, can be regular lives or can be anywhere between the extremes of bizarre and dull and boring. They really do not seem to have anything to do with any of the patient's symptoms and issues.

These falsely planted lives usually have a story of continuation in the Light, like a motion picture. But they are vague and meaningless and have nothing to do with the patients' symptoms. They interfere with the therapy and create unnecessary confusion. Patients' symptoms are relieved only when they recall and relive their own past lives and resolve the problems and issues.

Patients have described different ways Satan and his demons feed them false lives to confuse and delay their healing. They are as follows:

Feeding a past life of an earthbound entity through a patient's soul part and its connecting cord: Here a demon has a soul part from the patient's brain. The demon takes an earthbound entity and its memory and shoves it through the patient's soul part and its connecting cord to the patient's brain. The patient then recalls it as his or her own past life, while it is really the memory of the earthbound entity.

Printing or typing a story on a patient's soul part which is transferred to the patient: Here a patient describes a demon with a device like a typewriter. The demon has a soul part from the patient's brain that the demon puts in the typewriter as you would a piece of paper and then types a story on it. This false information (a story of the demon's own making) travels through the cord and into the patient's brain, where, consequently the patient recalls it as his or her memory.

Feeding a story into the patient through a device like a walkie-talkie: Here a demon sends a small type of receiving device into the patient through the patient's soul part, which is in possession of the demon. The demon has a walkie-talkie type of device, through which it speaks and transfers false lives into the patient; the patient then receives and recalls those false lives as his or her own past lives.

Projecting a life on the patient's soul part, which is used as a movie screen: Here a demon uses a patient's soul part as a movie screen. Using a device like a movie projector, the demon projects a story of its own making or a past life of another entity. These images and memories travel through the patient's soul part and its connecting cord to the patient, who receives them as his or her past life.

John, a thirty-five-year-old male, came to me with multiple problems. We did many sessions releasing his possessing demon and human spirits. Then we proceeded to explore other reasons for his problems. He was a good subject and went through many past lives. We both realized there was something very odd. Most of the past lives he recalled were complete but were very dull, and some were bizarre and did not seem to have any connection with his problems.

During one session, when he went to heaven after death, I asked him to look back in his past lives to check if those lives were really his. He did not see those lives that he recalled as his past lives. So I asked him to look back as he was recalling those lives and find out what was happening. He saw Satan feeding him false lives through his soul parts, which were in Satan's possession. We asked the angels to bring his soul parts from Satan and integrate them with John after cleansing and healing. After that, John was able to recall his past lives which were responsible for his problems.

Single Symptom Coming from a Single Past Life

Sometimes a single symptom is coming from a single past life. With the resolution of the traumas and issues from that one past life, the symptom can be completely cured in just one session. Following are some examples of such dramatic cures.

Premenstrual Symptoms (PMS)

Peggy, a thirty-year-old mother of two children, complained of having severe abdominal cramps and heavy bleeding during her periods. She felt irritable and depressed and had overwhelming sadness before and during her periods.

Under hypnosis, she regressed to another life in Hamburg, Germany, in 1941. She was a fifteen-year-old girl. She said that her parents were rich Germans. One day soldiers came and took her away in a big black car. Although she was a German girl they did not believe her and took her to a concentration camp and made her wear a Jewish star.

She described that several soldiers brutally raped her one by one, over and over, while she was there. She became pregnant when she was seventeen years old. The following is a part of the transcript of what happened to her at that time.

> **Peggy** [crying]: "I am seven months pregnant, but I look like I am nine months because I am so thin. I am so frightened."
>
> **Dr. Modi**: "Why?"
>
> **Peggy** [crying]: "They are going to torture me."
>
> **Dr. Modi**: "Move ahead and tell me what they are doing to you."
>
> **Peggy** [crying in pain]: "They cut me up. They cut my belly and are ripping me apart [crying and sobbing]. I am dying. [All of a sudden Peggy became limp and there was silence.] Then she said calmly, "I am dead. It is all over. I am free. I am watching my body from above."
>
> **Dr. Modi**: "What happened to the baby?"
>
> **Peggy**: "They strangled the baby and killed him. It was a boy."
>
> **Dr. Modi**: "What are your thoughts about what happened to you?"
>
> **Peggy**: "If I did not get pregnant I could have lived longer. Why did I have to suffer? I want the soldiers and

doctors dead. Being rich cannot protect you. I cannot hate those people. They are evil and do not even know it. It's over, nothing you can do. They are waiting for me. I am going."

Dr. Modi: "Where?"

Peggy: "Where you always go in between lives. Now I am here. It is peaceful."

She described being in the Light. From heaven, she recognized many solders and doctors who raped and killed her in that life are also here in this life in different relationships. After she forgave them she felt free from that life.

Later, after a couple of weeks, she told me that after that session, for the first time during her menstrual period, she did not have abdominal cramps or excessive bleeding and did not feel irritable, sad, and depressed.

She also said that during her pregnancy in this life she had a mortal fear of death and did not want to have a boy (the baby in that life was a boy). She was also cold all the time in this life, and that discomfort was relieved after that session. She described being cold in the concentration camp all the time because she was often kept naked and did not have enough clothes to wear. She also had a fear of being rich all her life.

Nine years later, Peggy reported that she is still doing well and her symptoms have not returned.

Sinus Pain

Albert, a forty-five-year-old male, suffered from constant pain in his sinuses for about twenty years. Each pain spot was a target for infection. He had sinus infections frequently and had to take antibiotics, which gave only short-term relief.

During a session, I asked him to close his eyes, focus on his sinus pain, and let that feeling take him back to the event that was the source of his problem. Albert found himself regressed to another life in Afghanistan in 1800. He described the traumatic event as follows:

Albert: "I am in the country with five other men. They are my comrades and fellow rebels. We are betrayed, ambushed, and several of our people are killed. The enemy has occupied the town in the valley while we hide out in the mountains. I am fastened down in a spread-eagle position. My former comrades are torturing me."

Dr. Modi: "Why?"

Albert: "They believe that I betrayed them. But I did not. I know who the traitor must be but they do not believe me."

Dr. Modi: "Describe to me what is happening."

Albert: "The leader of our group is standing a few feet from my right hand. One man is kneeling at the top of my head, grabbing a handful of my hair to hold my head steady. Two others are standing on each side of my body holding their instruments of torture. [looking anxious and scared]

Dr. Modi: "What is happening?"

Albert: "The daggers in their hands have metal blades about eight inches long. They have sharp edges and sharp points. Now my former friends are shoving the daggers through my face and nose into my sinuses.

"They are wiggling them around and twisting them. It hurts! My bones are cracking and breaking! [squirming with pain] The blood is pouring from my face and it is going down my throat choking and killing me."

Dr. Modi: "As they are torturing you what are your thoughts?"

Albert: "I am angry. They are torturing and killing me unjustly. I will never be in a situation like this again. I will always keep this pain as a reminder so I can remember never to be in a compromising situation. I will never forget it."

After recalling, reliving, and releasing the traumatic event, including his last thoughts, decisions, and promises and forgiving his tormentors, he felt free from his pain immediately after the session. Later Albert reported that the pain points in his sinuses in the current life were the same as the spots where the daggers broke through the bone.

His longstanding sinus pain was completely alleviated after just one session. Nine years later, he is still doing well and his sinus pain has not returned.

Allergies to Hay, Wheat, Weed, Pollen, and Corn

Pam, a twenty-five-year-old housewife, was allergic to hay, wheat, weed, pollen, and corn. These allergies caused sinus problems and headaches most of her life.

Under hypnosis, when I asked her to go to the source of her problem, she found herself in a life as a nineteen-year-old female in 1032 in Russia. She was married and had a three-month-old baby girl. She remembered at the age of twenty years running through wheat fields with her baby because soldiers were coming after them. She described the scene as follows:

> **Pam**: "There is a war and nobody is there to protect us. We are in a wheat field and we are running toward the bridge, but my baby and I do not make it."
>
> **Dr. Modi**: "What happened?"
>
> **Pam**: "A soldier cuts me down with his sword. I fall on my baby and she gets smothered in the wheat field because I could not move."
>
> **Dr. Modi**: "What happens then?"
>
> **Pam**: "I am lying in this wheat field with my face down. As I try to breathe, goldenrod, wheat, pollen, grass, corn, and dirt go in my nose and sinuses. It is itching and burning and it is hard to breathe and I die."

After death, from heaven, she forgave that soldier for killing her and her baby. Pam understood the connection between her feeling responsible for her and her baby's traumatic death and inhaling the dust, weed, corn, and wheat pollen while dying, and her allergies to these agents. They are the reminders of the loss of her baby and her traumatic death experience.

After that session, she was free from her allergies. Nine years later, according to Pam, she is still free of them.

Multiple Symptoms Coming from a Single Past Life

For some of my patients, one past life was responsible for multiple emotional, physical, and relationship problems. Just dealing with this one life and resolving all the issues and traumas from it dramatically improved or relieved many of their physical and emotional symptoms and relationship problems.

Case of Donna

Donna, a twenty-one-year-old female, had multiple symptoms off and on most of her life, more so during the two years before she came for the treatment. She had depression, anxiety, difficulty in sleeping, early morning awakening, poor appetite, inability to gain weight, and suicidal preoccupation with feelings of hopelessness and helplessness.

She also expressed having multiple fears: fear of being abandoned, of rejection, of losing control, of going crazy, and of bugs. She also could not watch concentration camp movies. Physically, she had back pain, aches and pains all over her body, and pimples.

During a session, under hypnosis, she regressed to a life in Germany as a seventeen-year-old girl in 1939. Her name was Becky. She recalled going for a walk and when she came back the whole town was empty. Nobody was there, including her family. She did not know what happened to them. She went to the train station, where German soldiers captured her and took her where her mother and sister were.

They were taken to a big flat area where kids and grownups were separated and sent to different concentration camps. She recalled being beaten and abused and her back was broken. She and others had very little to eat. The place had bugs and roaches that were constantly biting. At one point doctors poured acid on her face to see if it would make the skin lighter. It burned her face and caused blisters.

After several months, her mother and then her sister died. She felt guilty about not being able to take care of her younger sister. Becky died a few months later of starvation.

After that session, Donna's depression and nervousness improved a great deal. Her fears of rejection, of being abandoned, of bugs, of losing control, and of going crazy were all alleviated. Her back pain and pimples improved. She was able to eat better and had gained weight. She was able to sleep well and was not suicidal. All these problems came from the life in a concentration camp.

Case of Amanda

Amanda, a thirty-eight-year-old female, came to me because of severe depression, suicidal preoccupation, and inability to function at home and at work. She had headaches, jaw pain, sinus problems, throat infections, and drainage.

I asked her to focus on her thoughts and feelings and let them take her to the source of her problems. She regressed into a lifetime in Nebraska in 1919. Her name was Betty.

Betty was forced by her husband's family to take care of her sick mother-in-law. Her mother-in-law was up all day and night screaming and constantly calling Betty for one thing or the other. Betty became very resentful because nobody was helping, or listening to her. She was feeling depressed, tired, and helpless and could not stand her mother-in-law's screams.

Betty took a rifle and went into the woods. Her mind was fuzzy and tired. She wanted to end it all. So she put the rifle in her mouth and shot herself and died. Her last thoughts were "I have to get away from everybody. This is the only way I will find any peace. I cannot stand the screaming. I want to be released from this hell on the earth. I will never allow myself to be used like this again."

After the death of her body she found herself out of her body looking down at her body. Her mouth, sinuses, face, and head were all blown into pieces.

Lessons: From heaven, Amanda understood that the lessons she needed to learn from Betty's life were that she should pray and ask God for help, wisdom, and strength. She should never commit suicide but face and resolve her problems the best way she can. She has done a great deal of damage to her soul by committing suicide.

From heaven, she saw that when she was in the woods committing suicide, her soul and body were all dark, because they were filled with demons. Also, there were many dark demons who were lingering around her telling her "Go ahead and kill yourself. This is the only way out." They gave her the strength to commit suicide.

Problems and symptoms coming from Betty's life: Amanda saw many symptoms coming from Betty's life. They were depression, suicidal preoccupation, temporomandibular joint pain, sinus problems, headaches, throat infections, and drainage.

After that regression, most of Amanda's symptoms were relieved.

Case of Susan

Susan, a forty-year-old female, had severe premenstrual symptoms, which she described as follows:

"Before my periods I get horribly depressed, irritable, and emotional. I feel an overwhelming sense of sadness and loneliness. Everything hurts, even my hair. All my joints become extremely painful. My knees swell and big cysts pop out on the back of my knees. Sometimes the pain is so bad that I cannot walk. I have severe cramps, headaches, and backache. I get constipated. I have severe bloating and I gain about ten pounds. I feel very tired and drained. I take Ansid and Nuprin. This helps, but not much."

About an hour before the regression, Susan began to feel severe pain in her vagina and inside of her thighs. An overwhelming sadness crept over her and she felt extremely tired and drained. Her period was not due for about two weeks, but that was how she felt during her periods. It was as though she had already tuned into the event responsible for her PMS. I asked her to focus on her feelings and let them take her back to another time to the source of her problem, when she felt the same way.

Susan regressed instantly to another life in Spain. It was around 1701. She was a twenty-eight-year-old gypsy female who was in a hospital. She had run away from her family to be with her lover. She was pregnant. One day while riding a horse she fell and landed on her stomach, knees, and face. She felt the fall killed the baby she was carrying but did not abort and had not told anybody.

She became extremely sick due to the infection and was running a high fever. She had severe pain all over and was bleeding heavily. Her insides ruptured and she died, feeling alone, sad, and responsible for her baby's death. Her last thoughts were "I should not have gone horseback riding. I killed my baby."

From heaven, she saw that she lost many soul parts to the baby, her grandmother, and her lover. Many of her soul parts were with demons in the darkness. She saw that demons used those soul parts to reactivate the memory of her physical and emotional feelings and guilt about killing her baby, which she felt when she was dying. They were all transferred to and experienced by Susan here in her body. All those soul parts were brought back, cleansed, healed, and integrated with Susan with the help of the angels.

About two weeks after the session, Susan had her period. There was a dramatic change in her. She did not have any bloating, cramps, headaches, back pain, or any other pain in her body. There was no swelling in her knees and she did not overeat. She didn't feel depressed or irritable. She no longer felt the overwhelming sense of sadness and loneliness. Her frame of mind was very good.

Single Symptom Coming from Multiple Past Lives

Sometimes patients claim they are dealing with an emotional, physical, or relationship problem in this life and have experienced it in many past lives. They find that several lifetimes ago, they did something negative that they need to correct. The problem they now face is a consequence of that life, which they call a connecting or a karmic life. Unless they correct the problem, it will keep on coming back, life after life, until it is completely resolved. Now, in this life, the patients get another chance to come to grips with the problem, resolve it, and break the chain. In these cases, instead of dealing with every lifetime, the patient can go to the very first life, when the problem began, and a few other key lives in between, to resolve the problem and break the cycle.

A Case of a Hearing Problem

Josh, a forty-five-year-old male, had a hearing problem that started about twenty years before, when he worked in a pipe mill. According to Josh, the noise level was terrible and constant, and as a result his hearing gradually went downhill. Josh could hear bass noise all right, but he had a hard time with high-pitched sound and soft-spoken people. He got frustrated that other people could hear things that he could not, and he had to ask people to repeat themselves. He was prescribed a hearing aid but could not use it. Because of his hearing problem he withdrew from people and became a loner.

During a session, he described his feelings about his hearing problem as follows:

"I feel like I am not a whole person."
"I feel inferior."
"I feel aggravated and disgusted."
"I want to shy away from people."

After a few repetitions of these phrases Josh regressed to a time in this life when he was thirty-one. He was in the steel mill working on pipe. He described noise so intense that he felt agitated. It was so bad that he blocked the noise by imagining he had cotton in his ears or that his ears were covered.

Then he regressed to the age of twelve in this life, when he began to use guns to hunt. The loud crack of the gun made his ears ring and sometimes for days he couldn't hear people because of the ringing in his ears.

First Past Life: Then I asked him to move back to another time, to the source of his hearing problem. He regressed to another life in 1660 as a forty-year-old male on a pirate ship. His name was Adam. They used to go to the islands to rob and kill people. At this time they were fighting pirates on another ship by firing the cannon. He couldn't stand the cannon's noise. It made him feel as if it were going to burst his ears. One day a cannon accidentally exploded, and Adam was blown apart.

Second Past Life: Josh regressed to another life in England as a twelve-year-old boy who volunteered to ring the church bell three times a day. The bell was so loud that he suffered with headaches and ringing in his ears. Within a few months he became deaf in both ears. He never got married and lived alone. He felt cheated and did not want to be around anybody. He died at the age of forty-five of a heart attack. His last thoughts were "I wish I could hear one more time."

Third Past Life: Josh regressed to another life as a fifty-year-old male, an American Indian living in 1430. He was a leader and he and his people raided a village and killed many people senselessly. One of the villagers shot him with a bow and arrow, which went through his right ear and came out of the left ear and he died.

From heaven, Josh was very surprised to learn that in his current life, at the age twelve and later while working in the pipe mill, the sound did not produce any real physical damage to his ears as he thought and he did not lose any soul parts from his ears in this life. He saw that his hearing problem came from the traumas he suffered in many previous lives. It was also a reminder of the senseless killing in the lives as a pirate and also the Indian chief.

The demons had many soul parts from both his ears which he lost during the traumas to his ears in those past lives and were restimulating in Josh the memories of the painful noise of cannon firing and exploding and bell ringing. The sounds of guns firing and the pipe mill in this life were reminders of those traumatic memories.

He also saw that demons were blocking his hearing by clamping the cords, which were connecting the missing soul parts to his ears. All the soul parts to both his ears were brought back, cleansed, and healed and were integrated with Josh with the help of the angels. According to Josh, his hearing has improved a great deal. At times he is able to hear sounds that others cannot hear. He is more communicative, social, and outgoing.

As we look at this case, we can clearly see that Josh's hearing problem had its roots in many traumas of his past lives, which followed him and were manifesting in his current life. Through recalling, reliving, releasing, understanding, and resolving those traumas from those past lives and bringing and integrating the lost soul parts with him, his hearing was restored to normal.

A Case of Smoking

Using regression therapy, I began to realize that almost every emotional, mental, and physical symptom can have its roots in one or more past lives. I was very surprised when my patients found the source of their smoking habits in one or more past lives, too.

Sue, a forty-year-old librarian, began to smoke cigarettes when she was in her freshman year of college, as a way to calm down during her finals. Later on, she began to smoke pot so she could fit in with her "hippie" friends. When she came to me she had quit cigarettes three months earlier but continued to smoke pot.

During the first session, I firmly told her that if she wanted to do this therapy she would have to quit using pot because it damages the protective energy shield around us and opens us for possession. She followed the instruction and did not use pot but started to smoke cigarettes again and was unable to stop that habit.

As she thought more about it, she realized it was not just the nicotine or the marijuana she was addicted to, but it was the act of smoking and inhaling the smoke and the feeling of the smoke going down through her lungs that she was addicted to. This gave her comfort and warmth. She associated the act of smoking with room to think, a minivacation, a creative space, a time to brainstorm and for creative planning, a time to get in touch with her spirituality and great insights. She also felt that smoking has a "grounding" quality and if she were not grounded she would float away.

She knew that there was a deeper reason for her smoking, besides just a habit or addiction, but she did not know exactly what. Before each regression she sat in the waiting room and smoked and tuned into her physical or emotional feelings from a life connected with the symptom that we were planning to explore. Under hypnosis, she discovered many past lives as the source of her smoking problems.

First Past Life: I asked Sue to focus on her thoughts and feelings about smoking and let those thoughts and feelings take her to the source of the problem. Sue immediately regressed to a past life in North America when she was a sixteen-year-old female. Her name was Chavil. She was the "appointed one" who was selected for the wisdom council because of her ability to see things. In this council they smoked belladonna, mushrooms, and certain plants that produced a heightened state of awareness that they considered the next step up.

The council was small and the meetings were intimate. The council met once or twice a month and rituals lasted for days. Often the council people shared the same visions. They believed that by doing these rituals they sustained the world and kept the dark spirits away. This spiritual quest was augmented by love-making between spiritual partners as a selective breeding to produce visionaries who would maintain and protect the culture and the world as they knew it.

At the age of twenty-three, Chavil became pregnant and had a child by her spiritual vision partner. Her son also joined the council at the age of sixteen and had a son by another member of the council, producing another gifted child. Chavil later died at the age of sixty.

From heaven, as she looked back in that life she understood the lesson that smoking was not necessary for the vision and the knowledge. She was born with it and already had the gift.

Second Past Life: Sue regressed to another life as a source for her smoking problem. It was 1757 and she was a twenty-year-old male whose name was Shalil. He was by himself in an open space away from the town. He was on a vision quest. He was fasting and praying for guidance. He was sitting by the fire performing a ritual of smoking some hallucinogens, chanting, and throwing some stuff in the fire that sparked and produced smoke, which he inhaled. He expected some revelation to come from this ritual. He did this for seven days but nothing happened.

He returned to his tribe. Everybody knew he failed. He felt ashamed and humiliated. He died later at the age of sixty-three feeling depressed and bitter, wondering why God did not bless him with the gift of vision.

From heaven, he got the understanding that he was searching for something that he had all along and he did not need to smoke or perform rituals to get it. All he needed was to have trust and faith in himself and God.

Third Past Life: Sue recalled another life connected with her smoking as a medicine man, a Sioux Indian, in North America. He healed people with herbs and potions. Smoking herbs was a part of a healing ritual.

He was killed because he could not heal and save the chief's child. He was burned alive. He died feeling confused and angry at God because he felt forsaken by God. From the Light (heaven) as he looked back he understood the lessons as follows:

"Cosmic decisions are not made by man but by God. Do not place such faith in humans but turn to God. The tribe invested

too much power and faith in the healer, but he was not God. Another important lesson that he understood was that smoking was not necessary to contact God."

From heaven, Sue also saw that she had lived many lives (about 250) as a priest, priestess, or some other kind of a religious figure and smoking and inhaling were important parts of the religious rituals to contact God in most of those lives.

Sue also understood that smoking cigarettes makes the aura (energy field) porous and opens it up for negative spirits to come in. She also realized that marijuana and other drugs create holes in the energy field, allowing the earthbound, demon, and other entities to come in. It also causes the Light to leak out. It is like feeding the Light into a sieve, and as a result the shield cannot regenerate.

Cluster of Symptoms Coming from a Cluster of Interrelated Past Lives

On occasion I find that a cluster of patients' physical and emotional problems comes from a cluster of past lives that are all interconnected. This situation is hard to deal with and it is difficult to know whether you have succeeded in the treatment or not, except when all of a sudden patients realize that they do not have those problems anymore.

Andrea, a thirty-eight-year-old married female, mother of three children, came to me because of multiple symptoms. She was depressed, anxious, hyper, and restless and had mood swings many times a day. She had racing thoughts and chronic low energy level and felt foggy, confused, and blank at times. She had difficulty in sleeping even as a child. She slept only two to three hours a night and had early morning awakening. She had constant conversation in her head and recurrent stomach problems. She had panic attacks several times a day and had fear of going crazy, fear of failing, and fear of water.

She described herself as a person who was a perfectionist with trouble in making decisions and had severe obsessive-compulsive behavior. She washed clothes in the wash cycle four to ten times, then another full cycle and washed dishes two to three times before loading the dishwasher. She had to shake clothes ten times before hanging. She checked doors three times before leaving in the morning and twisted door locks six times. While changing bedsheets, she measured them on either side from the bedframe so they would hang exactly the same. She folded clothes in a way so that they fit the corners of the dresser drawers and separated clothes by color and put white clothes in front and dark clothes in the back. Hangers had to hang the same way. Everything had to be just perfect and in order. If not, then she had to repeat it all again.

Andrea was very secretive about everything and about her obsessive-compulsive behavior. She spent a great deal of time and energy repeating things until they were "right." She was also very overprotective of her younger brother and did everything for him, creating problems in her marriage. She felt her husband made her feel inferior and according to him she could not do anything right. They had poor communication.

I prescribed Desyrel at bedtime for her depression. I made a relaxation tape that helped her a great deal with the sleeping problem and anxiety. During the next several sessions, I did individual and marriage counseling with her and her husband. It improved their relationship, but most of her other symptoms continued, so we decided to use hypnotherapy. During the next several sessions we released many earthbound and demon spirits from her and retrieved and integrated many fragmented soul parts. Afterward, many of her symptoms improved a great deal except for her perfectionism, obsessive-compulsive behavior, panic attacks, indecisiveness, secretiveness, fear of losing control, lack of self-esteem, and feelings that she was being constantly watched and controlled, especially by her husband. So we decided to try regression therapy.

She was a Roman Catholic and because of her religious beliefs she did not believe in past lives, but because of the severity of her symptoms, she was willing to try. She was a good hypnotic subject and often because of the intensity of her emotions was able to regress to the source of her problems with bridge techniques. In the next several sessions, under hypnosis, she found several past lives as the source of her crippling problems.

First Past Life: Andrea was a fifteen-year-old female in North America in 1709 and her name was June Fernmoore. Her mother taught her to do things in a certain way and made her do them over and over till she did them right. Her mother always pointed out what she did wrong and not what she did right. Her mother died when she was fifteen years old. June felt sad and promised herself that she would do things the way her mother had wanted her to. All of that life she did things over and over and checked and double-checked everything. Everything had to be in order and perfect. Other people were pleased with her but she was not happy with herself. She was tired and worn out and she died at the age of forty-four of pneumonia.

Her last thoughts were "It was a useless life. I wasted time doing the same things. If I could do it all over again, I would do it differently. I kept myself preoccupied with unnecessary chores, rather than feeling the emotion that I was not good enough." From the Light she recognized her mother in that life as her mother in the current life.

Second Past Life: Andrea regressed to another life as a twelve-year-old girl in Atlantic City. Her name was Linda. She was on the beach with her parents and a little brother, Patrick, who drowned in the water. She was supposed to watch over him. She felt guilty and responsible for his death, which had caused her parents much grief.

At the age of twenty-eight she got married and had a son, Patrick, named after her brother. However, this did not fill the void. Linda died at the age of forty-eight of breast cancer, missing her brother and promising herself to do a better job next time and not to make the same mistake.

Third Past Life: Andrea was a young girl in an orphanage in London. Her name was Maggie. Chores as an orphan were never done well enough, and she was punished over and over. Later she became a seamstress. She repeated activity in sewing. Maggie remained isolated, serious, and unhappy. She never married and died in a blizzard. In this life also she realized that she did not hurt anyone but did not help anyone, either. She hid her emotions behind work.

Going through these lives gave Andrea a better understanding of her obsessive-compulsive behavior and she was less anxious about it, but she still continued with this behavior.

Fourth Past Life: During one session, Andrea was extremely upset with her husband and was repeating the following phrases over and over.

"I feel like a prisoner."
"I feel trapped."
"I do not like to be told."
"I do not like to be watched over."
"I have no control over anything."
"My freedom is restricted."

After three to four repetitions, Andrea regressed to a life in Germany in 1943. Her name was Julie. She was twelve years old and was a prisoner in a concentration camp with her seven-year-old sister. She and others were digging a trench. A guard was watching over them to see that the work was done well and correctly.

One day the guard shot a woman because she was sick and could not dig. Later, as Julie passed by the woman's body, she learned it was her own mother, who had been kept in a separate barrack. She had not seen her since they were brought to the concentration camp.

Although she was distraught, she could not show it. She feared the guard and was determined not to allow the same thing to happen to her, at least not while she had any control of her life. She was determined to do it right. Her thoughts were "I will keep on going. I am not going to let that happen to me. I feel panicky fearing it will happen anyway, but I will not let anyone see how I feel."

In the barracks nobody talked to each other. Everybody was very secretive. Nobody trusted the other. One day, while getting her food ration, Julie tripped and fell and spilled her food. She was put in a dark solitary box that measured 4 feet by 6 feet. There was no light or window and she was kept there for a long time without food. She tried to curl up and sleep but could not. She listened to every sound, and was afraid of bugs. She felt as though she were going crazy. She had no control over her life. After a long time the guards took her back to the barracks, where she saw her sister, who was crying. They both cried and she promised her sister that she would always be there for her.

According to Julie, every day a train came and people were selected to board the train and they never came back. She heard the rumor that they were killed. She felt panic and fear every day that it might be her turn next. She slept very little during most of her stay in the concentration camp because of the fear of what would happen next. When would it be her turn?

After about eight months in the camp, she, her sister, and others were taken to the train, where they were herded in like cattle. She lost her sister in the crowd and was upset and panicky and could not find her. They were taken to another building, a gas chamber, where she and others were killed.

Julie's last thoughts were, "I am scared. I had no choice. It was made for me. I did not do anything to deserve this. I am angry about being trapped in a situation. I have to accept my fate. I can't do anything. I will never be in this situation again where I have no control."

From heaven, Andrea recognized her sister then as her younger brother in the current life. She felt responsible for him and did everything for him out of guilt in this life too, even though he was grown up.

Problems coming from Julie's life: From heaven, Andrea saw the following connections and problems coming from Julie's life:

- Feelings of being controlled and watched and of being a prisoner.

- Obsessive attachment with her brother: She did every-thing for him out of guilt.
- Panic attacks and generalized diffuse anxiety: All of those eight months she lived with these feelings and dread of what would happen next.
- Obsessive-compulsive behavior: By repeating and sticking to the details while digging the trenches and doing it right, Julie survived her situation. She promised herself that she would not end up like that woman who was shot (her mother).
- Perfectionism: Trenches had to be so wide and so long. If you did not do it right, you got shot like that woman.
- Feelings of isolation: Her parents were not there with her. They were separated in the concentration camp. She felt alone and isolated. She had to figure out everything on her own.
- Fears: Her fear of going crazy, fear of unknown, and fear of failing came from that life.
- Secretiveness and not being able to trust anybody: In the barracks everybody was secretive and did not talk to each other because they could be punished or killed if they did.
- Insomnia: All those eight months in the concentration camp she stayed awake, listening for the train and worry-ing about what would happen next.

During the next session, Andrea reported her panic attacks and fears were improved. Her obsessive-compulsive behavior was also improved. She described it as follows:

"Now I wash clothes to clean, not to count. I wash dishes to knock off surface dirt. I do not shake the clothes. I check doors to lock only. Beds are changed for sheets to hang reasonably. I find it easy to concentrate on daily tasks. I work more efficiently and get more things done in a day. I feel more confident in making decisions and am able to speak what is on my mind. I am sleeping more peacefully. I do not have obsessive concern about my brother and do not feel guilty about it."

Fifth Past Life: During this session we began to explore problems of her being indecisive. I told her to focus on those thoughts and feelings and let them take her to the source of the problem. Her thoughts were:

"I am not sure about the decisions I make."
"It is difficult to make a decision."
"I worry about making a mistake."
"I change my mind frequently."

After a few repetitions of these phrases, she found herself in a life in Philadelphia, USA, in 1863. She was a thirty-two-year-old man. His name was Paul. He was an officer in the Union Army, a main player and planner in a battle between the Union and Confederate armies. Although a skilled strategist, Paul's indecisiveness crippled his every move.

Paul's underage son, Tyler, was also a participant in this particular battle. Paul allowed him to join the army against his wife's wishes. Tyler was shot and killed by enemies. Paul felt responsible for his son's death and fled the army without notice. He returned home to a distraught and emotionally distant wife to live out his remaining years.

He died at the age of sixty-five of pneumonia, thinking about the wrong decisions he made, judging himself harshly and never forgiving himself for his mistakes. He promised himself that he would not make these mistakes again.

Sixth Past Life: Andrea regressed to another life that was also a source of her perfectionism and indecisiveness. She was a twenty-three-year-old man in Norway in 1556. His name was John and he was a captain in charge of a cargo voyage from Norway to England. There were eighteen other people on board, including his first mate, Steven, who had more sailing experience than John. A severe storm came up and he was too proud and stubborn to take the advice of the more experienced first mate, Steven. He jailed Steven to quiet him and retain control.

The ship was destroyed, and all the crew members drowned. John died feeling panicky and responsible for everybody's death. His last thoughts were:

"It was all my fault. I endangered everyone's life by not listening to Steven. Next time I will do it right. I will listen. I will do it differently. I will not make the same mistakes again."

From heaven, she recognized her firstmate, Steven, as her husband now.

Problems coming from John's life: Andrea saw many problems coming from John's life: indecisiveness, fear of making mistakes, perfectionism, fear of taking authority, obsessive-compulsive behavior, and the fear of water. She also saw part of her problems with her husband coming from this life. She resented the fact that he knew more and is right most of the time.

During the next session, Andrea reported feeling much better. She was not repeating chores over and over and she was feeling calmer. Andrea was more able to accept those situations over which she had no control. She was more willing to listen to others and was able to make decisions easily. She was sleeping well most of the nights and did not have racing thoughts and fear of going crazy. She was not as secretive and was able to relate and communicate better.

As we look at Andrea's problems it seems that they began in 1556 with John's life, where, because of his wrong decision and judgment, all his crewmen on the ship died. He died feeling panicky and responsible for the loss of their lives; and promised himself that he would never make the same mistakes again and next time he would do it right. This determination led to Andrea's obsessive-compulsive and perfectionistic behavior, life after life, including the current life. After she recalled, relived, and released those past life promises, decisions, and emotional and physical problems, there was a great deal of improvement in her crippling lifelong problems. All those past lives and all her symptoms were interconnected.

Suicide

Patients who are preoccupied with or have attempted suicide in this life report under hypnosis a similar theme in one or more past lives. They recall committing suicide in one or more past lives, instead of facing and dealing with their problems. They say the negative consequences from suicide have absolutely devastating effects on the soul; it literally shatters it.

Subsequently, during the review of their past lives from heaven, they understand that suicide in those lives did not solve anything but created bigger problems for future lives. As a result, they must plan, with the help of a guide, another life in which they will have to cope with similar problems without taking a shortcut again by committing suicide. If they commit suicide in the current life again, they will have to plan still another life in which suicide once again will be a great possibility.

The burden of a suicide is great. Not only does the soul carry the responsibility of taking its own life, but the ripple effect of suicide on family and others carries its own price as well.

Nicki was a thirty-year-old married female who felt that depression had taken over her life. She was constantly drained and tired. She had no ambition or initiative to do anything. She was about forty pounds overweight, adding to her feelings of depression and withdrawal. She felt lonely even when she was around people at home and at work. She found herself overeating every time she felt lonely. She had uncontrollable crying spells for no reason. At times she had suicidal thoughts and had visions of driving her car down a hill.

Under hypnosis, she recalled a life in Atlanta, Georgia, as a forty-two-year-old male who weighed about 320 pounds. His name was Joseph. He owned a general store. People, especially kids, made fun of him because of his weight. They called him names like "fatso," "tub of lard," etc. Kids used to steal from his store, but he could not chase them.

He never got married and felt depressed and lonely most of his lifetime. The more lonely he felt, the more he ate. One day at the age of forty-eight, he was trying to talk to a lady who came to the store, but she insulted him by saying she did not want anything to do with a guy who was fat. He was very hurt and felt rejected. He took a gun and shot himself in the right temple. His last thoughts were "I need to end my misery. I will not be treated this way again. I will never feel that useless again. I will never be this overweight again."

From heaven, as Joseph reviewed his life, he got a very clear understanding that he should not have taken an easy way out by committing suicide. He saw that he should have worked hard to cope with his problems and that real happiness does not come from food, other people, or from the way we look. He also understood that he had done a great deal of spiritual damage to himself and he would have to face and reexperience similar problems again without taking a shortcut by committing suicide.

From heaven, Nicki saw that in that life Joseph had lost many soul parts from his head, brain, sinuses, and eyes, which were in possession of the demons in hell. They were restimulating the feelings of depression, loneliness, and suicidal thoughts in Nicki by massaging those soul parts.

Symptoms and problems coming from Joseph's life: From heaven, Nicki recognized the problems coming from Joseph's life were depression, feelings of loneliness, suicidal thoughts, weight problems, headaches, sinus problems, and feelings of being fat, ugly, and sluggish.

From heaven Nicki also saw two other past lives when she committed suicide:

1. In England in 1411 when she was a man who was accused of being unfaithful to the king. He felt humiliated and committed suicide by plunging a sword through his heart.
2. In South America in 1702, she was a female and her husband was killed by another man. They were fighting over her. She was devastated and as a result committed suicide by jumping from a cliff.

Nicki was surprised to learn that in heaven, before coming to earth, she planned that as Nicki, she would go through similar problems that made her commit suicide in Joseph's life—like weight problems, depression, loneliness, and suicidal preoccupation—and that she had to learn to deal with them without committing suicide again. After the session, most of her symptoms were relieved.

Murder

According to my patients' reports, the damage from committing murder is extensive. During regressions to past lives in which they killed somebody, when patients look back from heaven, following their past life deaths, they fully understand the burden they carry for cutting short another life. It requires careful planning from heaven to repair the damage. Basically they have to return as many times as necessary with the person they killed until the two can live in a loving relationship.

The sad part is that, although in heaven people have a perfect understanding of what they did and what they need to do to repair the damage, when they come back together in another life on the earth they forget the plan. They end up hurting each other, lifetime after lifetime, rarely understanding why.

The irony is that although they understand and forgive each other in heaven, what is done on earth has to be undone only on earth. Murder is a tough one to resolve.

Patients state that Satan and his demons know everything about their problems and plans. On earth, the demons, through the patients' captive soul parts, restimulate and exaggerate their negative emotions and actions toward each other, which came from those past lives, creating more problems between them.

Working out murder: My patients say they plan to work out the negative action of murder in many different ways.

1. They plan to come back with the person they murdered in the past life, in a close relationship as a spouse,

parent, child, or a sibling and get a chance to make up for their negative actions. They get an opportunity to learn to love and forgive each other.

2. They plan to come back together in a life where they get a chance to save the person's life whom they murdered.

3. Some patients plan to have the action of murder work out on their own body. They plan to die in such a way that they correct and balance for the previous murder. They plan to suffer in the same way they made the other person suffer.

4. Some patients plan to correct the negative action of murder through good works and caring for other human beings.

Bob, a forty-five-year-old white married male, had frequent headaches since he was a little boy. During these headaches he had blurred vision, mostly in the right eye. He also had had severe colitis off and on since he was a little boy.

During a session, under hypnosis, he regressed to a life in China in 1264. He was a thirty-year-old man named Khan. He was a psychic and had the gift of knowing the past and the future and was hired by the king because of this gift. Most of the time he knew who the king's enemies were and had them killed by poison. The more he succeeded in predicting the future accurately and helped the king by getting rid of his enemies in secret, the more he was rewarded. Over time, he became more arrogant and hungry for power and control. Somehow the queen found out what Khan was doing. As a result, he secretly poisoned her, too. When the king found out that he was responsible for his wife's death, he ordered him to be killed.

He remembered being brutally beaten with chains and killed. His head and right eye were injured as he was being killed. After his death, when he went to heaven and reviewed his life, he painfully recognized how he had abused his gift of being a psychic for his own aggrandizement. He realized how he had hurt many people by cutting their lives short by murdering them. He also realized that he would have to make up with those people for murdering them in future lives.

During the next session, he regressed to another life, where he saw himself as a twelve-year-old boy who had brown skin. His name was Gana. He was a servant for a family who lived in tents and traveled from place to place. He described the place as a desert that was very hot.

He found out that the enemies of his master had poisoned the water in order to kill the master and his family. He was very loyal to his master and drank the poisoned water to save his master and his family's lives. He died feeling a severe burning pain in his gastrointestinal tract.

After his death, from heaven, he saw the connection between the two past lives. He recognized his master and his family members as people he poisoned in the life in China. He also realized that some of these people were in this current life, too. By drinking the poisoned water and saving their lives, he made up for poisoning them in the Chinese life. He also recognized that he had planned for Gana's life in heaven. He planned to drink poisoned water to save the lives of people he had poisoned in Chinese life.

After these regressions, his long-standing migraine headaches and colitis were completely relieved.

Symptom Formation

Over the years, doing past life regression therapy with my patients, I realized that the mechanism of symptom formation from past life traumas is the same as from present life traumas.

We use the defense mechanism of repression to repress most of our earlier memories, normal and traumatic, in our subconscious minds. Normally we are consciously aware of only the memories that are needed to function properly every day. Those memories, which are not needed at any given time, are stored in our subconscious minds. We do not remember them all the time, but when we need them for any reason we can always get in touch with our subconscious minds and retrieve those memories. Our subconscious minds act as a storehouse, or a memory bank, in which we have deposited and stored all our day-to-day memories. They can be ordinary or traumatic, from the current life and from all the past lives from the beginning of time.

Many people wonder why, if they have lived other lives, they do not remember them. If we remembered everything that has ever happened to us in this life and other lives, consciously without the benefit of repression, our conscious minds would be too cluttered with all those unnecessary and sometimes painful memories. We would not be able to focus and function properly in our day-to-day living and we would be overwhelmed with all those memories, especially the traumatic ones. We would become overburdened and dysfunctional from too many unnecessary memories and painful emotions and physical symptoms. In that case we would either freeze and become catatonic, so we would not have to deal with those mostly painful, traumatic memories, or become a full-blown psychotic, unable to deal with anything.

So our minds create a protective mechanism of repressing and storing the memories that are not needed for our day-to-day functioning. We put a barrier of repression between the subconscious and conscious mind. As long as this mechanism of repression is strong and working well, we function in a healthy way.

Any time this repression becomes weakened, as by a sudden shock to the psyche or chronic stress, memories can emerge from our subconscious minds to the conscious minds, bringing their emotional, mental, and physical problems. What develops depends on what types of memories are surfacing.

My patients, under hypnosis, consistently tell me that their subconscious minds contain the memories not only of their current life, but also of all their past lives from the beginning of their existence, no matter how boring, mundane, important, or traumatic they are. Nothing is erased or forgotten. All the memories are recorded or stored in our subconscious minds.

Weakening of repression: Repression can be weakened by different types of traumas.

Any event, trauma, or situation that can cause unexpected shock to our minds and bodies can jerk open the barrier of repression. If the door to the subconscious mind is forced open, every memory will be pushed out into our conscious minds or close to our conscious minds, from this life and from many other lives. Most commonly, the memories of the traumatic events will emerge because of their intensity, affecting us emotionally, mentally, and physically, and we feel we are unable to handle life.

Many of my patients tell me that all their lives they were able to function well and cope with any and all of their problems, but after a sudden traumatic event they are not able to cope with anything. Every little thing upsets them and they are no longer able to function well, emotionally or physically.

Looking back over years of my psychiatric practice, including my psychiatric residency, I especially remember working with patients who had psychotic breakdowns after using marijuana, speed, LSD, and other mind-altering drugs, including alcohol. They talked about having unusual memories and sometimes mystical experiences that did not make sense to them or to us.

Now I understand that these drugs broke open the barriers of repression, causing all those memories to surface from the current life, from past lives, and from between lives in heaven. This occurrence was usually so overwhelming that patients became psychotic and acted and behaved in strange and irrational ways.

Working with my patients, I realized how dangerous these drugs are. Not only do these drugs and alcohol break open their repression, allowing traumatic memories to surface, they also weaken their shields, allowing many earthbound and demon spirits to come inside them, making the whole problem even worse.

Any type of chronic stress can also weaken the repression gradually and slowly. Memories are allowed to surface from the subconscious mind to the conscious mind slowly, leaving patients chronically anxious and depressed.

Sometimes a trauma from a past life can surface from our subconscious to our conscious minds because of an association with a current life situation, a person, or a place, causing emotional, mental, or physical problems.

Lanette, a female patient, was locked in a bathroom at the age of ten and was not able to open the door. This incident brought back memories and feelings of being buried alive in another life, causing her a fear of closed spaces after that incident in this life. After recalling, reliving, and releasing the traumatic event from the current and past life, she was free of her claustrophobia.

In any situation, when the repression is weakened, the traumatic memories leak or are pushed out from the subconscious mind, close to the conscious mind, but not totally into the conscious mind. As a result, patients feel the emotional and physical symptoms, but do not have clear memories and understanding associated with them consciously. Unless these memories and traumas are resolved and healed, traumatic memories will continue to cause emotional, mental, and physical problems. In therapy, these memories are brought out to the conscious mind, with or without hypnosis, and by recalling, reliving, and resolving the trauma, the symptoms can be healed.

My patients state that different emotional and physical traumas in a past life can also cause soul fragmentation. These soul fragments can go out to different places or people or are grabbed by Satan and his demons, creating weakness and holes in our souls. This weakness in our beings or souls caused by the soul loss makes us more open for infestation by human and demon spirits.

According to my patients, Satan and his demons use those fragmented soul parts to create emotional, mental, and physical symptoms in different ways as follows:

- By touching and massaging those soul parts, they can restimulate the memories and symptoms of those past life traumas.

- They can send demon, earthbound, and other entities, dark energies, and devices through the connecting cords that connect the soul parts with the main body of the soul.
- They can also insert negative thoughts, ideas, attitudes, and visions through the connecting cords, exaggerating the problems.

The unresolved emotional, mental, physical, and relationship problems and issues from our past lives, including our last thoughts, promises, and decisions, are brought back in the current life with our souls, which contain all the memories from the beginning of time. These unresolved emotional, mental, and physical residues from past life traumas can create similar problems in our current life.

With past life regression therapy, those past life traumas that are causing emotional, mental, and physical problems in the current life are brought to the patient's consciousness. They are solved by recalling, reliving, releasing, and resolving the emotional, mental, and physical residue of the trauma, and retrieving and integrating the lost soul parts, allowing healing and alleviating the symptoms in a short time.

Symptoms Caused by Past Life Traumas

Over the years, treating patients with regression therapy, I have come to realize that many of their problems are often related to the unresolved physical, emotional, and mental residues, including their last thoughts, decisions, and promises coming from past life traumas and deaths. They are carried over to this life with their souls creating the symptoms, which need to be resolved. Some of the emotional, mental, physical, and relationship problems coming from past life traumas are as follows.

Psychological Symptoms

Depression and emotional turmoil: In many of my patients, depression and related symptoms stemmed from the traumatic events in their past lives. Memories of rejection, loss of a loved one, or any type of physical, mental, or emotional trauma in a previous life can cause depression in this life. Seasonal depression or depression during a certain important religious day is often due to a trauma around that season or religious day in a past life. In the current life either a person, place, or an event triggers the memories of those traumas from past lives, causing depression.

Fears, phobias, and panic attacks: Sudden traumatic death and other traumatic events in past lives can cause fears, phobias, and associated panic attacks in the current life, when similar situations are faced. Because of a sudden traumatic death, those last emotional, mental, and physical feelings were not resolved. They are often carried over to the current life with our soul. Those memories are often triggered and restimulated by similar events in the current life. The interesting thing is that whatever we are afraid of has already happened to us. The following are some of the phobias and their causes in past lives as described by my patients.

Fear of heights: Falling from a cliff, tree, or a high place.

Fear of water: Death by drowning.

Fear of fire: Being burned in a fire.

Fear of closed spaces: Being trapped in a small place and not being able to breathe, being buried alive, locked in a prison cell with no window, etc.

Fear of writing: Here patients describe that in one or more past lives they were traumatized or killed because of their writing. As a result, they promised themselves never to write again, a promise that was carried over to the current life.

Jesse had a severe writing block. Under hypnosis, he regressed to a life in Rome, to the year 1500. He had been stoned to death because he was writing about God. His last thoughts were "I will not write any more. Because of my writing, I was killed."

Fear of speaking: Patients often recall past lives when they were traumatized and killed because of what they said.

Sonny had a fear of speaking in front of people. He recalled several lifetimes when he was traumatized and killed because of his speaking, where his tongue was frozen and pulled out. He was also decapitated and hanged in other lives. He promised himself in each life "I will never speak again. I will not tell them what they do not want to hear. It is not worth getting killed over."

Fear of failing: According to my patients, this can be caused by memories of failing in one or more past lives, when they made a wrong decision. As a result, they either got killed or somebody else was killed. They then promised themselves that they would never fail again or would never get involved in anything where they might fail. These promises are often carried over to the current life and are creating the problem.

Fear of success: It can be due to memories of a past life where they were extremely successful and as a result were killed or tortured.

Arnold, a thirty-year-old patient, had a fear of success. During a session, he regressed to a life when he was an extremely successful businessman. People thought he must be a witch to be so successful, and as a consequence he was burned to death. As he was dying he promised himself that he will never be in this situation again.

Eating disorders: Anorexia, bulimia, and obesity often have roots in one or more past lives. Patients usually recall one or more lifetimes when they starved to death and as they were dying their last thoughts and promises were "I will never be hungry again. I will never feel hunger pain again." In this life those feelings and promises are brought back with their souls and as a result they find themselves eating even before they feel hungry. They do not want to feel the hunger again.

Other times, patients state that in one or more past lives they were thin and beautiful, and as a result they were raped or killed. So, they promised themselves "I will never be beautiful again. I will never be thin again. I will never let anybody hurt me like that again." They bring those thoughts and promises with them and act on them in this current life.

During the therapy, after recalling, reliving, releasing, and resolving the traumas of the past lives and understanding and releasing their last thoughts, feelings, and promises they made to themselves, and retrieving their lost soul parts, they are able to lose weight with dieting and maintain it.

Deedra recalled a past life that was responsible for her weight problem. She was a fifteen-year-old girl living in Ireland. There was a famine and she had very little food to eat. As a result she was always hungry. One day three men broke into her home. They raped her and made fun of her because she was too skinny. As they were doing so her thoughts were "I will never be thin again. I will never be hungry again. I will never let anybody hurt me again."

Sexual problems: Sexual problems can also have their roots in past lives, according to my patients' reports.

In females: Frigidity, lack of sexual desire, pain during sex, and other sexual problems have to do with being raped or tortured sexually in one or more past lives.

Jamie, a thirty-eight-year-old female, had a history of dyspareunia (pain during intercourse), which created problems in her marriage. Under hypnosis, she regressed to a life in Israel in 435 B.C. as a twenty-seven-year-old female who couldn't have children, so her husband was very angry and abusive toward her. He would beat and rape her. He would take sharp objects and insert them in her vagina, saying that she was of no value because she was a barren woman. She would bleed and have pain and infection in her vagina.

One day she was trying to get away from her husband but was caught by the towns people, who stoned her. She died promising herself "I'd rather be dead than be abused like this. I will never be under the control of any man. I will never let anybody abuse me like this."

After that session her dyspareunia was relieved

In males: Impotency and other sexual problems in men can be caused by some type of traumatic incidents in one or more past lives. Patients report that they were killed because they had sex with somebody, or they made somebody pregnant and as a result she killed herself or they both were killed. Usually it is not a simple question of morals. It is a question of life and death. These problems are usually relieved by resolving and releasing those traumatic memories and promises.

Many incest and sexual abuse problems also come from one or more past lives. The abused and the abusers have misused each other sexually in one or more lifetimes. It can be stopped through past life regression therapy with one or both of them individually. Treating even one person can break the cycle.

Dawn, a twenty-five-year-old female, recalled being abused by a family friend. She was very upset and angry with him and had a very hard time forgiving him and moving ahead with her life. During one session, after regression to a past life, when she went to heaven after the death of her body, I asked her to go to her planning stage for her current life. She was surprised to find out that she planned to be raped by this family friend because she raped him in a previous life, when she was a wealthy man and he was a female servant working for him. This helped Dawn in understanding the reason for her rape, which was for balancing and erasing her negative action from that past life.

Premenstrual symptoms (PMS): Patients find different reasons for their PMS symptoms in one or more past lives. Some describe these symptoms as the result of some type of sexual trauma or suffering and dying during childbirth.

June, a thirty-two-year-old married female, had severe PMS symptoms. About three to four days before her periods she became extremely depressed, angry, irritable, and sometimes even suicidal. She felt this way more when she was around her husband and believed she was ugly and useless. She had severe cramps and heavy bleeding. Under hypnosis, June recalled a life in London, England, in 1570, when she was raped by a man. She felt ashamed and humiliated. She did not want to face anybody after that incident, so she committed suicide. Her last thoughts were "I will get even with him someday for what he did to me."

After the death of her body, when she went to heaven, she recognized the man who raped her in that life as her husband in the current life. She understood why she felt so irritable and angry with her husband and chose to forgive him for raping her in that life. After that session, she was free of her PMS symptoms, and her relationship with her husband improved a great deal.

Relationship problems: According to my patients, their likes and dislikes toward different people and relationship problems can also have their roots in one or more past lives. Relationship problems may sometimes seem out of proportion to the circumstances in the present life. They can manifest in every aspect of life, as between husband and wife, parents and children, brothers and sisters, neighbors, boss and employee, coworkers, teachers and students, and others.

Katy was a thirty-five-year-old female who came to me because she and her husband were having marital problems and, as a result, she was depressed. She also had PMS symptoms with irritability, depression, and anger three days before and during her periods.

Under hypnosis, she discovered that she and her husband had been with each other in a rocky and destructive relationship in many lifetimes. Over several sessions, she found the following lifetimes and what happened between her and her husband.

1. Life in England: They were marrie,d but she was cheating on him so he stabbed and killed her. Her last thoughts were "I will chase him life after life for what he did to me."
2. Life in France: Her husband was a female prostitute. She was a man and wanted to marry the prostitute, but she turned him down. Out of anger he choked the prostitute to death.
3. Life in China: He was trying to rape her so she stabbed and killed him.
4. Life in Brazil: They were brother and sister and their parents paid more attention to her. He was very jealous and angry with her.

After she recalled, relived, and released the trauma and forgave him and herself during each life, their relationship improved dramatically. She told me that not only her feelings and attitude toward him changed, but even his attitude toward her changed although he was never in therapy. Her PMS symptoms, which came from a lifetime when she had been raped, were also relieved.

Perfectionism, indecisiveness, and obsessive-compulsive behavior: These can also come from past lives. Patients say that in one or more lifetimes they made a wrong decision or did not do things right, and as a result either they or others were hurt or killed, causing them a great deal of emotional turmoil. In that life they promised themselves that next time they would never make that mistake again; they would try harder or keep on trying until they do it right.

Danny, a forty-year-old man, had problems making decisions and taking any responsibility at home and at work. He was a perfectionist; no matter how well he did, he was not satisfied. He also did not like any conflicts.

Under hypnosis, he regressed to a life in which he was a ruler of a small state. He decided to go to war to fight for their land. Many of his people were killed and his state lost the war. He believed he had the blood of all his people who were killed on his hands. He loved his people. He felt defeated and tortured by the thoughts of his people starving in the future. He remembered making the following decisions and promises to himself:

"I will not take that much responsibility again. I will not care about people that much again. I will never trust my judgment again. I will not make similar mistakes again."

In this life he was still following the decisions and promises he made to himself in that life. After this regression his boss became sick and Danny was placed in charge of his department. Before, even the thought of being in that situation would cause severe panic attacks. After that session, he had no problems and was very much at ease with the responsibility and with making decisions, and even enjoyed it.

Workaholism: According to my patients, problems of workaholism can come from a lifetime where they could not provide enough for their family, who died of starvation or some other type of tragedy, because they did not have enough money. While dying they promised themselves to work hard and make enough money so they and their families would not have to suffer ever again.

Addictions: Drugs, alcohol, cigarettes, and any other addictions can have their roots in past lives, too.

Arnold found out the reasons for his smoking cigarettes in his past lives. In one past life he was a shaman. Smoking was an important part of the healing ritual. It was supposed to be an important way to contact the spirit world and communicate with the divine.

In another life, he had a tobacco factory. Business was not good. By the time he died he had lost his business and family. He died poor. His last thoughts while dying were "Smoking is good for your health. I wish people smoked more. I lost everything because people did not smoke."

Physical Symptoms

Physical symptoms can also be alleviated through past life regression therapy. These symptoms include musculoskeletal symptoms, immune system diseases, and psychosomatic conditions. The body is usually reliving unresolved traumas that are carried over from other lifetimes. My patients have found the sources for the following physical symptoms in their past lives and different reasons for them.

Headaches: These are caused by being shot in the head, head being crushed, clubbed, beheaded, hanged, etc. They can also be caused by memories of brain diseases such as infections, tumors, and aneurysms.

Neck and shoulder pain: These are caused by hanging, strangulations, decapitation, being clubbed, shot, stabbed, or choked, and other injuries to the neck and shoulders.

Back pain: It can come from an injury to the back by falling, shooting, stabbing, beatings, etc.

Gastrointestinal problems: They can be caused by being shot or stabbed in the stomach, poisoned, having infections, burning in a fire, inhaling smoke, etc.

Sinus problems: They can be caused by an injury to sinuses, torture by putting nails in the sinuses, lobotomy performed through the nose, sinuses freezing in cold weather leading to death, drowning and water going into the sinuses, suicide by shooting with a gun into the mouth and sinuses being blown out, dying with sand, dust, or pollen going in the nose and sinuses, etc.

Arthritis: It can be caused due to traumas to different joints where joints were being torn apart during a torture, being injured in an accident, being frozen, having infections or inflammation, and other types of traumas in a past life.

Sally had arthritis in her feet. She found that in a past life in China she was a princess. They bound her feet out of custom and she was never able to walk. She lived in pain all her life and she had to be carried everywhere. She was a helpless object of beauty. After she recalled, released, and resolved that life, the arthritis in her feet was relieved.

Skin sensitivity and diseases, including acne: These can be caused by being burned in a fire, torture by being poked with hot needles, acid being poured to torture, skin infection, starvation causing skin diseases, being burned by boiling water, dying in hot weather under a scorching sun, etc.

Asthma: According to my patients, asthma is usually caused by having constricted breathing and gasping for breath while dying, as in drowning, burning in a fire and choking from smoke inhalation, being hanged, being strangled, being decapitated, being choked, dying on a dusty road and inhaling dust, etc.

Allergies: There is often a connection between the allergies and allergens. Usually these allergens are associated with a memory of a traumatic event.

David had allergies to milk and milk products because in his past life all his cows died of some disease and he lost everything. He died on the street cursing those cows.

Don was allergic to milk and milk products. He regressed to a life when he was being put in a dungeon and had only spoiled milk to drink.

Jody traced the cause for her allergies to chickens to a life where she had to kill her infected chickens.

Jim was allergic to dust and hay because he died in a dusty barn filled with hay in one of his past lives.

Terrance traced the reasons for his allergies to cats, dogs, and birds to a past life when he used to torture and kill animals, including cats, dogs, and birds.

Fred had allergies to grains because in his past life he lost his farm, where he grew grains, rice, corn, wheat, etc. Crops failed and he died on the streets thinking about his farm.

Circulation problems: According to my patients' reports, poor circulation in their hands and feet is caused by being hanged, beheaded, hands and legs being cut off, hands and feet being tied and circulation being cut off, etc.

Olivia, a twenty-five-year-old female, had poor circulation in her hands and feet, which became black and blue and very painful at times. She also had a rash over her body from time to time. Under hypnosis, she recalled a life when she was a female who was accused of being a witch. She was tied to a pole. Her hands and feet were tied tightly, leading to poor circulation and pain. She was finally burned to death.

After she recalled, relived, released, and resolved the trauma, the circulation in her hands and her skin rash improved immediately. She did not have black-and-blue hands anymore.

MY LIFE BLUEPRINT

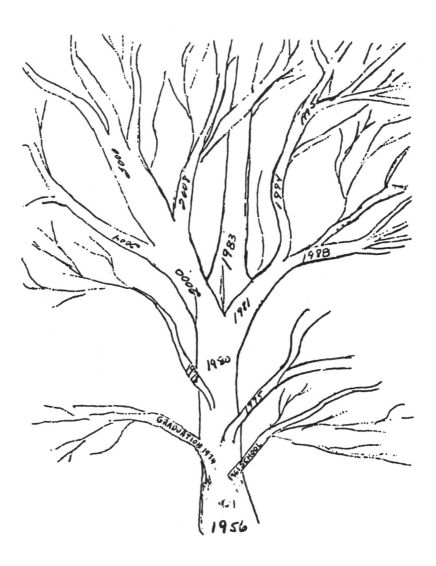

Drawing by a patient. Each branch represents another path or choice in life. Larger branches are the larger choices in life. Smaller branches are the smaller choices in life.

Summary

Working with hundreds of patients with past life regression therapy for about eleven years has given me a completely new understanding about psychological and physical illness. To summarize what my patients have told me under hypnosis: everything we have ever touched, sensed, smelled, felt, heard, experienced, and done is recorded in our subconscious mind. That is, everything not only from the current life, but also from all our past lives and between-life experiences in the Light (heaven) and everything from the beginning of time.

It is possible to recall any of those memories, any time we want to and need to. Many of my patients have even regressed to the time of their creation and to the creation of the universe and beyond. Vivid details are consistent from patient to patient and will be discussed in detail in future publications.

According to my patients' reports, the subconscious mind, which in fact is our soul, not only has the knowledge of the source of their emotional, mental, and physical difficulties and conflicts, but also provides solutions for the problems and even the healing. Based on my research and my experience with my patients, about 70 percent of the secondary symptoms and 30 percent of the primary symptoms come from past lives. Fears, phobias, sexual problems, and personality disorders often have their roots in past lives. Physical symptoms such as musculoskeletal symptoms, psychosomatic symptoms, and autoimmune disorders also have their origins in past lives.

We use the defense mechanism of repression to repress most of our earlier memories, normal and traumatic, in our subconscious minds. If we remembered everything that has ever happened to us in this life and other lives, consciously without the benefit of repression, our conscious minds would be too cluttered with all those unnecessary and sometimes painful memories. We would not be able to focus and function properly in our day-to-day living and we would be overwhelmed with all those memories, especially the traumatic ones. We would become overburdened and dysfunctional from too many unnecessary, painful memories, emotions, and physical symptoms. We would therefore either freeze and become catatonic, so we would not have to deal with those mostly painful, traumatic memories, or become a full-blown psychotic, unable to deal with anything.

So our minds create a protective mechanism of repressing and storing the memories that are not needed for our day-to-day functioning. As long as this mechanism of repression is strong and working well, we function in a healthy way. Any time this repression becomes weakened due to any circumstances, as by a sudden shock to the psyche or chronic stress, memories can emerge from our subconscious minds to the conscious minds, bringing their emotional, mental, and physical problems. What develops depends on what types of memories are surfacing.

Some of my patients describe having spontaneous memories from their past lives. Usually they recall vivid scenes and have a knowledge that it is their past life. These past life memories often are fragmented and may contain a traumatic event. As a result, they can be confusing and frightening. Young children can sometimes spontaneously recall events from a past life, but are often discouraged by their families from talking about them and gradually they learn to block those memories. These memories can be initiated by a person or place, an event, emotional feelings, or a physical pain or sensation. Sometimes they can be triggered by sight, sound, smell, taste, or touch. Some of my patients report having a spontaneous past life recall while they were using hallucinogenic drugs. Other patients have reported having spontaneous past life memories while meditating.

Many people dismiss the idea of past life therapy, thinking that they have enough problems in this life, so why should they dig out more problems from another life? According to my patients' reports, most of our current life problems and conflicts have roots in one or more past lives. Our unresolved emotional and physical problems, last thoughts, decisions, and promises are carried over with our souls from lifetime to lifetime into the current life. By recalling, reliving, releasing, and resolving the unresolved traumas, issues, and conflicts from past lives, they often can heal many emotional, mental, and physical problems and other conflicts in the current life, in just a few sessions. Sometimes, in only one session, the patient's problems can be resolved and healed.

Based on my patients' reports, multiple psychological and physical problems can come from a single past life. Conversely, a single psychological or physical symptom may have its roots in multiple lives. Other times, a cluster of emotional, mental, and physical symptoms may come from a cluster of past lives, which are all interrelated.

Under hypnosis, patients who are preoccupied with or have attempted suicide in the current life, report a similar theme in one or more past lives. They recall that, instead of facing and dealing with their problems, they committed suicide in one or more past lives. The consequences of suicide have absolutely devastating effects on the soul; it literally shatters it. The burden of suicide is great. Not only does the soul carry the responsibility of taking its own life, but the ripple effect of suicide on family and others carries its own price as well.

Patients describe making plans in heaven for their current life, where they will have to face problems similar to or worse than those that caused them to commit suicide in past lives. If they commit suicide in the current life again, they will have to plan still another life in which suicide once again will be a great possibility, until they face and deal with their problems without taking a shortcut by committing suicide.

Murder committed in past lives is another issue that is tough to resolve. Basically, they have to return as many times as necessary with the person they killed, until the two can live in a loving relationship. The irony is that although they understand and forgive each other in heaven, what is done on earth has to be undone on the earth only. The sad part is that, although in heaven people have a perfect understanding of what they did and what they need to do to repair the damage, when they come back together in another life on earth, they forget their plan.

They end up hurting each other lifetime after lifetime, rarely understanding why.

Under hypnosis, my patients recall living many lifetimes in different parts of the world and sometimes on other planets. They describe living a variety of lifestyles being rich and poor, good and bad, male and female, black, white, Oriental, and of different races, religions, and cultures.

They had various roles in different lives as healers, teachers, priests, monks, kings, queens, torturers, killers, victims, beggars, etc. They undergo different types of death experiences, such as being hanged, murdered, choked, burned, frozen, dying in their sleep, dying when they were young or old, being aborted, or miscarried, etc.

Patients describe living good, bad, peaceful, or traumatic lives. During the regression, most of the patients remember very ordinary but traumatic lives because of the residue from the unresolved traumas that are carried over from one or more past lives to the present life, causing the emotional, mental, and physical problems and conflicts. Very few patients recall living a famous life. When they do, it sometimes turns out to be due to cross talk, as described earlier. Even if somebody had recalled a life as a king or a queen or a famous person, it was not because of the glamour or the prestige of that life, but because there was an unresolved trauma or issue that needed to be resolved and understood.

All my patients describe the same cycle of life. They exist first as a spiritual being. They incarnate into a physical body, not blindly, not randomly, but with a definite plan in mind. In the Light (heaven), they describe planning their life in detail. They claim to choose their parents, spouses, children, and other key people in their lives. Patients also remember choosing their occupations, skills, and talents.

They plan in detail all the important events. Over and over, my patients tell me that not only do they plan happy, good, and productive events, but they also choose negative events, circumstances, and tragedies, to balance their negative actions from the past lives or because they need to learn something from them to grow spiritually.

I was very surprised when some of my patients reported that I was also present in their planning stage in heaven, for their current life. They told me that they even planned to have psychiatric problems and planned to come to me for their treatment. One reason they give for planning to come for this type of treatment is often to resolve and heal the traumas and issues from past lives so they can be strong and less influenced by outside negative influences. Another reason for this type of treatment is to tap into their inner knowledge and understanding of the reality of the spiritual world and how it affects us. Also, they come to understand their purpose so they can be more productive and helpful in this life.

Some patients say they belong to a group in heaven and they, as a group, planned to have a divine purpose to fulfill on the earth in this life. There are many such groups from heaven, working together on earth to achieve divine purposes.

According to the patients, first they are spiritual beings in heaven. They incarnate into a body, live their lives, die, and return to the Light (heaven). This cycle goes on and on. Amazingly, most of the patients consistently recalled the same information about this cycle, regardless of their culture, religion, beliefs, or whether they were an atheist or an agnostic.

Some of my patients recalled past lives in which they did not do anything. They did not hurt anybody, but did nothing good for themselves or anyone else. In their review stage in heaven, about that life, the beings of the Light showed the patients their book with blank pages. The understanding they received is that they did not do anything helpful and productive in that life and they will have to come back and do it all over again. If they do not do anything good, they do not just stay in the same place, they do not just mark time, but they go backward spiritually. Each life has to be a building block, a forward process.

According to my patients' reports, our past lives influence every part of our current life. Our positive and negative relationships with different people around us, our fascinations, likes and dislikes, our gifts and talents, our choice of occupation, spouse, and friends, our dreams and our physical, psychological, and personality problems can all have their roots in our past lives. The mistakes made in our past lives follow us like a shadow and affect us in our current life. We must resolve and work out those problems in the present life and heal ourselves before they become rooted in future lives. Patients under hypnosis say that life has to be lived as good, loving, and productive and as perfectly as possible.

If we think of the soul as being on a spiritual journey, each life becomes a station along the way at which certain tasks are to be performed and certain lessons to be learned. When, for whatever reason, we fail to do what we planned, we carry that task or lesson on to the next life. In this way our baggage becomes heavier. At some point along the journey, it becomes necessary to stop and resolve or learn old lessons in order to lighten our load and venture toward our goal.

Patients report that during different traumas in a past life our souls fragment. These soul fragments can go outside the body to people or places and are also grabbed by Satan and his demons. These lost soul parts create holes and weaknesses in our beings, our souls, and in our bodies, which continue in future lives. These empty spaces and holes in our souls open us for more possessions and negative influences. Also, the soul parts lost in past lives, which are in possession of demons in hell, are used by them to create similar emotional and physical problems for us in our current life. They do so by reactivating the memories of those past life traumas, by touching and massaging those lost soul parts, or by sending the negative entities, devices, and negative energies through the soul parts and their connecting cords to the main body of our soul, creating different physical and psychological problems. They can also transmit negative thoughts, visions, and attitudes through the cords.

Unless the residues from past life traumas are resolved and healed and all the soul parts are retrieved, cleansed, healed, and integrated, we will always be a target for influences by outside entities.

Occasionally, some people become exceptionally fascinated with these past lives and seem to be more preoccupied with them than dealing with their current life. The goal of past life regression therapy is to recall, release, understand, and resolve the physical, emotional, and mental symptoms, and other issues that are coming from past lives and manifesting in the current life. After resolving those problems, and understanding and learning the lessons, we need to leave them in the past and live in the here and now in our current life.

Past life regression therapy is a very dynamic tool and can be used to heal patients' psychological and physical problems. It also provides a better understanding about ourselves and our purposes and can be used to tap into the awesome knowledge that is there within all of us and is our divine inheritance.

Chapter IV

Possession or Attachment by Earthbound Spirits (Entities)

The Cosmic Hitchhiker

Sometimes I feel that I am not the me I've come to know.
What makes it hard to understand, these feelings come and go.
Sometimes I'm just my usual self, as normal as can be,
At other times I act so strange I hardly think it's me.

At times I feel so loaded down with other people's woes,
To live each day exhausts me—well, I guess that's how it goes.
I can't bear to see folks suffer, it hurts me so inside;
I want to take their pain from them, and run away and hide.

And other times I feel that life is just too hard to bear;
I feel so sick, so tired and drained, it seems there's nothing there.
What happens to my energy, and why am I so sad?
When there is nothing really wrong, why do I feel so bad?

If I could take a looking glass and see inside my soul,
I'd find the answer to my pain, I'd find that my control
Is in the hands of all of those whose misery and pain
I've taken from them selflessly so they'd be whole again.

And so I am a puppet, a living marionette,
For all those souls whose pain I felt, whose grief I'm feeling yet.
And none of us is free to be the things that we had planned.
Because our souls are always at the other one's command.

To free myself, and free you, too, to realize our goals,
I must release you totally back to your rightful souls.
We cannot share our essences or trade our souls around,
We can share each other's sorrows, with love we can abound,

But we must not compromise ourselves, our souls we cannot sell,
And so, my cosmic hitchhiker, I must bid you "farewell."

—Jane

Possession or Attachment by Earthbound Spirits (Entities)

Earthbound Spirits (Entities): These are the human spirits who did not make their transition to the Light (heaven), after the death of their physical bodies and have remained on the earth plane. They are also known as disembodied or discarnate spirits. Over the years, different patients and their possessing human entities, under hypnosis, gave information about who they are, why they remained in the physical world after the death of their physical bodies, why they did not go to heaven, why they were attracted to my patients, what opened the patients for these spirits to come in, how they affected my patients, and how to release them to the Light. All of this information will be discussed in great detail in this chapter. Please read with an open mind.

Appearance of Earthbound Spirits (Entities)

When patients find earthbound spirits inside them, they describe their appearance, which varies from patient to patient and from spirit to spirit. They may appear to the patients in human form, wearing the same clothes and looking the way they looked just before the death of their physical bodies. Some patients describe the earthbound spirits as luminous souls in human form.

Sometimes they appear to the patients as if they are overlapping the patients' whole body. Other times patients see these earthbound spirits located in specific parts of their bodies, such as in their head, chest, or leg, because that particular part of the spirit's body is having some problems. For example, if an earthbound spirit's body died of a head injury, the entity still will feel

POSSESSION BY EARTHBOUND ENTITIES
(Compilation of drawings by different patients)

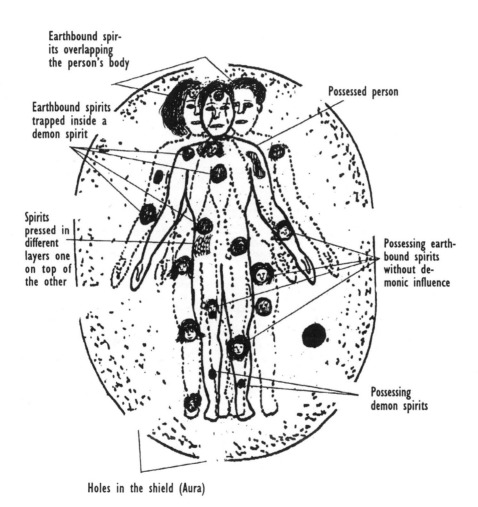

Earthbound spirits overlapping the person's body

Earthbound spirits trapped inside a demon spirit

Possessed person

Spirits pressed in different layers one on top of the other

Possessing earthbound spirits without demonic influence

Possessing demon spirits

Holes in the shield (Aura)

the pain in its head. So even though the spirit body may be overlapping the whole body of the patient, the patient becomes aware of that spirit as being present in his or her head.

Other times patients describe that the earthbound entities in them have human forms, but have a layer of darkness all around them. As a result, they look gray or black. This appearance is due to their being completely surrounded and infested by the demon entities, but not totally squeezed inside the demon. They are able to retain their full human form or may appear to shrink in size.

At times, patients describe that many earthbound spirits are squeezed in small balls and packed together in different parts of the patients' bodies. Sometimes, many of these spirits can be packed in one layer. There can be many such layers, one on top of the other.

Some patients describe that the earthbound entities in them are totally and completely surrounded, squeezed and consumed by dark demon entities. In these cases, at the beginning, as the patients look inside their bodies, all they see are black blobs, in different parts of their bodies, who claim to be demon entities. Initially, they cannot see any human spirits inside the black blobs. Only after the transformation of the demons into the Light are patients able to see the earthbound entities who were trapped inside the demons. According to the patients, these earthbound spirits are squeezed into small balls by the demons and as a result, lose their human shapes, forms, and memories. It is only after they are freed from the demon entities that they resume their normal human shapes and memories.

My patients tell me that if the earthbound spirits are outside the patients' bodies, they may appear to the patients in luminous human forms, or in their regular forms, wearing the clothes they were wearing just before the deaths of their physical bodies. If the entities have demonic presence inside them, they may appear to the patients as gray, black, or dark. They may also appear as angry, confused, evil, or cold.

According to patients, the outside earthbound spirits who are very confused after death most often appear in ghostlike forms.

Those earthbound spirits who have demon entities inside them will also appear as ghosts and people can see and sense their presence. Spirits who have strong demonic influence can often move things around or produce different manifestations.

Number and Location of the Possessing Earthbound Spirits

My patients describe having from one to as many as ten or even more—sometimes even hundreds—of earthbound entities in different parts of their bodies. One patient, as he looked inside himself, described seeing hundreds of human spirits. It looked like a "beehive" to him. Even when I work with so-called normal people, almost all of them find one or more human spirits inside them, even though they did not have any obvious physical or emotional problems.

Sometimes patients describe that both earthbound and demon entities are arranged in many, many layers in their bodies. When we release the first layer of entities, the patients feel clear and free of their original symptoms, but during the next session they report another layer of entities coming to the surface along with their physical and emotional symptoms. In these cases, it seems as if the patients have new entities coming in from outside, sometimes possible if the patient's shield is not strong for some reason. But in these cases of layering, the entities are already there, buried under each other.

Some patients describe having many such areas of layering in different parts of their bodies, depending on the body's weaknesses. According to the patients, this weakness is created by the present and past life traumas that created soul fragmentation and loss of soul parts, causing the holes in the soul. The weakness is in the soul due to the missing soul parts and thus in the body. The holes in the soul, created by the missing soul parts, become filled in by many layers of human and demon entities. Unless these weaknesses are healed by regression therapy and all the lost soul parts are retrieved, cleansed, healed, and integrated with the patients, these weakened areas due to missing soul parts in different parts of the body will continue to be infested by the outside human, demon, and other entities.

The layered areas in different parts of the body have different shapes and sizes, depending on the shapes and sizes of the weak areas in the body. These layered areas are also of different thicknesses, depending on the number of the entities within each layer and the number of layers.

In these cases, it seems like a never-ending and exhausting process for the patients and for me. Sometimes they tend to quit the therapy and continue to have emotional and physical problems.

But if they are determined to put their time and effort into freeing themselves and learn to shield themselves from future possessions, they can be free of the foreign entities.

LAYERING OF SPIRITS IN THE BODY
(Drawing by a patient)

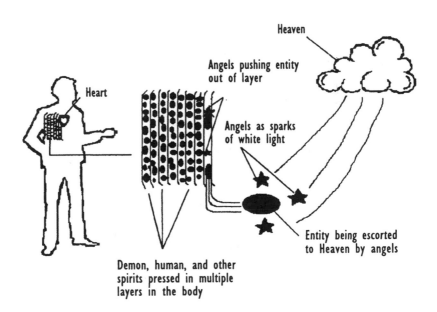

At the beginning, **Dave**, under hypnosis, could not see anything except darkness within himself, but was able to sense the presence of entities and receive the answers from those that were in his eyes blocking his vision. After he released many entities from his eyes, his vision opened up and he was able to locate more entities during each session and release them over many three-hour sessions. To both of us, it felt as if it would never end.

During one session, after a past life regression, during which he went to heaven, I asked him to look down in his physical body and see how many more entities were there. As Dave looked, he was surprised to see that he had many layers of these spirits still left in different parts of his body. He described these layers as thin layers of a pastry. He indicated having twelve layers in his brain, fifteen layers in his eyes, fifteen layers in his shoulders, four layers in the lower back and twenty-nine layers in his abdominal area. We requested angels of the Light to remove entities from each and every layer of his body. He described how the angels, very patiently and systematically, released the entities from each layer and helped them to the Light. Then the angels cleansed and healed those areas and filled and shielded them with the Light. We then proceeded to heal these weak areas by regression therapy and locating and retrieving and integrating the soul parts that he had lost during his current life and different past lives.

Age When the Spirits (Entities) Possess or Attach to People

Under hypnosis, different human and demon entities in my patients have claimed to join them at different ages from birth, throughout childhood and adulthood, until death. Some entities claim to attach to the patients even in the womb or follow and attach to some patients in more than one life.

Attachment during Birth, Childhood, and Later until Death

Tony, an entity in my patient whose body died at the hospital, said that he became confused and wandered around the hospital, not knowing what happened to him. In the nursery he saw a newborn baby crying. He liked babies and went to comfort this baby. Somehow he ended up inside the baby and couldn't get out.

Rob, a forty-five-year-old patient, had suffered from depression and suicidal thoughts occasionally throughout his life. He remembered being depressed and planning suicide even as a nine-year-old boy. He had attempted suicide twice. He also had a nervous stomach and had had nausea and vomiting from time to time since the age of nine.

Under hypnosis, he saw inside him a thirty-year-old female entity who had been stabbed in the stomach and killed. She joined Rob when he was nine and afterward he began to experience her stomach problems. He also had a female spirit who committed suicide and gave Rob the suicidal thoughts, and another one who died in a car accident. They all claimed to have joined him when he was nine.

After we released these entities to heaven, Rob's lifelong symptoms, including his depression, suicidal thoughts, nervousness, and stomach problems, were relieved.

Brian had a spirit of a drug addict who claimed that he joined Brian when he was experimenting with drugs at the age of sixteen. He admitted that he gave Brian the desire to use drugs and did not care what happened to Brian physically, emotionally, or financially.

Wanda had a spirit of a friend who joined her at the age of forty-five at a funeral home. She was distraught about his death and it opened her up for him to come in. He came in to comfort her, but then could not get out.

Attached When in the Womb

Some entities reported to have been with the patient's mother and then joined the patient in the womb. Other entities claim to be with one of the patient's family members before they joined the patient.

Linda, an entity who was in my patient Amelia, first insisted that this was her body. As the session progressed, the spirit, Linda, remembered how she came in with Amelia.

> **Dr. Modi:** "Linda, move back in time when you joined Amelia."
>
> **Linda:** "I do not see anything. It is dark. I am in a dark void."
>
> **Dr. Modi:** "Move back beyond that dark void. What are you aware of?"
>
> **Linda:** "I am on the other side. I am a soul. I am getting ready to be born as Linda. I am supposed to be born [crying] but something goes wrong. There is no body to go into."
>
> **Dr. Modi:** "Why? What happened?"
>
> **Linda:** "There is no body for me to enter. My mother had a miscarriage at six weeks. I did not know where to go so I attached to my mother. Then when my mom was pregnant with Amelia, I went from my mom to Amelia and attached to her when she was in the womb."

Attached in Many Lifetimes

Some entities claim to follow and attach to the same patient for many lifetimes because of love, anger, hate, jealousy, or desire for revenge. Sometimes they claim to attach to the patient even before they are in the womb.

Harry had with him a female spirit who claimed to be his sister in one of his past lives. Her parents died when she was young. Later Harry, who was her brother in that life, died of some infection. She was all alone and was forced into prostitution. She felt angry at this brother for leaving her alone. After the death of her body, she followed and attached to Harry for many lifetimes including this one, because although she loved her brother, she was angry with him for leaving her alone.

Who Are These Possessing Earthbound Spirits (Entities)?

Under hypnosis, patients often identify the possessing earth-bound spirits inside them as a family member, a miscarried or aborted fetus, a friend, an acquaintance, an imaginary playmate, a stranger, a past life connection, or an earthbound spirit who is working for Satan.

Family members: Often my patients describe having one or more deceased family members with them. The most common are grandparents and parents, then uncles, aunts, children, siblings, and other family members. Sometimes these family members come in because they love and want to help the patient. Sometimes they just do not know where to go, so they go inside the person who is open for them to enter. Other times they are angry with the patient and come in to take revenge. Sometimes patients invite these family members to come in and stay with them after the death of their bodies because the patients missed them and did not want to let them go. This phenomenon may occur consciously or unconsciously.

Bobbie, a forty-year-old female, had suffered with severe panic attacks off and on since she was six. During these attacks she felt chest pain, shortness of breath, fear of having a heart attack, and fear of dying. She was becoming severely depressed and was having a difficult time functioning. She also had dreams about her father from time to time. Under hypnosis, she found her father inside her, who had died of a sudden heart attack when Bobbie was six. Her father said that Bobbie invited him in because she did not want him to leave. After releasing her father to the Light, Bobbie reported that her symptoms improved a great deal.

Aborted and miscarried fetuses: Some of my patients have also reported having spirits of their aborted or miscarried fetuses with them. Here patients often complain feeling continued guilt or sadness, even though the incident had happened several years before. After releasing the spirits of these aborted or miscarried fetuses, the patients usually feel at peace and free of the guilt and sadness. These spirits of miscarried or aborted fetuses claim to stay with their parents because they love them and want to be with them or because they are angry at the mothers who aborted them.

Shelly, under hypnosis, found the spirit of her aborted baby trapped in a dark demon entity. I asked the demon how it came to hold this small baby as a hostage. The demon gave the following information:

> "When Shelly came to the clinic to have her abortion, I was there. We demons hang around those places, because these little ones are so easy to trap. When the spirit of her baby came out, it was confused. It did not understand why its mother did not want it. It was lonesome and scared. I went to it and surrounded and trapped it inside me. Then I brought it to Shelly, and the two of us entered her when she was grieving. I intensified the baby's feelings of hurt, rejection, and anger, which in turn intensified Shelly's feelings of guilt and sadness."

After releasing the demon and the spirit of her aborted fetus, Shelly felt free of her guilt and felt at peace.

Susan, a fifty-year-old female, had an abortion when she was twenty-five years old. Although it had happened a long time before, she still thought about it and felt guilty. She also had dreams about the aborted baby from time to time.

Under hypnosis, she saw the spirit of her aborted fetus, who said that he loved his mother and just wanted to be with her. After releasing the spirit of the aborted fetus to the Light, Susan felt relieved and no longer had any dreams about the aborted fetus and did not feel guilty. She felt at peace.

Acquaintances: Many of my patients reported having spirits of people they knew, other than their family members, with them as attached entities.

Rolanda had a history of depression for a long time. After a few spirit releasement sessions, her depression improved and she was able to function well.

About six months later, she came back because she was feeling depressed and tired after a family friend died of cancer. She was having difficulty sleeping and was having dreams about the friend who had died. Under hypnosis, she found the spirit of this friend inside her. After releasing this friend, her depression, insomnia, and tired feelings immediately improved. She did not dream about him after that.

Imaginary playmates: In psychiatry, when a child reports having an imaginary playmate, we consider it to be a product of the young child's imagination. But I have had many patients who reported their childhood imaginary playmates as being the possessing earthbound entities in them. These entities often claimed that they liked playing with my patients when they were young and then went in their bodies at some point when the patients were sick or upset or after they had surgery.

Tony had a child entity, Jimmy, who claimed to be Tony's imaginary playmate when he was eight. Later, he came inside Tony during a tonsillectomy when he was ten. According to Jimmy, Tony's spirit was out of his body watching the operation and was feeling panicky. Spirit Jimmy, who was with Tony trying to comfort him, came into Tony after the surgery and has been inside him since.

Joy described having an imaginary playmate when she was a little girl. Under hypnosis, she saw her imaginary playmate as a possessing entity. The entity was a five-year-old girl who had drowned. At first, she stayed around Joy and played with her. Later she joined Joy at the age of ten when she was sick. After that Joy began to have a fear of water, which was relieved after she released the entity.

Strangers: Many patients report having spirits of strangers with them. According to research, 77 percent of patients had earthbound spirits who were spirits of strangers.

Past life connections: Some of the human spirits in my patients reported that they have known my patients from another life, when my patients and the possessing entities were together, either in a loving or hateful relationship. Sometimes these entities claim to have followed and possessed the same patient in several lifetimes.

Harmon had a male earthbound spirit, Sal, who claimed to have known Harmon from another lifetime, when Harmon was his master. Sal was a very faithful and protective servant and they were more like good friends. After his death, Sal did not go to heaven and instead followed Harmon for many lifetimes, including this one, to protect his master. According to Sal, he had made Harmon suspicious of other people in all those lifetimes.

Lisa had the spirit of a woman who claimed she knew Lisa in a past life where they were very close. The spirit became very angry when Lisa married a man against her advice and then left her alone. She died feeling very angry and resentful toward Lisa. She followed and attached to Lisa during several lifetimes, including this one. This lifetime Lisa married the same man whom she had married in the former life. The attached spirit was determined to destroy their marriage in this life, too.

Earthbound entities who are working for Satan: An overwhelming number of the earthbound entities in my hypnotized patients reported that they were working for Satan. They claimed that Satan told them to go to the patient and create problems. Some of the earthbound entities said they went with Satan and his demons voluntarily because they wanted power or were angry with God. Most of them remembered being lied to and tricked into going with Satan. These entities also had a very strong demonic influence, which kept them earthbound.

Chuck, a thirty-year-old man who came to me for a weight problem, had many human entities who had died of starvation. One of these entities, George, said his body was crushed by a horse and later he died of starvation and thirst. The following is a transcript of the amazing account of what happened to him after the death of his body and how he ended up with my patient, Chuck.

George: "I am out of my body. I do not feel dead, although my body is dead. I am free of the hunger and pain that I was feeling before my body died. I do not know where to go, so I call someone to help.

"An angel with dark eyes comes to me and takes me through a dark tunnel where that angel turns dark and evil. He tells me to wait here. There are thousands of humans waiting here. They all look tired. The place is cold and damp. The cold goes clear through our bodies. I am feeling pain all over and I am hungry again."

Dr. Modi: "What happens next?"

George: "Someone comes. He is wearing a black robe and his face is covered with a black hood. He tells us that if we work for his master, we will be given eternal life and we will be in a better place."

Dr. Modi: "What do you do?"

George: "We all go with him because we do not like the place where we are. We want to be on the cloud. The dark being takes us in a big dark pit. We have to go with him. We have no choice. We feel like we are falling and falling. We yell but nobody hears us."

Dr. Modi: "What are your thoughts as you are going down?"

George: "Did I make the right decision? It does not feel right. I wish I could go back, but I cannot. We go to the bottom but do not hit the bottom. The place where we are is dark, but not completely dark. It is hot. It is like a big cave. We do not see the end of it. It is damp, cold, and hot. There is fire and a red glow all around.

"When you face the red glow your body is hot and the other side is cold. It is an evil place. There is no cloud. I am feeling hungry, thirsty, and in pain again. Everybody is moaning and groaning.

"We are taken over to a waiting area and we are told to wait there. More people in black robes with hoods come from a tunnel or a passageway and behind them there is this big, red glow and it gets brighter and brighter. It is something or someone."

Dr. Modi: "What does it look like?"

George: "He does not look like a man or an animal. He is big. He has horns like a buffalo, and has hair on his back. His head is big. Bigger than the rest of him, and he has black eyes.

"His facial features are big, his mouth and nose are big. The inside of his mouth is big. His hands are huge. The rest of him is comparatively small.

"He is saying that he is the master of evil and he is the Devil. He says that we chose to come and now we have to work for him. He has tasks for us and if we fail, the punishment will be severe. Now we are his children and we will never be able to leave."

Dr. Modi: "What happens then?"

George: "Then he leaves. I am feeling hungry and thirsty. Everybody is moaning again. The robed men take us to different places individually. One robed person comes for me. He says that I have to go to work. I have a job to do and I must not fail. I have to cause my feelings and pain in whomever I am sent to."

Dr. Modi: "How do you look at this time?"

George: "Dark. Looks like my body, but small. It is like my form shrinks a little bit. A nonsolid form like a ghost, but dark."

Dr. Modi: "What happens then?"

George: "Then I am sent through a tunnel and I can see outside again. It is like I am in and can see through somebody else's eyes. Like I am alive again and I can feel and hear a heartbeat, but it is not mine. I am inside this person."

Dr. Modi: "How do you go inside this person?"

George: "As I was in the tunnel, I was forced out of the tunnel. I was pushed hard toward this person and I go right through the body of this person who had an accident and was in pain. I could not stop myself and then I was inside of him.

"He is a young boy, eight years old, and he is in pain. Then I am floating inside his body and I started to feel the pain all over my body, the pain I felt when I was stepped on by the horses. I cannot breathe, I feel scared. Then the boy becomes unconscious. When I am on the bed, the little boy is on the bed too, like we are one. I cannot breathe, I feel scared. Then it goes dark and I am unconscious."

Dr. Modi: "How?"

George: "I do not know. Then we wake up. We both have a stiff neck and we both have a terrible headache."

Dr. Modi: "Is it your headache that you had when you were crushed, or is it Chuck's headache?"

George: "I don't know. We are disoriented. We have to lie down for a while until we are better and then we are allowed up. I am with him. It is like I am inside of him and I cannot get out. We grow up together. I am stuck. I cannot get out."

Dr. Modi: "What happens then?"

George: "Every once in a while those feelings of hunger, thirst, fear, and pain come out. I am still here in this boy, who is thirty years old now. I hear his name is Chuck."

Dr. Modi: "Check and see if you have a connection with Satan."

George: "Yes, a black wire or tube. There are others who are here. They were all sent by Satan, too."

We requested angels to cut their connections with Satan. After some therapy, George was ready to go to the Light and was released to the Light with the others who were inside. They all died of starvation too.

Ralph, a forty-nine-year-old male spirit in my patient, remembered that he had been choked to death by somebody. He saw himself in a spirit form and was totally confused and angry. He wanted revenge. As he called to somebody for help, he saw the Devil, who said that if he worked for him he would help him get revenge. As he went with him, Satan choked him with black stuff. He was told to go inside other people and do to them what had been done to him.

Ralph claimed that first he went inside another man and caused throat cancer by scratching and irritating his throat. After that host died, Ralph came inside my patient, causing him to cough and have an irritation in his throat.

Mark, an earthbound entity in my patient, gave the following account about how he ended up going with Satan and how he and others were tutored and trained in hell.

> **Mark**: "I died in a car accident. I could see my dead body down there, but I still felt just as alive as before. I felt confused. I thought when you die, you die, and that is the end of you. I did not know what to do or where to go. I saw the Light, but I did not go to it because I thought if I go to the Light then I will really die, and I did not want to die.
>
> "As I was looking around, a dark man dressed in a black hooded robe came to me and said that if I work for his master then he will help me live forever and I will never have to die. It seemed like a good idea. He took me to a dark, cold place. It did not feel good. I realized it was hell. On one side of hell there was fire and people were tortured and burned in fire. They were moaning and groaning. It was awful.
>
> "The man in the black hood said that now I belonged to Satan and if I did not do as I was told, then I would end up on that side where there is fire. I would be tortured and burned. I chose to stay on this side and follow the instructions."
>
> **Dr. Modi**: "What happens then?"
>
> **Mark**: "I and hundreds of other humans like me are taken to a room that is like a training center. There are instructors who are dressed in black and have evil, black, cold eyes. We have orientation-type sessions."
>
> **Dr. Modi**: "What happens there?"
>
> **Mark**: "One instructor is saying, 'Now you have to go back up on the earth and recruit people to come down here to work for Satan. We need people, we need souls. We

need to make our message known that the world is going to come to an end and everybody is going to come down here and work for Satan. Tell them that there is no such thing as heaven. Hell is the only reality there is.' Then we are taught how to enter in people's bodies and possess them."

Dr. Modi: "What are you taught about that?"

Mark: "We are told to look on earth for people who are in weakened condition, whose aura or shields are weak, uneven, and not bright and shiny. They will look depressed, nervous, unhappy, or sick in the hospital. We are told that people in the hospital, nursing homes, and funeral homes are easy to enter. So we often crowd in those areas. Then we are taught how to influence people we are in."

Dr. Modi: "What are you told about that?"

Mark: "We are given a list of things to do with people we are in. We are told to keep them sinful and not to allow them to see the good. Then they have to come down here. They will think that they cannot go to heaven because they sinned and then we can get them to work for Satan.

"We are taught how to keep people stirred up and fighting with each other whether they are individuals, couples, families, any two people, groups, religions, politicians, or the leaders of different countries. We have to make them constantly fight with each other and keep them agitated. We have to promote evil in the world.

"We are taught to break up marriages and thus break up families and society. To force people to physically, verbally, and sexually abuse spouses, children, and others.

"We are especially told to work on teenagers because they are impressionable. We talk them into using drugs and alcohol and being sexually promiscuous. We make them rebellious and fight with their parents,

209

teachers, and others around them. We just promote any type of evil in the world we can think of.

"We are told to push people into stealing, gambling, raping, murdering, and any kind of criminal and evil activity we can think of. We are also told to spread different types of sexual perversions."

Dr. Modi: "How do you make a person do all those things?"

Mark: "We just constantly whisper in their minds those thoughts and ideas, which they think are their own. We reinforce whatever negative qualities they have, such as anger, hate, jealousy, paranoia, fear, etc. We can even turn love into a negative, as in obsessive love. We constantly whisper new evil thoughts and ideas in their minds till they act upon them.

"There was an entire day when we were taught how to recruit people for Satanic cult worship. We were shown movies of what others are doing, such as animal and human sacrifice to Satan. They recruit lots of young people who are impressionable for this. We are also taught how to turn into a blob to hide inside people, so people like you cannot find us."

Dr. Modi: "How do you do that? How do you change into a blob?"

Mark: "We hide anywhere we find space. They told us that if we are in a situation where we need to change our shape, we can crouch down and if we think real hard about the Devil and pray to him for help, he will help us change into any form or shape so we can hide. Just as humans on earth pray to God, we who work for Satan pray to him.

"We are told over and over that the Light is dangerous and we have to stay away from it, otherwise we will die. When you asked the angels to put the Light around me, I thought you were going to punish me, too. I am sorry for giving you a hard time."

After some therapy and knowledge about his condition, he was willing to go to the Light and called out all the others who were hiding inside. They all were released and returned to heaven with angels and their loved ones.

Simon, an earthbound spirit in my patient, gave the following account about how they were trained in hell and how they create problems for humans.

> **Simon**: "I stand behind the person and I listen for a swear word like, 'go to hell,' 'damn you,' 'God damn it,' etc. It changes the person's vibrations. Then he says more swear words and gets loud and boisterous, which lowers his vibration and his shield opens up and I get in through him and come on the other side in front of the other person he is talking to.
>
> "I get behind the other person and when he swears, I touch him and whisper in his ears, 'Keep going, do not give up now,' and as his vibration falls, I look for a weak spot in his soul and get in his arm and make him hit that person and then hop out. If I stay there too long, then I will get stuck. Then I quickly jump to the other person and can get into his voice and change his voice right through the vocal cords. It is hard work, but we are taught well.
>
> "We can make the person angry and look through his eyes and go in the other person. The senses have more power—vision, smell, and hearing the words and thoughts. We can get in almost every one of you this way. I was trained in how to do this. There are all types of training schools."
>
> **Dr. Modi**: "Where?"
>
> **Simon**: "In hell. It is like a big black two-dimensional plane, a lot of office spaces and buildings, like a whole city, the city of hell.
>
> "They teach us math, science, physics, how the human body works, what works and what does not work, how to enter people, how to change their minds,

how to influence their thoughts, how to concentrate on the physics with the vibrations.

"We are taught how to look for key words. There are key words in each language, even though they may sound different, but it is the meaning, it is the feeling that is important. Feeling is where the vibration is. We learn to listen to the feelings. With negative feelings, you lose your soul parts, which in turn creates holes in the soul and thus in the body and we can enter them. This in turn lowers your vibrations.

"The real black beings, demons and black humans, can bounce in and out without much effort. Those of us who are not really black, we have to wait for the key moment."

Dr. Modi: "What are the different swear words that open the shield?"

Simon: "'Hell,' 'damn,' 'God damn it,' and 'Jesus' said in anger when you don't mean good by it. It is the feelings that accompany these words that opens the person. 'Fuck' is a very bad word. It also lowers the vibrations and opens the shield of a person.

Dr. Modi: "What else were you taught?"

Simon: "They teach us about the windows of opportunity, which ones to get in and which ones not to get in and where we might get caught and burned.

"Basically, there are two windows that you can enter. Window of negative energy, such as through negative emotions. The window of positive energy is bad because we can get burned and we won't get to come back.

"We are shown a movie about how demons affect people in churches. Only the strongest and best-trained demons can go to the churches. They stand outside the churches or temples or mosques, because they cannot stand the Light that emanates there. They scan the church for negativity from outside. Only the top graduate demons go to these churches. The little demons get burned there, so Satan sends his armies of powerful demons to the churches. They cannot get into the churches, but they can fire the black laser beams and twist people's thinking.

"They focus on the preacher. Most of the energy is concentrated on the preacher. They concentrate on changing the words. The demons use the Bible and know it very well. They look for the spot here and spot there.

"The Bible is mostly pure, but there are selected areas that are not, and when the preachers refer to them, the demons can fire the negative laser energy, right through the preacher to the congregation and then shake it up a little bit and people get scared and they disregard the inner soul and start to listen to the dark thoughts. Sometimes they are successful and sometimes they are not, because the Light beings are there too, like there is a white circle and a dark circle around."

Dr. Modi: "What type of words and phrases in the Bible are not correct?"

Simon: "'Fear of God,' is a big one. Any time the preachers mention 'fear of God,' the phrase sets in fear and panic in the people and opens them up. This is one of the bases of fear for all other fears. It is the mountain for all fears. When you fear God, then you fear everything else. Demons inserted that phrase in the Bible.

Dr. Modi: "What are the different things that were changed in the Bible?"

Simon: "Demons have changed many things in the Bible. There were many Adams and Eves. Many Christians think there was only one couple. They think what the Bible says is correct. They do not understand that what the Bible does not say is correct too. We did not let everything that came from the Light be in the Bible. If we had done so, then we would be in trouble and we would not have much to work with.

"When they were translating the Bible, we pushed them to change the words, which changed the meaning. We can slide in and change things. The reincarnation and past lives were taken out. The fact that you are in heaven and plan to come here in duality and do not understand was left out. The fact that you come again and again was left out. The fact that you plan both positive and negative actions was left out.

"Christians think that the Bible is the only book from God. We distorted the meaning in many places. Christians believe that you cannot go to heaven if you do not believe in Jesus. This is a trick we use to confuse people. The truth is that if you believe in God, then you can go to heaven."

Dr. Modi: "What else were you taught?"

Simon: "There are big labs in hell. We are taught how to make a bunch of devices. It is like a metal shop. We can make all different types of devices to create problems for people. There are telepathic devices such as a radio transmitter, which we can implant in the body. It is about the size of a grain of sand, and is used later to transmit the thoughts.

"There are different types of clip devices like the big black paper clip that holds a bunch of paper. It clips the spiritual flow of Light. We can create any types of devices to create different types of physical, emotional, mental, and spiritual problems for humans."

After some psychotherapy with Simon and education about his condition, he was released to the Light (heaven).

What Opens Us for Spirit Attachment or Spirit Possession?

As I started to locate and release the earthbound entities from my patients, I started to wonder: Why and how could these entities enter the patient's body? What opens a person up for the outside entities to come in? And why are some patients more open than others?

Under hypnosis, patients say that around their bodies they have an electromagnetic energy field, a type of shield that they call *aura*. It shields and protects their bodies from the outside entities. Some patients who are psychic report that they can see this energy field or aura around people, animals, and plants even without hypnosis.

According to the hypnotized patients, some people have harder boundaries around their auras, as if they are heavily armored. This boundary prevents outside spirits from entering them. Other people have soft, porous, and fuzzy boundaries or edges around their auras, making it easier for the outside spirits to enter their shields and the bodies. These individuals do not have much defense and protection against the outside entities.

Patients report that different physical and emotional conditions, behaviors, and situations can open their shields, allowing outside spirits to enter their bodies.

Conditions That Open People for Possession

Under hypnosis, earthbound spirits in my patients described different conditions that opened my patients' shields and allowed them to come in:

- Physical conditions, such as sickness, anesthesia, surgery, accidents, unconsciousness, etc.
- Emotional conditions, such as anger, fear, hate, depression, compassion, grief, etc.
- Drug and alcohol use
- Rock-'n'-roll music
- Video games
- Entities on board
- Occupations
- People with soft, fuzzy, and porous boundaries of their energy field

HEALTHY AURA (ENERGY FIELD AROUND THE BODY) AND SHIELD
(Drawing by a patient)

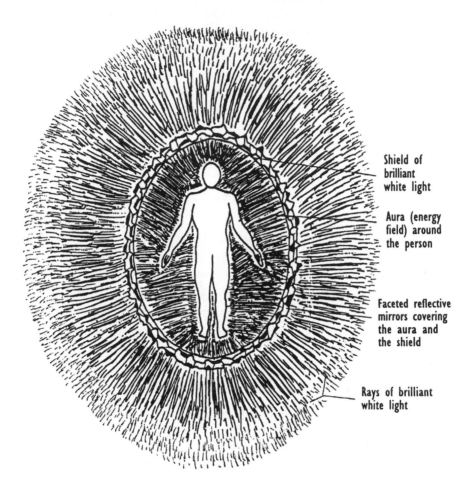

Shield of brilliant white light

Aura (energy field) around the person

Faceted reflective mirrors covering the aura and the shield

Rays of brilliant white light

Aura: The aura looks like a buffer zone around a person. It consists of a solid mass of white light about 18-20 inches thick. The mass consists of thin, densely arranged rays that look almost like a sheaf of wheat.

Shield: The shield appears as an oval-shaped protective mirror that looks faceted. Light reflects off the shield in many directions and for long distances.

- Missing soul parts and their connecting cords
- Entities coming in from another dimension
- Voluntary possession or invitational possession such as
  - Using Ouija board
  - Using automatic writing
  - Sitting in a séance
  - Channeling
  - Playing with conjuring games such as, Dungeons and Dragons, and Demons
  - Inviting a spirit to come on board voluntarily out of love

Physical Conditions That Open a Person's Shield

Entities in my patients often claimed that they entered the patients when the patients were physically ill, injured, knocked unconscious, sedated, or anesthetized. Some entities claim to come inside the patients while the patients are in the hospital after surgery or during an illness. They claim that hospitals are usually crowded with human and demon entities, waiting to enter people who are sick and open for possession. Chronic fatigue and exhaustion can also shrink the energy field, leaving a person open for possession.

Many of my patients describe being out of their bodies during surgery and watching the surgery from outside. They describe seeing many other spirits floating in the operating room and also throughout the hospital. These spirits sometimes come into patients after the surgery and bring their physical and emotional problems with them. These patients often report delayed recovery or having new symptoms that they did not have before surgery.

Jim had many human and dark entities in him. They all claimed to come into Jim when he became unconscious several years ago, opening up his shield.

Sam had an entity who gave the following information: "I had a heart attack. They rushed me to the emergency room but I was already out of my body. Doctors checked me and covered my body with the sheet. I felt confused and did not know where to go. I was wandering around the hospital. I saw this kid who was crying with pain. He just had surgery. I went to him to comfort him but got stuck there inside him."

Ashley had several human entities who all claimed to have come in when she had a car accident. According to them, the jolt of the accident opened her energy shield and they all came in and have been with her since then.

Callie, a thirty-year-old patient, had a female entity, Mary, who was twenty-seven years old. Mary gave the following description of what happened to her and how she ended up inside Callie.

> **Spirit Mary**: "They are operating on my body. I am watching from above [becoming upset]. Something is wrong. I am bleeding. All these machines are going crazy [looking panicky]. They are covering me with a ˙sheet and everybody is leaving. I cannot die yet. I am too young. This is awful. It is not right."
>
> **Dr. Modi**: "What do you do?"
>
> **Mary**: "I hear this one crying."
>
> **Dr. Modi**: "Who?"
>
> **Mary**: "Callie. She is having surgery in the other room. A C-section. She is out of her body and afraid that she will lose her baby. He has the cord wrapped around his neck. I go to her to comfort her because she is very scared. I cannot calm her down. After the surgery, I go into her to help her, but then I cannot get out. I get stuck."

Emotional Conditions That Open a Person's Shield

Some possessing human and demon entities claim to have entered the patients while they were depressed, angry, sad, fearful, hateful, or grieving. Even too much compassion can open the shield. Sometimes entities claim that the patients' doubts about the existence of earthbound or demon entities and past lives opened the shields, allowing them to come in.

Janice, a thirty-five-year-old female, was a good subject. We spent many sessions doing spirit releasement and past life regression therapy with a great deal of improvement in her physical and emotional symptoms. In spite of the fact that she herself reported seeing and hearing human and demon entities in her and recalled different past life traumas that were responsible for her symptoms, she constantly had doubts about them. During each session she came in with new human and demon entities. They all said that Janice's doubts about the existence of human and demon entities and past lives opened her shield for them to come in.

During one session, as we were releasing the human and demon entities from her, I asked her to look up inside the Light and call out anybody whom she believed and who could answer her questions. She saw Jesus as a being of Light with loving eyes. I asked Janice to ask Jesus any questions she wished.

The conversation went like this:

Janice: "Are these dark demon entities real?"

Jesus: "Yes. They work for the Devil. They influence people's thoughts, actions, and functioning. The Devil has been trying to control you for a long time because of the type of person you are, good and spiritual. Although Satan wants every soul, people who are good or spiritual or have a divine God-given purpose are a special target for him.

Janice: "Are these past lives real?"

Jesus: "Yes. People come down to earth again and again to learn lessons and grow spiritually. Jobs and purposes that are not finished continue to influence people in their future lives until they are resolved."

Janice: "Why is reincarnation not mentioned in the Bible?"

Jesus: "Scriptures of all the religions are given by God, but they all have subtle influences by the Devil and his demons. The idea of reincarnation has been taken out of the Bible by people who had demonic influence.

They did so to suit their selfish needs. Also, the Bible was translated from one language to another, and the Devil and his demons have managed to change the information in a subtle way by influencing the human translators. So, when reading any scriptures, only accept what feels right and ignore that which does not feel right. Trust your instincts and inner self. Do not follow everything blindly."

Jesus told her to be trusting and that she was guided to my office under his direction. It was necessary for her to get to such a low point so she would ask for help. After this session, Janice did not have any doubts and as a result did not open her shield for new entities.

Tracy had a spirit of her friend who said that he joined Tracy in the funeral home. Tracy was very sad and distraught about his death, which had opened her shield. He came in to comfort her, but then could not come out.

Jason had many human and dark demon entities in him. They all claimed that every time he had anger outbursts, it opened his shield and they came in. Then they would push him to become more angry and irritable, allowing more entities to come in. Jason had many, many layers of human and dark entities in him.

Joe often felt sorry for homeless people. Sometimes he used to invite them to his home and give them food and shelter. After the death of their physical bodies, they joined Joe. They all said that his compassion opened him up for them to come in. They did not mean any harm to him. They simply liked him.

Bridgit had a male entity who was mentally retarded. It joined her because she always had a great deal of compassion for mentally retarded people, and her compassion opened her shield up for him to come in.

Leona had many dark demon and human spirits who claimed to come in when she was watching a scary movie. They bragged:

"When people get frightened while watching a scary movie, their shields open up and we just come in. Many of us wait in the movie hall or at home to come in. Then we get them to watch more evil and scary movies and tempt them to adopt evil ways, and before you know, they are under our control."

Drug and Alcohol Use

Some patients, under hypnosis, reported that their use of drugs and alcohol opened their shields for outside entities to come in. According to them, drugs and alcohol make the shields porous and fuzzy or create holes in them.

Larry, an entity in my patient, was a drug addict who was beaten up and killed. He gave the following information:

"I was using drugs heavily and was also shooting heroin. I went to an apartment. There were a lot of people doing drugs. I tried to ask them for drugs but nobody could see or hear me. I saw this woman slumped against the wall. She was easy to get in because she was doing drugs. Everybody there had weaker light around them. After I got in her I continued to give her the desire to use drugs."

Rhonda had experienced multiple symptoms for two months. She had severe abdominal pain, nausea, aches and pains all over her body, difficulty in sleeping, and recurrent nightmares about dogs attacking her. When Rhonda called my office for an appointment, she doubled up with severe abdominal pain.

During a session, as she looked inside, she found the spirit of a little girl, Sue, who claimed to have joined Rhonda two months earlier when Rhonda was drinking. This little girl was attacked by dogs, her body was torn apart, and she was killed. After she joined Rhonda, Sue continued to feel stomachache, nausea, aches and pains all over her body, and the memories of the dogs attacking her. These feelings were transferred to Rhonda and became her symptoms. After releasing Sue, Rhonda was free of all her symptoms and did not have the nightmares anymore.

According to my patients, even nicotine and caffeine can make their shields porous, but less so than drugs and alcohol.

Rock-'n'-Roll Music

Some entities in my patients reported that they came in when the patients were listening to rock-'n'-roll music. One entity in my patient explained it as follows:

"Some of the rock-'n'-roll music is loud and cacophonous and the vibrations are so intense and invasive that they dissipate the shield, making the shield porous like a cheesecloth in people who are vulnerable, allowing outside entities to come in. Also, the flashing lights and loud music during a concert are so invasive and disharmonious that they cause the misalignment of the nervous system by interfering with the normal rhythm of brain waves and brain activity."

Video Games

Sometimes entities in my patients reported that their shields opened up when they were playing video games. The effect is similar to that of rock-'n'-roll music, but a stronger phenomenon occurs with video games due to the intensity of constant visual and auditory stimuli. One entity in my patient explained it:

"When children play with the video games at home or in a video arcade, they become mesmerized as they focus on the screen and the double-edged bombardment of repetitive auditory and visual stimuli opens their shields and leave them defenseless against the negative outside entities. Once we are in, we give them the desire to play more and more and influence them in a negative direction."

Entities on Board

If a patient already has one or more entities on board, it makes his or her energy field weaker, allowing more entities to come in.

Occupation

My patients mention that people with certain occupations are more vulnerable for possession: doctors, respiratory therapists, nurses, hospital employees, paramedics, undertakers, chiropractors, massage therapists, and people who do spirit releasement therapy. Different Light beings through different patients have repeatedly suggested to pray for protection faithfully every day.

Julia, a respiratory therapist, felt compassion for dying patients. This compassion opened her up for the entities to come on board with her after the death of their physical bodies. She had a collection of them with her and all of them said the same thing; "She liked us, she felt for us, so we came in."

Sheila was a nurse who had suffered severe headaches off and on for many years. She had a spirit of a young man who had a motorcycle accident. He died in the hospital in the intensive care unit. He joined Sheila as she was working there. Her compassion opened her up for him to come in. He said, "She was kind and I wanted her to take care of me."

People with Soft, Fuzzy, and Porous Boundaries of Their Energy Shields

According to patients, people who are psychics and other people who are more spiritually developed normally have soft, fuzzy, and porous edges around their auras. This makes them more open for possession by outside entities. Also, many of the psychics want to help people, and sometimes their compassion opens them up for entities to come in. Some entities claimed that a few psychic people who are arrogant and think they have all the answers open themselves up for the outside entities to come in. Their ego and arrogance make them easy targets for negative influences.

Those people who are less spiritually developed also have softer shields with porous edges. Those in between seem to be fairly protected because of harder boundaries of their shields.

Fay had many human and demon entities. They all said: "She was easy to come in. It was like just sleeping with her. She just does not have any firm boundaries. We can walk in and out of her anytime we want."

223

Grant was a clairvoyant and an excellent psychic and was very compassionate, and that trait opened him up for many entities to come in. They all said: "He was easy. We can just get in and get out of him any time we want." This caused him many physical and psychological problems. After locating and releasing all his entities, I taught him how to create a protective shield around him to avoid any further infestation by outside entities. This worked well for him.

During one session, he told me that he went to a Civil War cemetery. At the cemetery he saw hundreds of spirits of soldiers who were talking to him. They all were sad, confused, hurting, and crying with pain and felt trapped. He wanted to help them. He kept on telling them to look up and go to the Light. Some went, but most did not. They were confused. After he came home he continued to see and hear those soldier spirits who were knocking on his shield and saying, "We want to go home, we want to go home."

Under hypnosis, he saw hundreds of them around him, knocking at the shield and saying, "We want to go home, we want to go home," but they could not come in. His protective shield was effective. As he looked inside himself he saw one soldier in his hand who said his name was Christian. The following is a transcript of what happened during that session.

Dr. Modi: "Christian, what happened to you?"

Christian: "I am a lieutenant. I was shot in the Civil War. A lot of us did not go up. We did not want to be dead. We wanted to stay here and continue. We all are hurting with pain. We are confused and we do not know where to go. Nobody sees us or hears us.

"When this man came, he was glowing. We all noticed him and he was able to see us and hear us. He kept telling us to go to the Light, but we did not know where. He had a strong shield around him so we could not come in. Only I snuck in when he touched my tomb. His compassion opened him for me to come in. We all wanted to go to the Light, but we did not know how."

Dr. Modi: "Okay, Let me help you. Christian and all the others who are here, look up and tell me what you see."

Spirit Christian: "A big circle of Light and a crowd of people and angels in it. They are our loved ones."

Grant: "I see many black hands from outside the Light coming. But the angels of the Light are pushing them away. They are the deceivers, the dark demon entities. The angels are surrounding the whole place and all the entities with the Light."

I asked all the entities to hold the hands of their loved ones and angels who were in the Light and go home to the Light. As they were going, Christian asked if he could call his buddies and other soldiers who were still stuck at that cemetery. I said, yes. To my surprise, Grant saw hundreds of soldiers coming from that cemetery and going into the Light.

Grant was amazed and said: "Oh, Dr. Modi, you should see this. Hundreds and thousands of them are going to the Light with the angels. Some of them who were beheaded are being put together and healed by the angels, and they are going happily with their loved ones. It is a very emotional reunion for them. As they go to the Light, their color is changing. They are becoming brighter and dark blobs are falling out of them. Some of the soldiers are still at the cemetery. They are too attached to the nearby bar and try to hang around the ones who drink. They are too dark and not ready to go yet."

Entities Coming in through the Missing Soul Parts and Their Connecting Cords

Sometimes, even when the shields are strong and completely intact, patients find new entities coming in through the missing soul parts that are in possession of Satan and his demons in the darkness. Patients often state that Satan and his demons are shoving human and demon entities into them through the missing soul parts and their connecting cords, which are in their possession.

Nora had many human and demon entities infesting her whole body. It took several sessions to free her from all her possessing entities. When she was all clear we proceeded to do regression therapy. Initially she was able to see, receive, and describe the past life very vividly with emotions. After a few minutes everything became dark and she was not able to receive any information or images. So I asked her to check her body for any influence. She saw a gray-looking human entity in her eyes. He appeared confused and shocked. On questioning, he said: "My name is Albert. I was just floating around outside trying to find a body to possess. I was called in by Satan. It was like I was sucked in and taken to Satan. He had a soul part of this person in his hand. He punctured a hole in her soul part and pushed me through it and the cord, into this person's eyes and I am here. I had no control over it."

Albert was also surrounded by a dark demon entity. It was separated from Albert, was transformed into the Light, and then was sent to the Light. Albert was also sent to the Light. We requested the angels to bring all of Nora's soul parts that were with Satan and his demons, cleanse them, heal them, and integrate them with Nora. After that Nora was able to see and receive the information from her past life without any problem.

Entities Coming from Another Dimension

Sometimes patients reported new entities coming in, even when their shields were strong and intact. In these cases the entities (mostly demons) said that they came in from another dimension that had the same vibrations as our dimension. One time, after releasing such an entity, we asked the angel, who was helping us, to explain it. The angel said that demons and angels can travel freely between two dimensions whose vibrations are the same; thus the demons can enter into a person even when the shield is strong and intact. It can happen only from certain points between the dimensions. They suggested that every day we should request the angels to stay on guard around us in this dimension and in all the other dimensions.

Voluntary Possession or Invitational Possession

Sometimes patients reported being possessed by human or demon entities while playing with a Ouija board, channeling, doing automatic writing, or sitting in a séance. Playing with conjuring games such as Dungeons and Dragons and Demons can also open people up for possession. In all these situations, patients reported that they voluntarily called and invited an outside spirit to give them information and as a result opened their shields for possession.

Skip did automatic writing from time to time over several years. The entity who was writing through him claimed that he knew Skip from a past life. Skip was under the impression that this entity was a being of the Light, maybe a spirit guide. But during a session we found out that it was an earthbound entity in Skip, one who knew Skip from a past life and did not go to the Light. It joined Skip when he was trying to do automatic writing and called somebody to give him information, opening his shield. The entity used his hand to write messages for him and give him information from time to time.

Dave, a fifteen-year-old male, had a demon entity who claimed to come in when he was playing the game Dungeons and Dragons. The demon said that it came in because Dave called him in.

Sonya, an eighteen-year-old female, had a male entity who said: "I came in when Sonya and her friends were playing with a Ouija board. I was there and I started to move the planchet. Everybody, including Sonya, got scared; the fear opened Sonya up and I came into her."

Quinn had an entity in him who said: "I came in when he was playing with a Ouija board. He called out for somebody to come to provide answers to his questions. This opened his shield up and I came in."

Inviting an entity to come on board: Sometimes patients report that they have voluntarily opened themselves up and invited an entity to come in to stay with them. It is usually a loved one, but can be anybody else.

Leena, a twenty-eight-year-old female, had the spirit of a five-year-old girl, Tina, who gave the following description of how she came to be in Leena:

Dr. Modi: "What happened to your body, Tina?"

Tina: "I was sleeping. My daddy came home drunk. He was yelling and screaming. I started to cry. So he took my pillow and pressed it on my face and I couldn't breathe.

"They took my body to the hospital but I was already out. I followed my body. At the hospital there were many people who were just floating around.

"Then I met Leena, who was scared. Leena was having an operation; she was eight years old. She was out of her body and was scared and crying. I was just floating there. I went to her and we started to play with each other. After her surgery she invited me to come in with her and I have been here ever since."

Sandy had the spirit of her mother, who said that Sandy invited her in because she felt guilty that she was not with her mother when she died.

Arney invited his father in because he did not get a chance to say goodbye to him.

Looking at all the conditions reported by my patients that opened them for possession, I realized that every human being is open for possession. We all get sick, have emotions of anger, fear, hate, depression, compassion, sadness, and grief. We have accidents and surgery, and some drink and use drugs. My patients tell me that most of the time they are not even aware of the entities inside.

David, during one session, saw an angel who said, "None of the human beings can be totally and completely protected from the outside entities when they are on the earth, regardless of how spiritually developed they are in the Light."

In very rare cases I have seen people who have a special shield or bubble around them, completely protecting them. Under hypnosis, they report that they came from the Light with this special bubble, because they have some special purpose to achieve during this life. They are provided with this special bubble or protection shield from the Light, which is around their souls and around their bodies both, so they can be totally protected, internally and externally, all through the life from outside entities and influences, and fulfill their purposes.

Why the Spirits (Entities) Remain Earthbound

As I began to recognize, locate, and release the attached earthbound entities from my patients, I started to wonder why these earthbound entities remained earthbound and why they did not make their transition to heaven. So I began to ask these questions to the entities during the treatment.

The different possessing earthbound spirits in my patients gave various reasons why they were still stuck on the earth plane and why they did not make their transition to heaven:

- Ignorance and confusion
- Strong emotions—anger, hate, love, fear, jealousy, and the desire for revenge
- Addictions to drugs, alcohol, cigarettes, food, gambling, or sex
- Obsessive attachment to a person, place, or an object
- Past life connections
- Unfinished business
- Demon possession and influence
- Interference by Satan and his demons and earthbound entities who work for Satan
- Influence through missing soul parts

Ignorance and Confusion

One of the most common reasons that these possessing earthbound spirits gave as to why they did not go to heaven was their ignorance about what happens after death, what to expect, and where to go. Some spirits felt that death would be the end of their existence and that there would be nothing afterward. One male entity told me, "When you die your body goes into dust and that is the end of you." Some reported seeing the Light but ignoring it because they did not know that they were supposed to go to it. Some felt that if they went to the Light, then they would really die.

Some of these possessing earthbound spirits stated that they did not know what happened to them. They were supposed to be dead, but they did not feel dead. They felt very confused to find that they still felt as alive as before and still had all their problems. To their surprise, they felt the same emotional turmoil and pain they felt before the death of their physical bodies. They felt very confused about everything and did not know what to do or where to go.

Sometimes people who committed suicide saw the Light and their loved ones or angels in the Light, but they turned away because they believed they committed a sin and they did not belong in the Light, or that they would be punished in heaven. Almost always, earthbound entities who committed suicide had very strong demonic influence, which not only confused them and pushed them to commit suicide, but also continued to confuse them after the death of their bodies and kept them from going to heaven. They sometimes have other earthbound entities in them who committed suicide and who pushed them to commit suicide.

Although some of the people who commit suicide go to heaven, many of them stay earthbound. If they end up possessing somebody, then they make their hosts feel depressed and suicidal, too, in which case the host may also end up committing suicide.

According to my patients, people who died suddenly, as in cases of a sudden heart attack, murder, or a car accident, often do not even look back at their dead bodies and sometimes have no clue that their physical body is dead. They desperately try to communicate with people but nobody hears them or sees them.

They go to the funeral home and feel very confused about seeing their bodies in the casket. They cannot understand how it is possible. Out of their desperate need for communication and comfort, they end up possessing somebody who is open. It is usually a loved one or a friend who may already be open because of the grief.

Sometimes these entities are so confused that they insist they are in their own body instead of their host's body. Initially they totally deny the death of their body and refuse to accept the fact. These entities require extensive therapy to understand what happened to them.

Stanley, an entity in my patient, recalled:

"I am hovering over my dead body. But I do not feel dead. I try to talk to people but nobody could see or hear me. I feel confused. I do not know where to go. I do not believe in heaven or hell. I believe that whatever you have on earth is your heaven. And when you die, you are dead and that is the end of you."

Stephanie, a twenty-eight-year-old female entity in my patient, recalled being stabbed to death. She was confused because she still felt as alive as before. Following is the conversation with her.

Stephanie: "I do not think I will ever be allowed in heaven. I was a prostitute and I used to steal so I could survive. When I was a little girl I used to go to Sunday School and we were told that if we sinned, we could not go to heaven."

Dr. Modi: "Stephanie, look up and tell me what you see."

Stephanie: "What is that? It is awfully bright. It is coming down. It is not a spaceship, is it?"

Dr. Modi: "You tell me."

Stephanie: "Oh, it is beautiful! There are beautiful angels inside that Light. What are they doing here? They are right in front of me. They are pretty and smiling at me. People who look like that usually do not smile at me."

Dr. Modi: "Would you like to go with them?"

Stephanie: "Are you sure they want me?"

Dr. Modi: "Ask them."

Stephanie [looking up]: "Would you take me with you? I have been a terrible person. [Looking puzzled] They are smiling at me and saying, 'Yes we will.' I cannot believe it."

Dr. Modi: "What else would you like to ask?"

Stephanie [talking to angels]: "What do I have to do when I get there? [surprised] You are telling me that I do not have to do anything? I do not have to earn my way? I always have to earn my own way. Uh, that might be kind of nice; O.K., I will go."

The patient saw her holding the angels' hands and going to the Light.

Alice had the spirit of a ten-year-old little girl inside her, whose name was Becky. The following is a transcript of the conversation with her.

Dr. Modi: "Becky do you know where you are?"

Becky: "Yes, I am with Alice."

Dr. Modi: "What happened to your body, Becky?"

Becky: "I do not know."

Dr. Modi: "Move back in time, Becky. Find your body. What happened to it?"

Becky [crying]: "I do not want to. I do not want to die. [quiet] I can see my body. I fell and broke my back. (crying) My body is just there. It won't get up or move. I am afraid of Mom. She will be angry with me. I was not careful enough."

Dr. Modi: "Would you like to go to heaven?"

Becky: "No. It will be boring there. Nobody to play with. I like Alice. I want to stay here with her."

Dr. Modi: "Just look up and tell me what you see."

Becky: [surprised] "I see a bright Light. There is a playground. There are kids jumping ropes. I think I will go there. Looks like fun."

She held the hands of the kids in the Light and went happily to heaven.

Olivia had a spirit of a stillborn baby, who gave the following account of what happened.

"My mother is on the table in the hospital. I am just born. She is crying because I am not crying. I am not making any noise. I am confused. I do not know what happened. I heard this little girl crying. I went to her, touched her, and after that I started to cry, too. I was inside of her."

Strong Emotions

According to my patients, strong emotions such as anger, hate, jealousy, love, despair, fear, and the desire to take revenge are some of the common emotions that keep a spirit stuck in the physical world.

Anger: Strong anger about something or somebody can keep a person earthbound. Spirits often try to possess the person with whom they are angry or people close to that person, to create problems for them. Sometimes the earthbound spirits do not go to heaven because they are angry at God for what happened to them.

Valerie, a female entity in my patient, recalled that she killed her husband in 1901 so she could be with her lover. After a few years her lover killed her. She died angry and revengeful. She gave the following account: "After I died the Devil came to me and told me that he would help me take revenge and give me eternal life if I would work for him. I made a pact with the Devil that he could have my soul if he would help me take revenge and give me eternal life. The Devil took me to hell, a dark, cold place, where I saw a lot of people crying and suffering. The Devil stabbed and hurt me and wrote his name on me. Then he told me to go to this person and bring her soul to him and if I failed, he would punish me in the worst way."

Fear: In cases of fear, the entities say that they are afraid of being dead so they desperately deny the death of their body.

233

Some tell of having a fear of punishment and a fear of being sent to hell because they did something wrong. Some have a fear of the unknown so they desperately cling to life even if it means living in somebody else's body or living through somebody.

Peter was a male entity in my patient. We tried to release him during a session, but he refused to go to the Light. He expressed the fear that he would be punished and sent to hell, because he killed his family and then killed himself. He felt that for people like him, there was no place in heaven. I explained to him that according to what others have told me this was not true. He had a hard time believing me, so I asked him to look at the Light and call out anybody from heaven whom he could trust. He called for Jesus and was shocked and surprised to see him in the Light.

> **Dr. Modi:** "Tell me what he looks like."
> **Peter:** "Just like his pictures, except he is all Light. His eyes are very loving. They look like an ocean of love and Light. [looking surprised] He isn't angry with me!"
> **Dr. Modi:** "What would you like to ask him?"
> **Peter:** "I just want to know if I will be forgiven."
> **Dr. Modi:** "What does he say?"
> **Peter:** "He is smiling and reaching for me. I think it is O.K. I am going with him. Bye."

Guilt: Some earthbound entities feel guilty about things they did and feel that they do not deserve to go to heaven or if they go to heaven, they will be punished and will be sent to hell.

Bill, an entity in my patient, felt guilty because he cheated on his wife and gambled and decided not to go to the Light. He felt he was a bad person who did not deserve to go to heaven.

Hate: Hate can be a fueling emotion that keeps the entities earthbound. Here the entities describe that they go after the person they hate and possess that person. Sometimes they say that if they cannot possess the person, they will possess somebody who is close to the person they hate, such as a close family member. Through them they can hurt that person.

JoAnn had the spirit of her aborted fetus, who gave the following information:

"I am angry at my mother. I do not know why she got rid of me. I hate her for what she did to me. After I came out of my body I saw this man dressed in a black robe who came to me and said he would help me in taking revenge on my mother. Then the man in the black robe brought me here in her. I constantly made her feel guilty about getting rid of me."

After freeing the spirit of the baby from that dark entity, the baby became less angry and hateful and was willing to go to the Light after some therapy.

The desire to take revenge: Some spirits claim they are with my patients because they want to take revenge on them and try to create problems for them.

Sean, an entity in my patient, was a homosexual. After he died of AIDS, he possessed my patient. He had hated her because she did not want to have anything to do with him because he was a homosexual. Now he was determined to take revenge on her. He was determined to give her AIDS by possessing her. He refused to leave her during the session until she apologized to him. After that he felt better and went to the Light feeling peaceful.

Love: Many times spirits in my patients reported that they are here because they love the persons they possess. They can be a spouse, parent, child, or a good friend. No matter how loving the intentions are, this possession is always a mistake, because the spirits' physical, emotional, and mental problems are transferred to the hosts, causing them discomfort and problems. According to my patients, possession by a controlling and authoritarian parent or a jealous spouse can be very detrimental.

Beth had the spirit of her miscarried baby, who said: "I did not know why I could not continue. I loved my mom. I wanted to be with her. After she lost me, she was sad. I tried to talk to her and tell her that I loved her, but she could not hear me. I went in her to comfort her, and have stayed with her since then."

Addictions to Drugs, Alcohol, Cigarettes, Food, Sex, and Gambling

Addictions are some of the reasons the spirits in my patients give for not going to heaven. People who are addicted to drugs and alcohol may have one or more addicted spirits with them. Usually these spirits do not care what happens to their hosts or to their health or finances. All they are interested in is getting what they are addicted to. One of the reasons patients who are addicted find it hard to stop is because it is somebody else who is desiring through them. According to my patients, drugs and alcohol make their shields weaker and porous, enabling more outside entities to enter easily.

Larry, an entity in my patient, gave the following account:

"I loved gambling. I gambled all my life. After the death of my body, I did not go to heaven, because I wanted to stay here and gamble. I do not know how I ended up with this person. I cannot even get her to buy a lottery ticket."

Lucy had an entity who died of complications of diabetes. She gave the following reasons for not going to the Light.

"I had diabetes and doctors put me on a strict diet. I was constantly craving food, especially sweets. I used to hide and eat. I loved to bake, then I ate what I baked. Since I am in this girl, I can eat everything I want, and I do not have to gain weight or be sick."

Joe, a spirit in my patient, gave the following information: "I was an alcoholic and I was shot in a gangster fight. I could see my body lying there dead, but I didn't feel dead. I did not know exactly what happened. I wanted to get those gangsters, but I could not find them. I needed a drink to think straight. So I went to the bar. I tried to talk to my friends, but they could not see or hear me. I tried to reach for a beer glass, but I could not hold it. My hand just went right through it. I was getting more and more angry. I needed a drink fast! I saw a friend who was drunk. I went to him and tried to put my hands on his shoulders, but somehow I found myself inside him. Since then I have been here, drinking through him."

Harold, a spirit in my patient, said: "I was a drug addict. After the death of my body, I saw the Light and angels, but I was not ready to leave. I needed drugs desperately. A man in a black suit came to me and said that if I worked for his master, he would get me the drugs. He took me to a dark, cold place, which was hell. His eyes became mean and evil. He told me to go to this person and I could live in him, then I would be able to use drugs through him. After I went into him, for a while I could not make this person use anything, but gradually I succeeded in pushing him into using pot and alcohol."

Obsessive Attachment

Attachment to a person, place, or an object can also keep a person earthbound.

Jane, an earthbound entity in my patient, gave the following account of why she did not go to the Light.

"I was a good Christian and I believed that after my death I would go to heaven. After the death of my body, I saw the Light and angels in it. But I decided not to go in it because it seemed too final and I was not ready to die. I wanted to see my grandchildren grow. I loved them and did not want to leave them."

Dolly always had a feeling that there was something in her home. During one session, under hypnosis, Dolly saw an older female entity who was clinging to her, but was not in her body. This entity gave the following account of why she was there.

"The house this person lives in is my house. My husband and I built it, and I am determined to stay here. I am not going to let her stay in my house. She'd better understand that this is my house and I am not going anywhere."

After some education about her condition and some psychotherapy, she was released to the Light. After that, Dolly did not feel any presence in her home.

Past Life Connection

Some possessing spirits claim that they have known the patient from another life, in which they were in a loving relationship or

237

they hated each other. According to these possessing entities, an early death with unexpressed feelings and emotions, guilt about leaving the other alone, promises to be together forever, jealousy, anger, hate, and the desire to get revenge are some of reasons for them to follow the people into another lifetime and possess them. Sometimes the same entity claims to possess the same person in several lifetimes.

Here the spirits describe leaving after the death of their host. They remain earthbound and wait for the host to return from heaven. Then they attach to the host anytime, in the womb or after the birth.

Flora had six earthbound entities who were tightly clinging to her. They knew Flora from a life in A.D. 300. One entity was her husband, and five entities were her children in that life. They were very close to each other. They all loved her and stayed earthbound to take care of her in that life. They followed her for more than thirty lives and attached to her because they loved her and wanted to take care of her.

Cindy had severe temper outbursts and mood swings. She had in her a spirit of a deformed boy who was determined to hurt her. On further questioning, he said that he was the brother of Cindy in the seventeenth century in London. He was deformed and retarded. Cindy, who was his sister in that lifetime, made fun of him and was very cruel to him. He died at an early age feeling angry and hateful toward his sister. He attached to her in that lifetime and three more life times, including this life. In one lifetime he made her commit suicide.

This possessing entity had a demon entity in him that made him angry and hateful. After the demon entity was released, he did not feel angry and hateful toward Cindy and had no desire to take revenge. He was willing to go to heaven and was released to the Light.

Unfinished Business

Some entities in my patients claimed that they did not go to heaven because they had some unfinished business to take care of. It could be a project, or a business deal, or anything else. Here they possess a person through whom they can finish the project.

Taylor had with him the spirit of his father, who said that he did not go to the Light because he had to take care of some unfinished business. He was building a home and died before he could finish it. He was hoping that through his son he could finish it, but he did not succeed.

John, an earthbound entity in my patient who died in 1950, gave the following reason for remaining in the physical world:

"I was doing some very important research but I died of pneumonia. I saw my body down there but I did not feel dead. I went to the lab. I had an awful lot to do. It was important research. My colleagues in the lab could not see me or hear me. I realized that I must be dead. I stayed in the lab around the people who took over my research. I continued to tell them what to do and how to do it. Although they believed it was their thoughts, it was I who was giving them the idea about how to do it. Then I do not know how I ended up with this person."

Demon Possession and Influence

According to my patient reports, one of the most common reasons that human spirits stay earthbound is demon possession. It is really the demon entities inside the earthbound spirits who are afraid of the Light. These earthbound entities with demonic influence claim that the Light burns their eyes and they cannot stand it. So they turn away from the Light. The demons inside these earthbound entities also feed them thoughts exaggerating their anger, hate, guilt, and fear, keeping them from going to heaven.

Max had a female entity, Katy, inside who said: "I died of stomach cancer. I knew I was supposed to go to the Light, but every time I made an effort to go to the Light, I felt like something or somebody was holding me down and I could not go up. And somehow I ended up in this person."

Max saw inside Katy a large demon entity who bragged about giving her cancer and keeping her from going to the Light. After releasing the dark entity, Katy was able to go to heaven.

Sometimes during past life regressions patients recall that after the death of their physical bodies they remained earthbound for a long time, sometimes for hundreds and thousands of years. They recall being completely covered, trapped, and consumed by a dark demon entity. At times when this happened they would forget about God and the Light. They would even forget who they were and the knowledge they had. In time, when they somehow remembered God and the Light and prayed for help, they were immediately rescued by angels or beings of the Light. The demons have only as much power as hosts give them.

Sissy, under hypnosis, recalled a past life as a priestess of a nomadic tribe of cave dwellers. There was no food and everybody was starving. She recalled fasting and praying on her knees, asking the goddess to enter her body. Their belief was that when the goddess entered her body, she became the goddess and she could save her people. Instead, she was tricked and was totally possessed by a demon who trapped and consumed her completely inside it. After her death, she was aware only of the darkness around her. But she could see her flame of Light in it. That dark being kept her trapped in it on the earth plane for a long, long time and she could not go to the Light.

I asked her to move ahead in time, when she made her transition to the Light, and to look back from heaven into that life, and tell me what really happened after she died.

From heaven, she looked back in that life and realized that she remained trapped in that dark demon, in the cave, for about 400 years. Although she was aware of her own Light, the soul, she forgot to ask God for help and to rescue her. Finally, a stranger in the cave tumbled over her bones and prayed for her soul to be rescued. As a result, she was rescued by the archangel Gabriel, who took her to heaven, after about 400 years.

From heaven, she realized that she forgot about God and never asked for help, but was rescued by the angel because somebody else prayed for her soul. She understood that she needed to learn the lesson that it is all right to allow your heavenly guides, angels, and helpers to walk with you and guide you, but never allow them to enter you. Every soul has its own purpose, and it is wrong for someone to come into your body. A heavenly being will never enter you, because they know better, but your asking this opens you up for possession and dark beings are always ready to enter you. She did not succeed with her purpose because she went along with the organized religion and did not use her inner spiritual knowledge. She also learned that somebody else's prayers to rescue lost souls are very important, and we should pray daily for the lost souls.

Amir recalled a past life in the jungles of South America when he and his tribe members were trapped by an enemy tribe and eventually died, feeling angry and vengeful. After his death, his spirit was taken to hell by dark beings who offered to help him in taking revenge on the enemy tribe members if he worked for Satan. He agreed to do so. His soul was surrounded, trapped, and consumed by a demon. Then they went and possessed different enemy tribe members, causing them different problems:

- They entered an enemy tribe member, who became so angry and frustrated (almost out of his mind) that he jumped in his canoe and paddled downstream to an enemy cannibal tribe, where he was killed and eaten by them.
- They possessed another enemy tribe member, who became so influenced that he thought that he was invincible. He attempted to fight a huge wildcat, but was immediately destroyed by the cat.
- They possessed and influenced men to fight over women, causing several deaths and severe injuries.
- They possessed and caused a great deal of sickness and death, transmitted via insects, not only to warriors, but also to women and children.
- They caused deaths by possessing and influencing medicine men and women to use poison berries in their medicines.

241

- They possessed and influenced children heavily, causing them to wander into the depths of the jungle, where they were killed.
- They influenced tribe members to attack other tribes, resulting in death and destruction.
- They influenced women to steal other women's possessions—pottery, bone jewelry, etc., resulting in turmoil, fights, and sometimes critical injuries and deaths.
- They possessed a tribe member and influenced him to sleepwalk into crocodile-infested water, where he was immediately destroyed by crocodiles.
- They influenced some tribe members to become so fearful of certain wild animals that on hunting trips they would panic and fall victim to these animals.

After about 220 years, they were inside a person who was sick from a disease that he and the demon had caused. The sick person visited a healer who healed with her healing hands. As God's Light went through the healer's hands to the sick person's body, a part of this Light cracked open the dark demon shell around him just enough to allow a small ray of Light to enter. This act allowed him to remember that he was a lighted being. He went to the Light and the dark demon could not stop him.

Mitch recalled a past life when, after the death of his body, his spirit was trapped, covered, and consumed by a dark demon. Then they entered many people over the years, causing them many problems and diseases, leading to their deaths. Then they entered a man, made him drink, and gave him desire to rape a young girl on the street. As that man tried to force the girl, she prayed to God for help. As a result, a bright Light with many angels in it appeared. The Light penetrated the demon, transforming it into the Light, and rescued his trapped spirit and took both of them to heaven.

The possessed man became confused and upset when he became aware that he was trying to rape the girl. He walked away from her and thus the young girl was saved as a result of her prayers.

Roberto recalled a past life in which, after the death of his body, his spirit was trapped, covered, and consumed by a dark demon spirit. Together they entered many people and caused them a variety of problems. While in a person's body, there was severe thunder and lightning, which cracked open the dark cocoon of the demon around him. His trapped spirit could see the Light and he remembered that he was a being of the Light. He then willed himself to come out of the demon and went to the Light (heaven).

All of these examples prove that even when earthbound spirits are completely trapped, consumed, and controlled by the demon, they still have free will and, through their or someone else's prayers, they can be rescued and helped by God and his angels. Demons have only as much power as we give them; with the help of God and his angels, we can be more powerful than Satan or his demons can be.

According to the hypnotized patients, even when they were completely under the control of Satan and his demons in hell, all they needed to do was ask God for help. Every time, they were instantly rescued from Satan and his hell. They claim God loves everybody unconditionally and does not reject or punish anyone. It is we who judge ourselves and punish ourselves and reject God. Nobody ever has to go to hell to be punished by Satan or his demons, regardless of what we have done in our lives. God gives us free will. God, his angels, and other beings of the Light cannot interfere with our free will. But anytime we ask God and his angels for help, they are instantly there.

Iris, under hypnosis, recalled a past life when she committed suicide. She gave the following account of what happened to her after the death of her physical body:

"I guess I am dead, but I still feel awful. I feel weak and my body hurts. I feel guilty about what I did. It is all dark and cold. I cannot see anything or hear anything. I am falling fast and cannot stop it. I am scared. I do not know what is happening. I feel as if I am being tied up and cannot move. I am cold.

243

"Somebody tells me to come with them and it will be warm. I am in hell. There is a fire and they are going to throw me in it. I am terrified. I scream, '*God help me!*' but I do not think He will help because I was bad. [surprised] I am not trapped anymore, as if I do not have those chains around me. A sunbeam comes like a falling star and there are angels in it, but I cannot move. Angels are reaching out for me and telling me that I can go with them to God, but I believe I was bad and cannot go. They tell me that God is not angry with me. I feel as if something is pulling on me like a piece of taffy, as if I am being pulled between the Light and the dark. Darkness is holding onto me because of my guilt. Angels are telling me to tell the dark one to leave me alone. When I do, the darkness falls away and angels are taking me to heaven. I am afraid that they will kick me out of heaven, but they do not. I feel pure love and healing.

"They take me to see three people who look very wise, like sages. I figure that now I will be in trouble, but they are loving toward me, too. I do not understand. I asked them, "Is this my judgment?" They tell me that they do not judge me and are not angry with me. It was I who was judging myself and was hard on myself. They just feel sad for me about what happened and they love me."

Joy recalled a life as a man who was respected and trusted as a spiritual leader by his people. He wrote a lot of spiritual material, which came to him through inspiration from heaven. He dedicated his whole life to writing spiritual material. At the age of fifty-two, he became sick with a disease. For months he could not digest and hold down food. He prayed for help, but his condition became progressively worse. He died feeling forsaken by God and felt angry at Him. He gave the following account of what happened to him after the death of his body:

"It is dark and cold. I am angry at God and feel abandoned by Him. I do not know where I am. I cannot see or hear anything. I am being pulled and dragged down. It is as if somebody has strings tied to me and pulling me down with it. They took me to this place that is dark and cold. It must be hell. It feels like I was there for a long time. I feel angry and forsaken.

"The demons take me to the fire. They look like black amorphous things. I am supposed to talk to somebody else. He is awful looking. His face is contorted and ugly. His eyes have fire in them. He is Satan. He is telling me that I belong to him and I must do as he says or he will throw me in the fire. It feels as though Satan cannot reach me. He is trying to fast-talk me, but something in my memory does not believe him.

"It is like I have my own little fire but it does not burn and it has its own memory, and I started to think about it. I feel there is something else besides 'bad.' It is almost like realization, and I start to remember God and the different spiritual things I wrote. I see a distant Light above me. It looks like it is coming for me. I realize that God has not forsaken me. As the Light comes closer, Satan gets nervous. He is threatening me. The closer the Light gets, the faster he talks. I begin to remember the song 'The Lord Is My Shepherd' and the minute I say it out loud Satan disappears.

"Light wraps me and takes me up, and I realize that I was not forsaken. Gates open and the angels and music come pouring out. It's the most magnificent sound I have ever heard. We move in. It is like a long procession of angels. The further we go, the brighter it gets. Now we all stop and I realize that I cannot look up because it is so bright.

"I feel I am in the presence of something awfully big, but I cannot look at it. It is God. He tells me that I was not forsaken, that every trial has a purpose and it helps us to grow spiritually. If we keep our faith and trust in Him, we can succeed and evolve spiritually. During my death, I denied and rejected him, but He did not reject me. He does not forsake us. Our anger does not faze Him. He loves us just the same. He tells me that while on earth we cannot be completely protected, no matter who we are. We have to have faith in Him and remember to ask for help. Our faith in Him preserves and shields our Light.

"He tells me I was chosen to be His voice and to write, and I have done well, but I am not finished yet. I will do it many times in future lives."

Interference by Satan and His Demons and Earthbound Entities Who Work for Satan and Have Demonic Influence

An overwhelming number of earthbound spirits claim that they did not go to heaven because they were interfered with, tricked, and stopped from going to the Light by Satan, his demons, and earthbound spirits who were working for Satan. The following are the accounts of different earthbound spirits.

Martha, an earthbound entity in my patient, remembered dying a long time ago and had no idea where to go. She wandered into a church, where the priest was praying for help for all the lost souls. She saw a column of bright Light and angels in it coming to her asking her to come with them. As she was ascending in the Light, a black hand grabbed her and pulled her away. She found herself in the darkness, where she was told to go to my patient and cause her problems.

James, who drowned, said, "After my death, I saw many dark-looking human spirits, who came to me and told me that I should not go to the Light. If I went to the Light, then I would really die. This way I could live on earth forever."

Alex, who died in a car accident, said, "I was confused. I saw the Light, but a dark-looking white man told me not to go to the Light because I would get burned. Then some dark beings told me how to possess people so I could live again. I did what I was told because I wanted to live again."

Bob said, "After my death I saw the beautiful Light, but Satan stopped me from going into it. He told me if I went to the Light I would definitely die. He told me that he would give me eternal life if I worked for him. Then he told me to come here with this person and cause him problems."

Lisa said, "I was raped and killed. After my death I was taken on a cloud. I thought I was going to the Light, but there was no Light there. I was tricked. People in gray clothes were dancing. We were just floating on the clouds. Then somebody pushed me down and somehow I ended up with this person."

Jim had a female entity who died of throat cancer and starvation. After her death she felt confused because she did not feel dead and did not know what to do. She saw beings on the cloud with brown gowns and mean eyes. They told her that she could go back to the earth and live again without pain and hunger, then told her to go inside Jim to live and eat through him again.

Julia recalled a past life in which she was unfaithful and promiscuous. After she died, according to her Catholic upbringing, she expected to go to hell and be punished because of how she lived her life. After her death, she saw Satan, who told her that she was bad and she had to come with him to hell. She was rescued by Jesus when she asked for help. Later, when she went to heaven, Jesus told her, "You should have prayed to God for help. Nobody needs to be punished in hell, no matter what they did. God is a loving and forgiving God and he does not punish anybody."

Influence through Missing Soul Parts

Sometimes, earthbound spirits claim that the dark beings prevented them from going to heaven by pulling down on their missing soul parts and their connecting cords, which they lost during different traumas. They also sent demon spirits in them through these missing soul parts and their connecting cords, who in turn blocked them from perceiving the Light and thus did not let them go to heaven.

Maya, an earthbound spirit in my patient, claimed that after the death of her physical body she saw the Light and knew that she was supposed to be in it, but could not go to it. She felt as if she had chains tied on her legs and was being pulled down and taken to the darkness. Then she was told by the dark beings to go to my patient and cause problems for him.

During the therapy, she saw that, due to the traumas in her life, she lost many soul parts, which were in possession of demons in hell. Through these missing soul parts and their connecting cords, they pulled Maya down to hell and prevented her from going to heaven.

Categories of Earthbound Spirits (Entities)

Over the years, different possessing human entities, through my hypnotized patients, have given many reasons for why they remain in the physical world after the death of their physical bodies, why they did not go to heaven, and why they were attracted toward my patients.

As I reflect on what my patients have said repeatedly under hypnosis, I find that these earthbound entities can be logically organized into the following nine categories. This list is based on a continuum ranging from entities that go to the Light easily, entities that have moderate problems, and entities that have serious problems in making the transition to the Light.

1. Those who die with a good deal of knowledge of the true nature of the universe expect to go back to heaven and expect reincarnation.
2. Those who expect an afterlife and God, but have no knowledge that they need to go back to heaven and do not expect reincarnation.
3. Those who lack the knowledge of heaven, afterlife, and reincarnation and have fewer emotions and less confusion and demonic influence.
4. Those who die with very strong emotions, mild confusion, and mild demonic influence.
5. Those who die with severe confusion, moderate demonic influence, and mild emotions.
6. Those who die with severe demonic influence, moderate confusion, and fewer emotions.
7. Those who have severe demonic influence and consciously hate God and deny and reject the Light, but do not voluntarily seek evil.
8. Those who have severe demonic influence, who not only hate God and reject the Light, but also consciously and actively seek and desire to do evil.

9. Those who are completely trapped inside a demon and are totally covered, consumed, and influenced by it.

In the first three categories, earthbound spirits have minimum demonic influence, confusion, and negative emotions, and only occasionally remain earthbound and possess somebody.

Category 1: This is the most normal and the most desired situation. Very few in this category remain earthbound and possess somebody. Here the entities have a good deal of knowledge of the true nature of the universe. They expect to go back to heaven and await reincarnation. They have minimum demonic influence, confusion, or negative emotions. They expect death to be an unpleasant experience, but feel they can survive it. They know that death is not to be feared and have an emotional acceptance of it. After the death of the physical body, these entities, within a very short period of time, look for heaven and go to the Light without any problems or interference.

These entities do not possess anybody except in very limited circumstances where it has been predetermined that this should happen in the hope of accomplishing some good.

These entities may have demonic influence, but their knowledge does not allow demons to stop them from moving into the Light. They can simply turn to the Light and say, "That is where I want and need to be, and the demons cannot stop me." As these entities go into the Light, any demons they have fall out of them.

Category 2: In this group are those who have a religious acceptance of the nature of death and who await an afterlife. But they do not expect to go back to the Light and do not have the knowledge of reincarnation. After the death of the physical body, they remain confused for a short period of time because things are not exactly the way they expected. But in a short period of time, they locate the Light and go back to heaven. They may have demonic influence, but they do not permit the demons to stop them from going to the Light. Chances of this group doing any possessing are rare, almost accidental. The person possessed is usually a loved one.

Category 3: Here entities do not expect an afterlife, heaven, or reincarnation. They are aware of the Light in most cases, but simply lack the knowledge or the feelings that they need to move on into the Light. When they die they become slightly confused because they feel that they are still alive. After a while they get used to the idea that their physical body is dead, that they continue to survive and it is time to look for the Light and go into it. Some from this group may become a possessing entity. They may try to live out their existence in a body, as they are accustomed to. But the chances of these entities possessing somebody are still much smaller than in the next six categories.

Category 4: This group includes people who die in the grip of strong emotions such as love, fear, anger, hate, jealousy, desire to take revenge, and desire for drugs, alcohol, food, sex, and power. They stay earthbound. They deny themselves the return to the Light. They may include any of the three preceding groups. Even the most spiritually developed person who dies in the grip of these strong emotions can end up in this category.

What happens to these entities depends on which emotion is keeping them in the physical world. They usually end up possessing somebody, depending on their emotions.

Category 5: After the death of their physical body, these entities feel terribly confused and upset. They do not understand why they are separate from their body. They are very confused about their bodies being buried or disposed of. They are lonely and desperately trying to communicate with people, but nobody sees or hears them. They cannot understand why there is no communication. They feel as real as can be. They cannot conceive that they have become a spirit. They wander around funeral homes and other places.

They do not know what to do or where to go. They see the Light, but do not perceive it because of the demonic influence. Many are so confused and influenced that they do not realize that their bodies are dead. Many of them appear as what we call ghosts. Sometimes they are perceived as ghosts and sometimes they are not because their emotions fluctuate rapidly, and they have no control over themselves.

These entities sometimes go to a human host. Other times they go to an object, such as a home, an automobile, or a piece of furniture. They are emotionally attached to the object, not physically. ("This is my car, my home, my room, my bed and I am safe here.") They stay there while they try to figure out what is going on. They are in great need of love, comfort, compassion, attention, and communication. When this entity finds anybody with compassion and open boundaries, it can move right inside the person.

The entity is like a person who is freezing. When it gets close to somebody who is warm like a fireplace, it just has to get close and it will gravitate directly toward the fireplace, the soul. Entities are not aware that they are doing any damage to the host. From the entity's point of view it is just seeking a warm, comforting place.

They try desperately to make contact with their hosts and that is where the damage to the hosts comes in. The hosts start to hear voices and experience the entities' emotional and physical feelings. They also have dreams about the entities' death and their traumatic experiences. Again, as far as the entities are concerned, they are just sitting by a warm fireplace. They are focused on the Light of the host, which is the soul.

Category 6: Here the entities are more thoroughly possessed by the demons. They have strong confusion and are less affected by their emotions. The demons manipulate and confuse the entities. The demons in them are afraid of the Light, so they keep the earthbound entities from going to the Light.

Category 7: These entities have severe demonic influence as described in category six, but they also make a conscious decision to hate God and deny and reject the Light. They have a grudge against God. These are the entities who blame God for the things that happened to them in their current life or a carryover from past lives. They may also feel guilty about something they have done wrong and are afraid that God will punish and reject them. So they decide to reject God before he rejects them. They choose on their own to remain earthbound. They may remain on their own for a long time without possessing somebody.

In their bitterness, they may try to possess somebody who is religious or spiritual and accepts God. They are there to cause problems for their hosts. The initial attack on their hosts is on the spiritual side, trying to interfere with their spiritual practices and trying to block them from the Light. As these entities become more and more upset, they will affect their hosts emotionally and physically.

What seemed like a good idea in the beginning may turn out to be an intolerable situation for these possessing entities. They cannot stand to be that close to the spiritually developed hosts. The love, the understanding, the prayers, and the Light that floods through the spiritual hosts are also absorbed by these possessing entities and they begin to heal. The spiritual nature of the hosts also helps to diminish the demonic influences in the possessing entities because the demons cannot stand their Light.

Category 8: These entities consciously reject God and the Light. They also actively seek that which is evil, negative, and destructive. These are the people who seek power, money, and evil ways to control and hurt others. They adopt evil as a part of their lives.

All types of evil people can be included in this category, including sadomasochists, rapists, murderers, and others. It is their natural personality, plus demonic influence, that pushes them toward evil. After the death of their physical bodies, they choose not to go to heaven. Instead they possess others, who in turn may begin to adopt the entities' evil ways.

Category 9: These earthbound entities are totally sur-rounded, trapped, and consumed inside a demon. They are totally controlled by the demons. They have lost all contact with the Light, sometimes even the memories of the Light. They are unable to think clearly or act on their own and are confused. Sometimes they do not even remember that they are human. They think they are the demon.

This is a more dangerous combination for the host than possession by just a demon or an earthbound entity alone. If the demon alone enters a host, it has less effect than a demon with an earthbound entity trapped inside. The demon uses the earth-bound entity inside it as a tool to get to the host. The trapped entity has no say as to who gets possessed, how long they stay, and when they leave. It is simply going along for the ride.

These entities fail to realize that they can be free of the demons. They reject Light and the knowledge that they have power over the demons. If at any time the trapped earthbound entity says that it wants to be free and wants to go to the Light and prays and asks God for rescue, it can be instantly free.

Treatment of Earthbound Spirits (Entities)

Treatment of earthbound entities depends on which category they represent. They all need to understand, however, that their body is dead. They are in somebody else's body and they are hurting themselves and their host by being there. They need to go to heaven, where they can rest and heal.

Categories 1, 2, and 3: Entities who belong to categories 1, 2, and 3, those who have a great deal of knowledge and who expect reincarnation or at least an afterlife, are easy to treat. These are the ones who are just a little bit confused and in whom there is little demonic influence. If any of them should end up in a human host, which is possible, all that is necessary is to direct them into the Light. They do not need any extensive treatment.

Those in categories 4, 5, and 6 are the most common types of entities that I find possessing my patients.

Category 4: Here the possessing entities have very strong emotions, less confusion, and less demonic influence. They die in the grip of strong emotions. We have to help the possessing entities deal with their emotions. Psychotherapy with these entities works successfully. After their emotions and feelings are processed and resolved, it is important to help them understand where they are and that they need to go to the Light. Then they are sent to heaven with a Light being.

Category 5: Here the possessing human entities are extremely confused and have moderate demonic influence and mild emotions. They most often appear as ghosts because they just do not know what they are doing and fluctuate back and forth rapidly. These entities also have to be helped extensively before they can understand where they are to go. Treatment is like doing psychotherapy with the spirits. They have to understand that their body is dead, that they are miserable, and there is a place where they belong. Then they are sent to heaven with a Light being.

Category 6: These entities have strong demonic influence, more confusion and fewer emotions. First, we need to deal with the demons who are inside them. Once the demons are released, a good deal of the confusion will dissipate. Their emotional level will stabilize, so that it will be easy to educate them about their condition and help them to heaven.

Category 7: These entities have rejected God, often out of strong anger, guilt, or fear. They feel that God will reject them for what they have done; therefore they choose to reject him first. They are often afraid that they will be sent to hell.

Again, the first step is to free them from all the demonic influences, dissipating most of their confusion. Then we need to deal with their emotional problems through psychotherapy. We need to help them to understand that everybody needs to go to heaven; there is no judgment or punishment and everybody is accepted with love. They need to understand that God is a kind and loving God and he does not reject or punish anybody.

If they still refuse to believe and do not want to go to the Light, I usually ask them to call out anybody from heaven whom they trust and ask them how it is up there. Usually the Light beings are able to convince them and take them to heaven.

Category 8: These entities hate and reject God because of what happened to them in their life. They willingly choose to work for Satan, sometimes making a pact with Satan.

Again, in therapy, the first thing we need to do is to work with the dark entities who are inside them and who are confusing and feeding them negative thoughts, guilt, anger, and fear. After the release of the demon entities, much of their confusion and anger will disappear. Then we need to work with their emotional problems and resolve them. We need to help them to understand that it is not God who caused their problems, but that they themselves, with the help of demons, have caused their own problems.

If they still are not sure and are afraid of going to the Light because of the fear of punishment by God, I ask them to call out anybody they trust from heaven who can help them. The Light beings they call are often able to explain the truth to them and help them to heaven.

Category 9: These Earthbound entities are completely trapped, surrounded, and consumed inside the demon. They have lost all contact with the outside world and with the Light, even with the memories of the Light and who they are. They are unable to think clearly. They fail to realize their power, that they can be free of the demon anytime they choose to ask God for help. They reject God and reject the knowledge that they have power over demons.

We first need to free them from the demon who is wrapped around them and trapping them in. These earthbound entities have to be educated about their condition, that they are trapped inside the demon and that they do not need to be there. They can take charge anytime and step out of the demon and the demon cannot do a thing about it.

Often, in the beginning, they appear to the patients only as black demonic blobs and the patients cannot see the human entities inside. Only after the demon entities are transformed into the Light can the patients see the human entities inside.

After they are freed from the demons, they are then helped with their emotions. Any unresolved emotions and issues are dealt with, then they are sent to heaven.

To release the earthbound entities from the patients, we do not need to do extensive therapy with the entities and resolve all their problems. We just need to give them enough understanding so that they can be released to heaven, where they can rest and heal.

Degrees or Extent of Possession by Earthbound Spirits

According to my patients, earthbound entities cannot take total control of the patient's mind, body, and soul. They can only be the guest entities inside the patient's body. When the human will is weakened, when the human mind is stupefied, as in cases of drug and alcohol abuse and other physical and emotional conditions, it is easier for the possessing earthbound entities to take partial control of that person's functioning for a short period of time.

A good example of partial control can be seen when people, after a few drinks, sometimes even after one or two drinks, change completely. There is a dramatic change in their person-alities, in what they say, and how they act. These people often have amnesia for that time period. It is not a total possession. In this case the host still has his or her own will, still has perception, and can exert influence on his or her own body. It is as though the main personality or the main part of the soul, which is the condensed part of the soul inside the body, withdraws into a room and closes the door behind. Then the strongest of the possessing earthbound entities takes over and motivates the body.

The main condensed part of our soul is in the chest, head, or neck. The soul is also present throughout the body, maintaining the functioning identity. So even though the central, condensed, main part of the soul has its eyes closed and another possessing earthbound spirit takes over and controls the body for a short period, that spirit cannot have full control. The soul is all over the body too, and is still acting as that person, even though there is somebody else giving the commands.

Factors upon Which the Effects of Possessing Earthbound Spirits (Entities) Depend

The effects of possession by earthbound entities depend on several factors.

Age when possessed: If the patient is possessed by earthbound entities in the womb or after birth and during childhood, it is very hard to differentiate the personalities and problems of the possessing spirits from the host. The host accepts these problems and personality traits as his or her own.

If possession occurred during adulthood, the before-and-after changes are more pronounced. In these cases, patients describe the changes as, not feeling the same since the accident or surgery.

Strength of a person: If persons are physically and emotionally strong, the possessing human spirits can exert very little influence on their hosts. In these cases, people are not even aware of any problems or possessions, although they may have one or more entities on board with them.

Any time the host is going through a physical illness, surgery, emotional trauma, sudden shock or unconsciousness, drug and alcohol use, or an accident, that person is weakened. The entities who were dormant inside the host suddenly become active, experiencing

257

their own physical and emotional traumas. Then the host starts to experience different emotional, mental, and physical problems.

At the same time, new entities can also come in because of the weakened energy field of the host, and the host starts to experience different emotional, physical, and mental problems.

Number of possessing entities: The higher the number of possessing entities, the wider the range of emotional, physical, and mental problems. Most often there is transfer of control back and forth between the host and the spirits. Also, possessing entities weaken patients' energy field or aura, leaving them open for more entities to come in.

Demonic infestation of possessing earthbound entities: If the possessing earthbound entities are infested and influenced by demon entities, the symptoms experienced by the possessing entities are more intense and severe, and the intensity and severity are transferred to their hosts.

Mechanism of Symptom Formation Due to Possession by Earthbound Spirits (Entities)

According to my patients, earthbound entities affect every aspect of their life—physically, mentally, and emotionally. They state that sometimes earthbound entities overlap and cover the body of the host completely, that is, legs upon legs, arms upon arms, body upon body, and head upon head.

The feelings, thoughts, emotions, and memories of the spirit are transferred over to the host and the host begins to experience them. They are incorporated by the host as his or her own symptoms. This transfer can be terribly confusing and damaging for the host. The possessing spirits are pretty miserable too because they are still feeling those painful experiences, in what they think are their own bodies, as if they are frozen in time.

If the possessing earthbound entities have demonic influence in them, then they create even more problems for their hosts and all the symptoms are intensified. The demon who is inside the possessing earthbound entity then finds itself with two humans to play with. It continues to torment the possessing earthbound entity and that torment is carried over to the human host. This demon also attacks the host directly.

Sometimes a human entity is totally surrounded, trapped, and consumed by a demon that totally controls the human entity. The patient can see only the demon blob in one or other parts of the body and not only experiences the symptoms of the trapped human entity, but also the symptoms caused by the demon entity.

The host can experience the possessing spirit's symptoms in different ways. The following are some examples of how physical and emotional symptoms can be transferred from a possessing earthbound entity to its human host.

1. If the possessing spirit died of a **gunshot wound** in the stomach, the patient can have a whole host of physical and emotional symptoms, such as discomfort or tightness or a knot in the stomach, nervous stomach, abdominal pain, nausea, vomiting, diarrhea, constipation, hyperacidity, gastritis, esophagitis, ulcer, or irritable bowel.

2. If a possessing spirit had **broken bones or crushed body parts**, it can manifest in the host as arthritis, fibromyositis, tendinitis, carpel tunnel syndrome, nerve irritability, aches and pain, numbness, tingling, or just an annoying discomfort in that part of the body.

3. If the possessing spirit died in a **fire**, the host can have skin conditions including sensitive or dry skin, acne, blisters, hives, red blotches, erythema, eczema, psoriasis, and different types of rashes. The host may also have asthma, laryngitis, or other types of lung conditions if there was smoke inhalation. The host can

also have symptoms of gastritis, colitis, burning feelings all over the body, hot flashes, intolerance of hot weather, and irrational fear of fire.

4. If the possessing spirit died of a **heart attack**, the host can have chest pains, shortness of breath, palpitation, dizziness, tightness in the chest, panic attacks, and irrational fear of heart attack and death.

5. If a possessing entity died of **hanging or choking or any type of injury to the neck and throat**, the host can experience irritability of the throat, pain in the throat, difficulty in swallowing, throat infections, thyroid problems, laryngitis, voice shutting down or changing, asthma, headaches, neck and shoulder pain, dizziness, and pain in the eyeballs. Sometimes the host also cannot wear anything close to the neck, and cannot button a collar.

6. If the possessing entity died of **old age**, the host can experience memory problems and feelings of having Alzheimer's disease. The host may feel older than his or her age, and may have all the signs and symptoms of old age, such as weakness, tiredness, lack of energy, eyesight changes, and other physical and emotional problems of the entity.

7. If a possessing spirit died of a **stroke and paralysis**, the host will experience weakness or even temporary paralysis of that part of the body, dizziness, fainting spells, aches and pains, speech problems, wobbly gait, and other problems the spirit has.

8. If the entity was depressed and **committed suicide by** taking an **overdose of sleeping pills**, the host can experience anxiety, depression, and suicidal thoughts, although he or she has no apparent reasons to feel that way. The host may also feel sleepy, lethargic, and weak and have a staggering gait, all because of the overdose of sleeping pills by the entity. The host can also have stomach problems.

If the possessing spirit **committed suicide by taking an overdose of amphetamines**, the host can experience depression, suicidal thoughts, racing thoughts, anger outbursts, hyperactivity, hypervigilance, restlessness, irritability, insomnia for days, paranoid ideations, impaired judgment, and hallucinations. The host can also experience other effects of the amphetamines, such as high blood pressure, tachycardia, headaches, skin rash, nausea, vomiting, and weight loss.

In most of these cases, physical examinations and tests are negative. When the immune system of the possessing entity is affected, it will also weaken the immune system of the host.

Symptoms Caused by the Earthbound Spirits (Entities)

Symptoms caused by possessing earthbound entities range from negligible to multiple. They can affect every part and organ of the host's body, from head to toe. They can be physical, emotional, and mental. Most of the time the hosts are not even aware of having any earthbound entities with them, and whatever symptoms they have due to possessing entities, the hosts attribute to themselves.

Physical Symptoms

Some of the physical symptoms caused by earthbound spirits in my patients are migraine headaches, dizziness, fainting spells, convulsions, hearing problems, ringing in the ears, vision changes, neck and shoulder pain, back pain, arthritis, chest pain, shortness of breath, asthma, palpitations, throat pain, difficulty in swallowing, nausea, vomiting, diarrhea, constipation, gastritis, esophageal ulcers, colitis, abdominal pain, obesity, anorexia, PMS, hot flashes, aches and pains in different parts of the body, different skin conditions, neuritis, numbness, weakness, tingling, chronic fatigue, allergies, etc.

X-rays and laboratory tests for these physical symptoms caused by the earthbound spirits are often negative, but patients' suffering is real and not their imagination.

John, a forty-year-old man, had intermittent chest pain for several months. About three months before he came to me, he was taken to the emergency room with chest pains. His EKG and other tests were normal. Heart catheterization also showed normal functioning. He also had panic attacks and depression.

During the session, under hypnosis, he found the spirit of a nineteen-year-old man inside. He was killed by being stabbed in the chest with a knife. After the spirit joined him, John started to feel the spirit's chest pain, panic attacks, and depression. After releasing the spirit, John was relieved of all his symptoms.

Jay was diagnosed as having an irritable bowel and had bloating, diarrhea, constipation, and cramping for several years. He had to take Bentyl and Lomotil for it. Under hypnosis, he found the spirit of a man who had died of colon cancer several years before. After his death, his spirit joined Jay, then Jay began to experience his symptoms. After releasing the spirit, Jay was free of his symptoms and they have not returned.

Tamara complained of feeling hot all the time. She found a spirit of a little boy who died of measles. He had a high fever when he died. After releasing the spirit of the little boy, Tamara was completely relieved of the hot feeling.

Jerry had severe headaches, stiffness, and pain in his neck, back, and shoulders, and aches and pains all over his body for several years. He had an entity who died in a car accident, injuring different parts of his body, including his head, neck, and back. After releasing the entity, Jerry's headaches, neck and back pain, and generalized aches and pains were completely relieved.

Dana was a thirty-year-old female from whom we released many dark and human entities. During one session, Dana felt tired, drained, and weak. She described feeling as if somebody had drained all her blood and looked like that, too, pale and weak. Under hypnosis, she found a spirit of a man who bled to death in a war and joined Dana two days before. After releasing that spirit, she felt more energetic right away.

Amanda, a forty-year-old female, suffered from multiple allergies for about four years. She was allergic to corn, wheat, beef, chicken, cabbage, carrots, apples, yeast, barley, beans, dairy products, orange juice, bananas, and more. She had panic attacks during which she felt jittery all over, and she had palpitations and shortness of breath, mostly after certain foods. She also had a difficult time swallowing.

Under hypnosis, she found an entity who had died of throat cancer. He said that he was allergic to all the foods and chemicals that Amanda had problems with and that he also had difficulty in swallowing. He also claimed to affect Amanda's immune system. After releasing him, her allergies, difficulty in swallowing, and panic attacks were improved a great deal.

Justin, a forty-year-old male, was diagnosed by his doctors as having fibromyositis. He had painful hip, knee, ankle, shoulder, elbow, and wrist joints. All his joints would become more painful and stiff under stress. Under hypnosis, he found the spirit of a seventy-year-old man who had severe arthritis in all his joints. After his death, he joined Justin, and Justin began to experience all the symptoms of the spirit, which were relieved after releasing the entity.

Daisy had convulsions every time a new spirit entered her. They were not typical epileptic convulsions.

Mona, a forty-five-year-old female, was admitted to the hospital for depression. The second day after her admission, she began to experience slurred speech, wobbly gait, and confusion. She was not on sleeping pills, pain pills, or tranquilizers, so the symptoms were not due to withdrawal reactions. She was examined by a neurologist, who did a CT scan and other tests and could not find anything wrong with her. Mona had in her the spirit of a woman who died of a stroke at the hospital. Being in the hospital stimulated the spirit's memory of the stroke and its symptoms, and Mona began to experience them. After she released the spirit, Mona's symptoms were relieved.

Scott, a forty-eight-year-old man, had severe migraine head-aches since he was a child. During these headaches he had throbbing pain on one or both sides of his head and eyes. He also had severe pain and stiffness in the back of his head and neck. Any physical activity aggravated his headaches. At times he got sick and threw up. He was intolerant to heat and his headaches got worse during hot and humid weather. Under hypnosis, he saw a young boy who had died of severe meningitis with stiff neck, headaches, nausea, vomiting, and high fever. Scott's head-aches and all the other symptoms were completely relieved after releasing the spirit of the young boy.

Dave, a thirty-year-old man, had severe sensitivity to sun expo-sure. He had severe rashes when exposed to the sun and could not tolerate hot weather. He also had an irrational fear of fire.

During the session, he found many human spirits who had died by being burned in fires and who were still experiencing the feelings of being burned. They were the ones who felt hot and were sensitive to sun and had skin problems. These symptoms were transferred to Dave, who in turn started to experience those prob-lems. After he released those entities, his symptoms were relieved.

Alex, a thirty-five-year-old man, experienced panic attacks with chest pains, difficulty in breathing, palpitations, and the fear of having a heart attack and dying. All his tests were negative. These problems started after his father died of a sudden heart attack. During a session, under hypnosis, he found in him his father, who was still confused about what had happened to him and was still feeling all his symptoms. After releasing his father to the Light, Alex was completely free of his symptoms.

Brad had suffered chronic laryngitis for a long time. Some-times his voice would shut off. He had two spirits in him who were responsible for his symptoms. One was a seventy-six-year-old female who had a stroke and was not able to speak because of paralysis. The second entity was strangled to death. After releasing these entities, Brad was relieved of his laryngitis.

Tim was a thirty-year-old white male who had a sore throat and bronchitis for about two and a half months before he came to me. He continued to have chest pain, cough, chronic fatigue, and sore throat. He had anxiety attacks off and on. He was not able to completely recover from bronchitis.

His doctor did a chest x-ray, EKG, thyroid test, blood tests including his blood sugar; all were within normal limits. His doctor could not understand why he was not recovering. He could not find any reason for his physical symptoms and referred him to me.

Under hypnosis, he found within him many spirits who had died of some type of lung problems such as pneumonia, asthma, tuberculosis, bronchitis, and lung cancer.

After he released these spirits, Tim's symptoms were relieved and he was able to function better. All of these spirits said that they had been with Tim for a long time, since he was young. But since Tim was strong physically and emotionally, they could not affect him much until he had bronchitis. Tim's bronchitis stirred up and stimulated the memories and feelings of these spirits about their lung problems, which continued and kept him feeling sick, even though Tim's bronchitis was cured.

Psychological Symptoms

Almost any type of psychological problems can be caused by earthbound entities.

Depression: Depression and its associated symptoms, such as chronic fatigue, difficulty in sleeping or sleeping too much, and poor concentration and memory, are the most common symptoms caused by earthbound entities.

These possessing entities do not have their own physical bodies. They use and drain their hosts' energy, causing chronic fatigue. Patients often complain about having no energy. They say things like "I feel like I am a walking dead person," "I literally have to drag myself out of bed," "I am always dragging myself," "Everything is an effort for me," etc.

If the possessing human entity died of old age, the patient will complain about feeling old, depressed, tired, and sleepy, having aches and pains, vision problems, confusion, and other problems.

If earthbound entities were depressed before the death of their bodies because of the emotional, physical, or situational conditions, it is transferred to their hosts, the patients.

While the patients are trying to sleep, the possessing earthbound spirits are constantly thinking and feeling their emotional and physical symptoms, and thus keeping the patients awake. If the possessing spirits died in a drugged state, sedated or under anesthesia, they can cause their host to sleep excessively.

Recurrent dreams and nightmares: Repetitive dreams and nightmares often turn out to be due to the possessing earthbound entities. These entities are still suffering from the memories of their traumas, which their hosts, the patients, in turn experience in their dreams and nightmares.

Neela, a forty-year-old female, had had severe abdominal cramps since she was a little girl. These cramps were so bad that labor pains during her deliveries did not seem all that bad. She also had had a repetitive dream since age eight about being pregnant and giving birth.

When she looked inside, under hypnosis, she found the spirit of a woman who died during childbirth and joined Neela when Neela was eight. After she released her, Neela's longstanding, severe abdominal cramps were relieved and she did not have the dreams of being pregnant and giving birth anymore.

Fran lost her brother in a car accident. After his death, she started to have repetitive dreams and nightmares about how the accident happened, although she was not present when it occurred. She also had vivid flashbacks and visions of the accident. She started to smoke the same brand of cigarettes and had cravings for foods that her brother liked. She was very depressed and had difficulty sleeping.

Under hypnosis, she saw her brother's spirit inside her. It was her brother who was having the memories of his accident, which Fran experienced in her dreams and visions. After she released him to the Light, most of her symptoms were relieved.

Poor concentration and memory: These are the other most common symptoms caused by possessing earthbound entities. Under normal conditions, it is not unusual to have trouble remembering the day-to-day events of our lives. Imagine having two, three, ten, or more other people inside one body thinking and remembering all their own life events at one time. As a result of such a situation, patients have thoughts and memories that are foreign to them. They usually describe having difficulty in concentration and therefore in memory, because everybody is thinking at the same time. The patients have those intruding thoughts in their minds, causing difficulty in focusing and concentrating on what they are doing. Their descriptions: "I used to have a memory like a computer; now I feel like I have Alzheimer's disease." "I have gaps in my memory." "I feel spacey." "My memory is so bad that people call me a space-head or scatterbrain."

Suicidal thoughts and preoccupations: Suicidal thoughts and preoccupations can also be caused by possessing entities who were depressed and suicidal or who committed suicide. After the death of their bodies, they continue to feel depressed, hopeless, helpless, and suicidal. These thoughts and feelings are transferred to the hosts, who start to feel depressed and suicidal. Releasing these spirits usually frees the patients from their long-standing depression and suicidal feelings. Sometimes relief occurs in just a couple of hypnotherapy sessions.

Ben, a forty-five-year-old man, had depression, suicidal thoughts, panic attacks, and pain in his head, neck and, shoulders. He tried physical therapy, Tenz unit, and cortisone shots without much relief.

During a session, under hypnosis, he saw inside a male spirit who claimed that he committed suicide by hanging himself because he was severely depressed. His depression, suicidal thoughts, headaches, and neck and shoulder pain due to hanging were transferred over to Ben after his spirit attached to him. After he released the spirit, Ben's symptoms were improved.

Panic attack: It is the third most common symptom caused by the possessing earthbound entities. It is manifested by a

267

sudden onset of intense apprehension, fear, or terror, often associated with feelings of impending doom, fear of losing control, a fear of dying or of going crazy. These feelings are often accompanied by physical symptoms such as dyspnea, palpitations, chest pain or discomfort, choking, dizziness, feelings of unreality, numbness, hot or cold feelings, sweating, and shaking. These attacks last anywhere from a minute to hours. Although the patients know that these fears and feelings are irrational, they cannot stop them.

Often in these cases, patients under hypnosis find that these feelings and symptoms are not their own, but belong to the possessing spirits. The spirits are reliving their traumatic experiences over and over as if they are freeze-framed or locked in time. These panic attacks are hard to cure with traditional therapy, and even with medications, because they are not the patients' symptoms to begin with. Releasing these possessing spirits from the patient often relieves the panic attacks.

Candy suffered from depression and a fear of men and was afraid of dying. She also had severe panic attacks, during which she felt sick, could not breathe, was weak all over, and felt like something drastic was going to happen and she was going to die. Under hypnosis, she found that she had the spirit of a ten-year-old girl who remembered being raped, brutally tortured, and killed.

After she released the little girl, Candy's panic attacks, depression, fear of men, and fear of dying were relieved in just one session. She was able to sleep and eat better.

Fears and phobias: Phobias are also often caused by the possessing earthbound spirits. It is the spirits' traumatic death experiences that are transferred over to the patients. If an entity died of drowning, the host will start to feel the fear of water. If the entity died in a car accident, the host will start to feel the fear of driving a car. If an entity died of a sudden heart attack, the host will begin to have an irrational fear of heart attack and dying.

Dexter, a thirty-two-year-old man, had a fear of driving, a fear of bridges, panic attacks while driving, depression, and suicidal preoccupation. He was treated periodically with medication and talk therapy with some improvement, but the symptoms returned.

During a session under hypnosis, he found the spirit of a man who had committed suicide by driving his car off a bridge. After he released that entity, Dexter's fear of driving, fear of bridges, panic attacks, depression, and suicidal thoughts were completely relieved.

Callie had a fear of fire and a fear of a furnace blowing up and could not watch concentration camp movies. She had a spirit of an eighteen-year-old man who was killed in an oven in a concentration camp. He joined Callie when she was a baby. After releasing the spirit, Callie was free of her fears.

Nina had a fear of water and had dreams about drowning. Under hypnosis, she found the spirit of a man who had drowned in a boating accident. After she released the spirit to the Light, Nina's fear of water was relieved and she no longer had the dream of drowning.

Sexual problems: Some patients have reported possession by an older entity, which caused lowered sexual desire in them. In older persons, possession by a young adult can cause increased sexual desire.

Russell, a sixty-five-year-old man, began to have frequent, uncontrollable, sexual urges for about three months. Sometimes, he had an erection even when he was not thinking of sex. Under hypnosis, he found a spirit of a young man, who was eighteen years old and joined Russell about three months ago. He bragged about giving uncontrollable, sexual urges to Russell. After releasing the spirit of that young man, Russell was relieved of his symptoms.

Homosexuality: In some of my patients, possession by an entity of the opposite sex has caused confusion in their sexual identity, especially when the possession occurred before puberty. A female spirit in a man may desire sex with a man, and this desire and attraction may in turn become the desire of the male host toward another male. The host may think he is a homosexual, when in fact he is only acting on the spirit's desire.

Transsexualism: A possession by an entity of the opposite sex, who is unhappy being stuck in a wrong body, may push the host to have a sex-change operation.

Gail had a strong urge to chew tobacco, wear men's clothes, and have a sex-change operation. Under hypnosis, she found the spirit of a man who was very uncomfortable being in a female body and admitted giving Gail the strong urges to have a sex-change operation. Her urges were relieved after releasing the entity.

Transvestitism: An entity of the opposite sex can force the host to wear clothes of the opposite sex.

Mood swings: Mood swings, racing thoughts, and other symptoms of manic depression can be caused by possessing earthbound spirits. Having many spirits of different people, who are experiencing different emotions, thoughts, and feelings all at the same time, can cause the host to switch back and forth between different moods, emotions, and feelings that cannot be explained.

This gives the patients constant racing thoughts. The patients have thoughts and feelings that do not make sense and they do not seem to have any control over them. Because of these constant racing thoughts, these patients often have difficulty sleeping. Patients often say, "It feels like all the channels on a radio are on at the same time." They also report difficulty with concentration and memory.

Rhonda, a twenty-six-year-old female, had a history of depression, racing thoughts, sleeping problems, poor concentration and memory, and suicidal preoccupation. She was diagnosed as having manic depression and was taking Lithium for it. She was admitted twice to the hospital for treatment.

During a session, under hypnosis, she saw many human and demon entities who claimed to create problems for her. They were all released to the Light after some therapy. During the next session, Rhonda reported that she had no racing thoughts, was sleeping better, and had no nightmares. Four years later, I heard she was still doing well and was not taking Lithium.

Homicidal thoughts and impulses: These can also be caused by possessing earthbound entities who were homicidal when they were in their own body. Their thoughts and feelings are transferred to their hosts, who in turn start to have those homicidal thoughts, impulses, and behaviors.

Almost always, these homicidal earthbound entities are heavily infested with many dark demon entities who are giving them the homicidal thoughts and impulses and push them to act on them.

Adam, a forty-year-old male, had had homicidal impulses from time to time ever since he was ten years old. Full-blown murder plans used to pop into his mind, complete with means, methods, escape routes, and alibis. There was no motive, since all the impulses, except one, involved strangers. There was usually a strong impulse to carry out the plan.

Adam described the murder plans as being inside his head, yet they felt separate and distant from him. It seemed to him as if someone else were in his head making the plans and then explaining it to him in detail. He was always strong enough to overcome the impulses and to not follow through with the plans.

The first impulse came when he was about ten and he was helping his uncle, who was on his hands and knees driving nails into the floorboards. Adam was standing behind him with a hammer in his hand. Suddenly he heard a thought voice in his head laying out a complete plan for the murder of his uncle. It went like this:

"You hit him in the back of the head as hard as you can. Then you roll him off the platform so he lands on that machine down there. See that lever that is sticking up? You smear some blood and hair on it so people may think that this is where he hit his head. Then you wipe the blood off the hammer with the hay and nobody will ever know that you did it."

Along with the message came an impulse to carry out the plan. He fought the impulse because this type of thinking was completely foreign to him. Even at that young age, he knew it was the wrong thing to do.

271

He had many such plans. He was very upset. He could not imagine that any part of his mind could think like that because the thoughts were so contrary to his personality and beliefs.

Under hypnosis, when he looked inside his body he saw many human and dark spirits. One of them was a dark-looking, cocky white man who was belligerent. He said that his name was Giarmo. He was a mobster and a racketeer. He admitted murdering people in his lifetime and he in turn was murdered. Somebody shot him. He joined Adam when Adam was three years old. He bragged about giving Adam many excellent murder plans, but was disappointed that Adam was strong-willed and would not follow through with them.

When I explained to him that he needed to go into the Light, he flatly refused. He was afraid that in heaven he would be punished and sent to hell, because of the bad things he had done. When I told him that according to what other people have told me, it was not true, that in heaven there is no punishment, he did not believe me. So I asked him to call out to anybody from the Light he could trust. At first he said he did not trust anybody. But later, after considering, he said that the only person he could trust was the Virgin Mary.

I asked him to look at the Light and ask for her. All of a sudden he said, with great surprise, "By God, she is here and she is real."

I told him to ask her any questions he wanted to. He asked her, "Is there a hell?"

The Virgin Mary pointed at him saying, "That is hell, being stuck in somebody else's body."

Then he asked, "Will I be punished in heaven?" He saw the Virgin Mary stretching her arms toward him with love and asking him to come with her and explaining that there is no punishment in heaven.

He went to the Light with the Virgin Mary. As he went into the Light, Adam saw many black blobs, large and small, falling out of Giarmo's body. Adam has been free of those thoughts since then.

Symptoms of schizophrenia and psychosis: Some patients report that the possessing earthbound entities constantly try to communicate with them and sometimes suggest to the patients what to say and do. In those cases, patients report having constant conversations and internal dialogue in their heads. At times they can hear constant critical accusations or angry voices from one of these spirits.

When there are multiple possessing human spirits in a patient, the spirits may speak to each other constantly or to the patient, creating confusion and making the patient feel that he or she is going crazy. In some patients, some of these possessing spirits also carry on communication with outside spirits. The patients are aware only that they are hearing voices of different people talking to them.

Some of these patients are clairvoyant and clairaudient. They can hear and see the spirits or ghosts. Those of us who do not see and hear beyond our five physical senses think they are imagining things.

These patients state that they also have a softer boundary of their energy field, allowing spirits to come and go as they please. Some medications also create openings in their auras, leaving them vulnerable to more spirits coming in.

Milton, a forty-five-year-old man had severe headaches and pressure in his head. He felt as though something were contracting, expanding, and moving in his head. He also described having constant conversation and internal dialogues going on in his head, which were very distressing to him.

Under hypnosis, Milton found many earthbound human spirits in him. After releasing these guest spirits from Milton, he was relieved of all his symptoms.

Gloria had a spirit who died in a mental institution. Angry at the doctors and nurses, the spirit told how she hopped from one patient to another and made them do things that irritated the doctors and nurses.

Jill was a thirty-year-old female who, after a car accident, started to hear voices speaking in Russian, German, and other languages. She became paranoid and angry and had nightmares. She also became nervous, irritable, and depressed.

During a session, under hypnosis, she saw forty to fifty spirits of men, women, and children in her. Some of them claimed to have died in concentration camps in Germany. Those who could speak English reported that they all came in during the car accident. We did not have time to talk to each and every one individually. So I asked all of them to look up. Jill reported seeing the whole place filled with the bright white Light and many angels and other beings of the Light in it. Some of them were deceased loved ones who were in the Light. Jill also described seeing all those people going to the Light, hand in hand with their loved ones and angels.

After the session, Jill described feeling empty inside and that she could now breathe easily. In the next session, she reported that the voices in her head were gone. She was not angry, nervous, or paranoid, and she did not have any nightmares. She was able to sleep and function better.

Tod, a thirty-six-year-old man, had a history of depression, nervousness, irritability, and mood swings. His moods would fluctuate within hours from happy to sad to angry without any reason. He was obsessed with his weight and would binge on junk food and then would induce vomiting and used laxatives intermittently.

He also had psychotic symptoms, including auditory, visual, and tactile hallucinations, and believed something was crawling over him. He had paranoid ideations. He sometimes could not sleep for several days at a time, in spite of taking high doses of medication, and he constantly had racing thoughts. He felt as though he were on speed, even though he did not use the drug.

Tod was admitted several times to the hospital with suicidal preoccupation and attempts. He had a diagnosis of psychotic depression, manic-depressive illness, manic- or depressed-type schizophrenia, and borderline personality.

Most of the medication did not have much effect on him and I was worried that one day he would end up committing suicide. When I learned about entities and how they can affect a person, I began to wonder what might be causing Tod's problems.

During a session, under hypnosis, he found an entity who committed suicide by taking an overdose of amphetamines. That entity had joined Tod; afterward he began to have suicidal preoccupation and all the symptoms of amphetamine abuse: racing thoughts, difficulty in sleeping, headaches, eating disorder, auditory hallucinations, paranoia, and other psychotic symptoms. After he released the entity, Tod's condition improved a great deal.

I have worked with people who were diagnosed as having psychosis and schizophrenia. In some, symptoms were completely relieved after releasing the possessing spirit. Others, who do not have enough ego strength and strong enough boundaries to their energy field, keep being infested over and over by these spirits. These patients feel totally helpless.

Combat neurosis and psychosis: These are also described by my patients to be sometimes caused by spirit possession. According to them, people in war are often afraid, angry, hateful, vengeful, and under a lot of stress, which opens them for possession. The use of drugs and alcohol can further open their shields.

Also, in war people die suddenly by being shot or blown away by bombs. They sometimes do not even realize that their bodies are dead. They feel confused, angry, and vengeful and end up possessing others who are already open.

Patients report that feelings of dissociation and depersonalization, recurrent nightmares, and flashbacks of traumatic war scenes are often due to the possessing spirits who died in the war and who are still reexperiencing their traumatic death over and over, as if they were frozen in time. These feelings in turn are experienced by their hosts. Releasing these suffering spirits frees the patients from their suffering.

Dissociative identity disorder (DID) or Multiple personality disorder (MPD): Possession by earthbound entities plays an important role in multiple personality disorder cases. Multiple personality disorder and its psychopathology and treatment is described in detail later in chapter 9.

Relationship problems: These also can be caused by earth-bound spirits. Sometimes loving or possessive spouses become very upset when widowed survivors remarry and they deliberately create problems for the new spouses.

Becky gave a history of irrational anger toward her husband. Sometimes she would wake up from a dream and start to punch him. She was puzzled at her behavior. During a session, she found in her a female entity, Lil, who claimed that she knew Becky's husband, Paul, from another lifetime, in the 1700s. He was Lil's husband.

According to Lil, Paul was unfaithful to her and as a result she committed suicide. Since then she has been following, possessing, and tormenting him from lifetime to lifetime, including this one.

Lil admitted that it was she who was punching Paul and was angry at him, and that she was determined to hurt him the same way he hurt her. After she released Lil, Becky's behavior toward Paul improved.

Obesity, bulimia, and anorexia nervosa: Patients have described their possessing earthbound spirits as one of the reasons for their eating disorders.

Overweight patients often find one or more earthbound spirits who either died of starvation or were overweight before they died. They can cause their host to overeat. Some patients have in layers many of these spirits, who either died of starvation; suffered with obesity, anorexia, or bulimia; or were diabetic and therefore give patients cravings for sweets.

Sometimes these spirits in my patients have reported that they are the ones who make the patients wake up in the night or walk in their sleep and eat at nighttime.

Buffy had the spirit of a teenager who died of anorexia. She was making Buffy overeat, saying, "Now I can eat and I do not have to worry about gaining any weight; I do not care if she gains weight."

Mona, who had anorexia, had the spirit of a girl who was kicked off the cheerleading squad because she was overweight. She was dieting and died of anorexia. After her death she joined Mona while Mona was trying out for cheerleader. Afterward, Mona became anorexic.

Jolyn, reported having weight problems. She used to wake up in the night and eat. She had a female entity who claimed to make her eat in the.middle of the night. After releasing that entity, Jolyn was free of her symptoms.

Ben, a thirty-one-year-old male, had a weight problem. He especially had a strong craving for sweets. Under hypnosis, he found he had the spirit of a woman who died of diabetes. She admitted that it was she who had the cravings for sweets and was making Ben eat sweets. After he released her, Ben's craving for sweets was relieved.

Claudia gained a lot of weight after she had surgery and had a very hard time losing it. During a session, under hypnosis, she reported having many extremely overweight earthbound entities in her. Some claimed to weigh up to 450 pounds. All of them claimed that Satan sent them to Claudia and they all joined her after the surgery. They claimed to give her desire to overeat compulsively and constantly and made her crave sweets and fattening foods. They did not care if overeating created physical problems for her.

Obsessive-compulsive behavior: Some patients found spirits to be the reasons for their obsessive-compulsive behavior.

Sandy, a thirty-year-old female, had a strong obsession to set fires. She had inside her the spirit of a twelve-year-old boy who had a history of setting fires. After his death he joined Sandy and she started to have the same obsessions. The obsession was relieved after she released the young boy into the Light.

Drug and alcohol abuse and addiction: My patients have often found spirits to be the source of their drug and alcohol problems. Over and over, patients have told me that they had one or more addicts inside them who were satisfying their desires to drink or take drugs through them. They also reported that drinking or using drugs further weakened their shields, allowing more addict spirits to come in. This explains why drug and alcohol addicts find it so hard to stop the addictions.

Cyrus, a thirty-five-year-old man, suddenly started to have the desire to smoke pot. He started to use it frequently, even though he never smoked pot before. He had the spirit of a teenage girl who was a drug addict and wanted to smoke pot. After releasing the spirit, Cyrus did not have any more desire for pot.

Dale, a thirty-year-old man, gave the history that he never liked drinking, except socially. After the death of his father, Dale started to drink fairly heavily, especially the same brands of whiskey his father drank. He also started to notice a change in his personality, becoming almost like his father. During the session, Dale saw that his father was with him. After releasing his father to the Light, Dale was able to stop drinking and returned to his normal self.

Children: I find that children with all types of problems, such as hyperactivity, poor attention span, mood swings, violent temper outbursts, and behavior problems, have one or more entities. This is especially true if the changes occur after a sickness, surgery, accident, or the death of a loved one.

Cynthia, a twelve-year-old girl, was brought to me because over six months she had become very hyper, restless, fidgety, and argumentative. She was very disruptive in the classroom and was getting bad grades. Under hypnosis, she found in her many spirits who claimed to have come into her when she had a tonsillectomy six months before. After she released them, according to her parents and teachers, there was a dramatic change in Cynthia.

Summary

Many patients, under hypnosis, have reported that they have one or more earthbound spirits attached to them. If we look at my research in Chapter X, we can see that 92 percent of my patients had earthbound spirits in them. Eighty-two percent had more than one earthbound spirit, 50 percent had spirits of their relatives, and 77 percent had spirits of strangers with them.

Sixteen percent of my patients had spirits of miscarried or aborted fetuses.

Many of the entities in my patients reported that they were not even aware that their physical bodies had died, and that they felt confused. Some stated that they always believed that when they die they die and that is the end of them. But they became very confused when they still felt, after the death of their bodies, just as alive as when they were in their bodies, and did not know what to do or where to go. Some entities in my patients said that they knew of the Light (heaven) and where they were supposed to go, but were afraid to go to heaven because of the fear that they would be punished and sent to hell. Some stayed earthbound because they were angry and hateful toward somebody and wanted to take revenge on them, while others remained earthbound because they did not want to leave their loved ones.

Some earthbound entities reported that they did not go to heaven because they were too attached to a place, person, or an object. Others said they could not move on to the Light because of some unfinished business they still had to take care of.

Many of these earthbound entities in my patients stated that they were working for Satan and were sent to my patients by Satan to create emotional and physical problems for their hosts and to bring their souls to Satan. Some of these entities reported being tricked by Satan and his demons, or by Satan's human followers, to join them, while others went willingly because they were angry with God about what happened to them in their lives. Others simply went with Satan and his demons because they wanted power, and to follow Satan's evil ways.

Most of these earthbound entities in my patients reported having one or more human or demon entities in them who were responsible for their confusion, anger, fear of the Light, and reluctance to go to heaven. The demon entities in them were afraid of the Light, so they kept these human entities from going to heaven as well.

Some patients reported that earthbound entities were totally trapped and enclosed in a demon entity and were recognized only after the demon was transformed into the Light. Sometimes these earthbound entities, who were trapped inside a demon, seemed to forget everything about their identity and thought that they were the demon. Sometimes these earthbound entities did not even know that they were with my patients. They felt they did not have any choice of where they go and what they do. They were simply along for a ride inside that demon.

Patients report that the electromagnetic energy field around them, which they call an aura, protects them from outside entities coming in to them and affecting them. Any of the conditions that weaken this electromagnetic energy field around them allow outside entities to come on board. Some of my patients reported that their auras had soft, fuzzy, and porous edges, so the entities could just hop in and hop out without any problems. Other patients had harder edges of their shields (auras) and were difficult to get into. Only when something went wrong with these patients did their shields open up.

These guest entities in my patients reported attaching to them when the electromagnetic energy field around them was weakened—while they were using drugs and alcohol, were physically sick, were knocked unconscious, were in accidents, or were anesthetized for surgery or sick in the hospital. Others claimed to have joined my patients when they were grieving, sad, depressed, angry, hateful or vengeful, or were emotionally upset and distraught after the death of a loved one or other crises.

Sometimes these possessing earthbound entities reported that they joined my patients when the patients were trying to contact spirits to provide them with answers by using Ouija boards, doing automatic writing, channeling, or sitting in a séance. Other times entities came in when they were playing with conjuring games such as Dungeons and Dragons, or Demons. In all these situations patients voluntarily opened themselves for the outside entities to come in.

Patients reported that every physical and emotional problem these guest entities had before the death of their physical bodies became the patients' symptoms after these entities came on board with them. These earthbound entities were responsible for most of their acute emotional and physical problems.

In therapy, these lost souls are treated as secondary patients who are stuck inside the patients. We need to help them understand their condition and to help them to heaven. It is like doing psychotherapy with these possessing entities by helping them understand that their physical bodies are dead but their spirits are not. The body they are in is not theirs, but instead they are in the patient's body. They are hurting the patient and themselves. They are still feeling the physical and emotional problems they experienced before the death of their bodies, and those problems are transferred over to the patients and are also felt by them.

The possessing entities are also hurting themselves by not going to the Light, which my patients report is heaven, the place everybody needs to return after the death of their physical bodies. They need to understand that there is no judgment or punishment in heaven and that everybody is accepted with love, regardless of what they have done.

In the treatment, we do not have to cure these earthbound entities and we do not have to work with them extensively. We just need to give them enough understanding so they can go to heaven, freeing the patients from the associated symptoms that were due to these guest entities.

I firmly believe that before we conduct past life therapy we must deal with the baggage (earthbound and demon spirits and soul fragmentation) from this life. The reason is simple: if we do not free patients from possessing spirits, when we proceed to past life therapy we may be getting the past life of the patient, or we may be getting the life or past life of the possessing earthbound spirit.

The earthbound entities in the patients act like foreign bodies. If a patient has a splinter in a finger, the patient will experience pain, swelling, redness, and, in some cases, infection and fever. Now, all these symptoms can be treated symptomatically with warm soaks, aspirin, and, in cases of infection, with antibiotics. The pain, redness, swelling, infection, and fever will subside temporarily. But as long as the splinter is there in that finger, the patient will continue to have pain, swelling, and infection off and on. The only way the patient can be permanently free from these symptoms is by taking the splinter out.

Similarly, these foreign earthbound spirits in the patient can cause multiple emotional, mental, and physical problems and, like a parasite, use their energy. These problems can be symptomatically treated with medications, psychotherapy, physical therapy, or other treatments, and the patient will feel temporary relief. But as long as the entities are still inside them, they will continue to remember and suffer with their traumatic feelings and pain off and on, which in turn, the patient will also experience. The only way the patient can be free of these symptoms is by removing those foreign entities from the patient.

A patient, for example, may have an entity who was depressed and as a result committed suicide by hanging. After the entity comes on board in the patient, the patient will start to experience the entity's depression, suicidal thoughts, headaches, neck and shoulder pains, and throat problems, due to hanging. Now we can treat this patient's depression with antidepressant medication, psychotherapy, or shock treatment and we can relieve headaches and neck, shoulder, and throat pain with Tylenol or stronger habit-forming pain pills and shots, or with biofeedback and physical therapy. All can provide temporary relief, but as long as the entity is still inside the patient, he or she will continue to suffer with those symptoms off and on. The only way the patient can be permanently free of those crippling symptoms is by removing the possessing entity responsible for the symptoms.

These symptoms are not the patients' symptoms and the patients do not need to suffer with them. By removing these foreign, parasitic entities, the patients can be totally and completely free of their crippling symptoms. There is little or no need for medications or long-term talk therapy, which only work as a Band-Aid approach. In just a few sessions, sometimes only in one or two hypnotherapy sessions, patients can be relieved of their symptoms.

These possessing earthbound entities are like cosmic hitchhikers on the highway to heaven, who use us like a motel and come in as an unwanted houseguest, with their baggage of physical, emotional, and other problems. When they are released during the treatment, they take those problems with them, thus freeing the patients from the unwanted problems that were dumped on them.

Most of the patients are totally unaware, innocent, and unsuspecting of the possession. They interpret the problems and negative behaviors the entities bring as their own. Only when they release those entities do they realize they have fallen victim to these cosmic hitchhikers, and what a toll they have paid for carrying them around.

I do not know whether these earthbound entities described by my patients are real or not. I do not think we can prove their existence. As a psychiatrist working with patients who are suffering with emotional and physical problems, the only thing that is important to me is the result. And over the years, I have seen astounding results with spirit releasement therapy. In my experience, almost eighty percent of the presenting or primary symptoms, and about thirty percent of the secondary symptoms were caused by possessing human and demon entities, and releasing them released the patients' symptoms. Such percentages justify the continued use of this therapy.

Chapter V

Possession or Attachment by Demon Spirits (Entities) and Other Spirits

The Dark Deceivers

Who is that hovering there in the shadows?
Behind the screen of my consciousness?

Am I the only one here? or are there others
Who tease and taunt and try to drive me
To my own dark ruin?

Elusive beggars, caught between the darkness and the Light
Fraught with fear and false promises,

Free yourselves! Leave me now!
And find the feeble spark of your own memories.
Watch it grow until you become it,

Let it show you the golden path
That will lead you from a prison of darkness
And guide you—Home.

—Jane

Possession or Attachment by Demon Spirits (Entities) and Other Spirits

Protection Prayer

As I began to recognize and work with human and demon spirits in my patients, releasing them caused my patients to experience dramatic freedom from their physical and emotional symptoms. Some patients, however, reported that they continued to be influenced by human and demon spirits, even after we had released all the spirits.

Sam, a patient, reported that even after releasing the spirits from him he continued to be influenced by the other spirits. As he looked inside he saw new spirits again. As we were releasing these spirits, Sam said that the entire place was filled with the brilliant, white Light and there was a large angel with loving eyes, whose name was Urial. I asked angel Urial why Sam was continually infested by these entities and what could he do to protect himself.

> **Urial:** "Sam's aura, the energy field, is weak. He needs to pray for protection. Also, all human beings have their own guardian angels assigned to protect and guide them. But we angels cannot do anything unless you ask us for help. If you do not ask for help, we cannot help."
>
> **Dr. Modi:** "Why not?"
>
> **Urial:** "God gives everybody free will. We cannot interfere with your free will. If you do not ask us for help, we cannot help, but when you ask, we are instantly there to help you. We are just, a thought away from you and can be with you instantly. So tell everybody you work with and care for to ask for help and we shall be there.

"Request your angels to remove all the earthbound, demon, and other entities, dark shields, dark energies, dark devices, and dark connections from your body, aura, soul, and cord, and also from your home, workplace, places of recreation, cars, and everything in them and miles and miles around them. Then ask them to fill and shield you, your home, workplace, and cars with the brilliant, white, liquid Light. Request them to plug all the holes and tunnels in you and your surroundings and cars.

"As the angels do that, you should visualize a column of dazzling, shimmering, vibrant, white, liquid Light coming from above your head and filling your whole body, cleansing and healing every part, every cell, and every organ of your body. If you cannot visualize it, you can just imagine it and it will be so.

"Then imagine this brilliant, white, liquid Light spreading an arm's length all around you, below your feet, above your head, in front of you, behind you, and on both sides of you, creating a bubble of brilliant, white Light all around you. Then visualize this bubble of white Light covered by the reflective, spiritual mirrors, with the reflective mirror surface outside the bubble and covered with rays of shimmering, white Light all around.

"These demons are afraid of the Light. They think they will be burned and killed by the Light. So if you visualize or imagine yourself like a brilliant, blinding, hot, afternoon sun, several times a day, every day, you can keep them away from you.

"Also stay away from drugs, alcohol, and intense emotions, which can open your shield for these entities to come in.

"Similarly, visualize your home, workplace, cars, and places of recreation being cleansed, filled, and shielded by the brilliant, white, liquid Light and imagine them looking like a blinding, hot, afternoon sun.

Ask your angels to stay on guard around you and your surroundings as long as your soul exists. You should also pray for and protect your family members, friends, coworkers, and even the people with whom you have problems and their surroundings.

"All human beings have energy centers (chakras), which can also be infested and blocked by entities and negative energies. So you should routinely ask your angels to cleanse, heal, balance, and open up all your energy centers when needed and cover and protect them when not needed.

"Human beings also have many spiritual channels of communication with the Light (heaven), which can also be infested with entities and negative energies and can be blocked and have holes. So request your angels regularly to cleanse, heal, open, shield, and protect all your channels of communication with the Light (heaven).

"Use these protection prayers at least twice a day, every night before sleeping and in the morning after you wake up, and you will be protected. Remember, we do not come until we are called, so call upon us and we shall be there instantly. We are just a thought away."

Similar protection techniques were reported by many patients from different cultures and different religions. Amazingly, they were very effective with most of my patients. More specific protection techniques were given by the Light beings through different patients, which will be described in full detail later.

Based on what different Light beings suggested through different patients on how to pray for protection, I have prepared the following protection prayer and technique, which my patients and I have found very effective in protecting us from the negative entities, energies, and influences. It should be used every night before sleeping and in the morning after waking up.

Protection Prayer

"I pray to God to please cleanse, heal, shield, and protect me, all my family members, friends, coworkers, and all our surroundings—our homes, workplaces, cars, places of recreation, and everything in them and miles and miles around them from Satan, all of his demons, all human beings under his influences, and all the foreign entities, dark shields, dark energies, dark devices, and dark connections. Please fill, shield, protect, and illuminate all of us and our surroundings with your love and Light as long as our souls shall exist, and bless us, enlighten us, balance us, transform us, and guide us in the right direction. Please keep us loving, giving, caring, forgiving, and humble all the time.

"Please cleanse, heal, balance, and open up all of our energy centers and channels of communication with the Light (heaven) as needed, and cover and protect them when not needed.

"I form an intent not to be possessed and influenced by any spirits and reject all the works of Satan, his demons, and humans under their influences. I also form an intent to accept the works of God and achieve God's purposes by dedicating my life to God and to achieve my goals and purposes, which I planned in heaven for this life."

Protection Technique

"I request the protector angels of the Light (heaven) to please collect and remove all the foreign entities, dark shields, dark energies, dark devices, and dark connections from my body, aura, soul, cord, and all the energy centers and from all my family members', friends', and coworkers' bodies, auras, souls, cords, and energy centers, and from all our homes, workplaces, cars, and places of recreation and from everything in them and miles and miles around them. Collect them in the net of Light, lift them out, and help them to the Light or bind them in the space. Remove and destroy all the dark shields, dark energies, dark devices, and dark connections totally and completely.

"Please fill, shield, and illuminate all of us and all our homes, workplaces, cars, and places of recreation and everything in them and miles and miles around them, with the brilliant, white Light. Plug all the holes and tunnels in all of us and all our surroundings and cars. Please build an impenetrable shield of brilliant, white Light around all of us and around our homes, workplaces, cars, and places of recreation. Cover all the shields with reflective, spiritual mirrors and the rays of brilliant, vibrant, white Light.

"Please cleanse, heal, and shield all the foreign entities that cannot be removed and all of our fragmented soul parts that cannot be integrated at this time, with a triple net of Light and metallic shield. Cut all their dark connections.

"Please cleanse, heal, balance, and open up all of our energy centers and channels of communication with the Light (heaven) as needed, and cover and protect them when not needed.

"Please stay on guard around us and our surroundings. You have our permission to take any action on our behalf to protect us as long as our souls should exist. Thank you."

Now visualize or imagine a column of brilliant, dazzling, shimmering, vibrant, white, liquid Light coming from above your head from God and going through your head, filling and illuminating your whole body from the top of your head to the tips of your fingers to the tips of your toes, cleansing and healing every part, every organ, and every cell of your body. Now imagine this white Light spreading an arm's length all around you, below your feet, above your head, in front of you, behind you and on both sides of you. A wonderful bubble or shield of brilliant, white Light all around you, your family members, friends, and your homes, workplaces, cars, and places of recreation. Imagine these shields covered with reflective spiritual mirrors and rays of shimmering, white Light.

You, and only you, have a right to live in that body and shield. If anybody or anything tries to enter into your shield, you will be aware of it, even at subconscious levels of your mind, and you will have a right to say no to them. Instead of allowing them in your shield, you will direct them to the Light, or where they belong.

Just imagine yourself, your family members, friends, and co-workers and everybody's homes, workplaces, cars, and places of recreation like a blinding, hot, afternoon sun, several times a day.

Use this protection prayer and the visualization at least twice a day, especially at bedtime and in the morning after waking up, and in between when needed.

The Demons

The Darkness Within

The darkness within consumes me,
And I have no defense for its hunger,

There is no place to hide,
No way to protect myself,

And so here I am, wondering

Why?

—Jane

The terms *Satan* and *demons*: As I have explained, I personally like to call these beings *dark entities, dark beings,* or *negative energies* because of their dark appearance and negative actions. Many would consider these terms comfortable euphemisms, less direct words for the one considered offensive like *Satan* and his *demons*. Because this work deals with what my hypnotized patients tell me and represents as accurately as possible their case histories, it would be false and misleading to refer to these dark entities by my own labels. Instead, though it may disturb or offend some, I address them as they are named by my patients, who consistently call them *Satan* and his *demons*. None of this information is based on religion or spirituality. It is based only on the information given by my hypnotized patients.

After that session with Sam, many of my patients from different cultures and religious beliefs gave, under hypnosis, similar accounts and descriptions of the demons, and the same techniques freed them from the emotional and physical symptoms with which they were suffering.

My patients often tell me that these dark demon entities are very deceptive. They try to hide and do not want to be discovered at any cost. At first, when the patients look inside they often describe seeing nothing except darkness or a blank. There is no sense of power in the beginning. But as the patients begin to focus on that darkness or nothingness, they begin to see a shape, a form, or a movement in that part of the body.

Hypnotized patients often give a physical description of the demons that they find inside them. Based on my patients' reports, demons come in different colors, shapes, and sizes. They appear in different numbers and in various locations in the body.

Color of the Demons

Patients under hypnosis describe these demons as beings of different colors. Most commonly they appear to my patients as different shades of black, gray, brown, or red, or tinged with green, red, orange, or yellow.

These demons claim that their color depends on the vibration of the planet they inhabit. Demons on the earth appear mostly as black, gray, red, or brown. The higher the vibration of the planet, the lighter the color of the demon.

The more intense the black color of the demons, the more powerful they appear to the patient. The following are some of the descriptive phrases my patients gave to describe the color of the demons:

"Thick black smoke." "A black rock."
"A black piece of coal." "A yucky green color."
"A brown rock." "A gray blob."

"A fiery red blob." "Like black or brown chocolate."
"A yellow blob." "An orange blob."
"Black liquid."

Number of the Demons

Hypnotized patients mention having one or more demons in them. Sometimes their whole body is infested by hundreds of demons.

Patients describe it as . . .

"having freckles all over the body, both large and small"
"black and gray pebbles all over the body"
"like a beehive," etc.

Shapes and Forms of the Demons

The Dark Illusion

Then Satan came and said, "I am the Light."
And he glowed for one brilliant moment.

And as I watched, breathless,
His Light faded into nothingness

And he was consumed by his own
Dark illusion.

—Jane

Under hypnosis, patients describe these so-called demons as having different shapes and forms. Demons are reported to be round or pyramid-shaped or as having more complex geometric shapes. Sometimes they are described as amorphous blobs, having no particular shape. Sometimes demons appear as evil-looking animals or humanoid forms. They can take any form to scare people.

My patients use an array of descriptive terms for these demons: "a black rock," "piece of coal," "dark jaw with sharp teeth," "sinister eyes," "a dragon," "a gargoyle," "giant like Goliath," "like a monster," "a beast," "like a skeleton," "like a Dracula," "being who is part human and part animal," "a black ugly devil with horns," "black chocolate syrup," "thick black smoke," "black or brown rocks," "being in a black robe with the hood covering his face and eyes," "like a lizard, snake, bat, cat, spider," and "like mythological animals."

The demons look and feel very cold to the patient. If the demons have eyes, they appear to my patients as dark, black, red, evil, blank, empty, vacant, piercing, stern, cold, hateful, or sinister-looking. Sometimes these demons can appear to the patient as beings of the Light with white robes and loving eyes like an angel, or other beings of the Light, even as God. They can create an illusion of light in them and around them. They are even able to communicate in a loving way briefly, but they cannot stay in that form for more than a few seconds to a few minutes. They quickly change into black, evil-looking beings with the black, red, piercing, hateful, stern, blank, cold, evil-looking eyes. The illusion of light around them quickly disappears. Their hands, when touched, feel cold and bony to the patient.

Locations of the Demons in the Body

Patients report that these demons occupy different parts of their bodies. They are found in every organ and every part of the body, including bones, blood vessels, tissues, and the soul, causing different symptoms and diseases.

Sometimes they appear to exist in the patients' bodies in multiple layers, with the top layers hiding other layers. In that case, when we remove the demons from the top layer, patients appear to be completely clear after that session. During the next session,

POSSESSION BY DEMON ENTITIES
(Compilation of drawings by different patients)

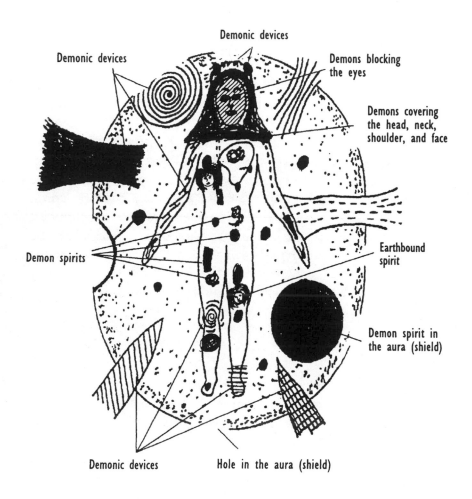

Demonic devices

Demonic devices

Demons blocking
the eyes

Demons covering
the head, neck,
shoulder, and face

Demon spirits

Earthbound
spirit

Demon spirit in
the aura (shield)

Demonic devices

Hole in the aura (shield)

however, patients see new demons inside causing a different set of new symptoms, which are called the tertiary symptoms.

In this case it seems that the spirits did not leave the first time, or new ones came in. Although that can happen sometimes, in the case of layering it is the next layer of entities coming up from the deeper layers of the body. They surface after the entities from the top layers are removed.

One patient can have many layers of entities in many different parts of the body. They can be of various sizes, depending on the size of the weak areas in the body. The layers are also of different thickness, depending on the number of layers and the number of entities within each layer. Usually there is a mixture of demon and earthbound entities and requires many sessions to release them. At times it seems like a neverending and exhausting process to the patient and to me.

Patients also report that demons have even infested their souls. Here they describe their souls normally as a white Light often found in the chest, head, or neck. They report that some soul parts are missing from their souls and those empty places are being filled and occupied by the demons. In that case, the soul may appear dark or patchy gray in color. Sometimes patients describe demons completely surrounding their bodies from the outside. Other times patients mention that the demons are in their auras or energy fields, covering the whole or a part of the energy field around them.

Size and Rank of the Demons

Under hypnosis, patients see these demons in all different sizes, ranging from tiny dots to giant-sized creatures. These so-called demons, speaking through the hypnotized patients, claim they are organized by their size and rank and by category. They are assigned duties on the basis of their abilities and their power. According to these demons, the larger demons command the lesser demons. Each is lied to about its status.

An overwhelming characteristic found when talking to these demons is their delusion about how powerful they are. This delusion is partly fed by Satan and partly it is self-induced. Often they will brag about being a higher demon in Satan's hierarchy. Sometimes they claim to be one of the top ten demons or an extension of Satan himself. After they are transformed into the Light, they realize that they are not who they thought they were and they are not as powerful as they believed. This they realize and admit only after their transformation into the Light.

According to these demons, lesser demons do not have much knowledge and power, while larger ones have a lot of knowledge. They sometimes describe themselves as being trained and specialized to cause certain illnesses and problems for humanity and other living beings, just the reverse of a doctor, i.e., they specialize in causing certain illnesses, while doctors specialize in treating certain illnesses.

Attitude and Behavior of the Demons When Discovered

The power of the demon is not immediately sensed by the patients. When the patient focuses on the demon, quite frequently there is a personification. The demon can assume a humanoid form that can be conversed with through the patient. Even if demons do not have this personification, we can still communicate with these black blobs.

Sometimes patients initially describe no feelings or hint of power, purpose, or intent of the demons. They report the primary aspect of the demons as being cold. They are cold to each other, cold to humanity, and cold to the universe. People feel cold in their presence.

When spoken to, demons appear to be quite proud and arrogant and very willing to tell, even brag, about what damage they have done to the patient. Usually the more the demons talk, the more anger and hate come to the surface. Patients describe demons as very angry and hateful beings. They hate their hosts;

they hate humanity; they hate each other; and they hate Light and the beings of the Light.

To the patients they come across as cold, ugly, sly, sneaky, underhanded, hostile, angry, arrogant, hateful, evil, and belligerent. They lie a great deal. They are described by the patients as having foul mouths and cursing a lot. Everything that is negative in a human personality is expressed through these demons. Patients gave the following descriptions of the demons' behavior and attitude when they are discovered:

"It is growling and screaming obscenities."
"It is scared and angry."
"It is hissing, spitting, kicking, and screaming."
"It is scared because we found it."
"It is very arrogant and it is just laughing and laughing."
"He is cursing up a storm."
"He is swearing and spitting."
"He is fighting the Light."
"He is punching my stomach to death."
"He is jumping up and down with fear."

Patients describe demons as intensely powerful, but unable to use their full power against humans. I have seen many cases where a demon wanted to force a patient to act and say things, but the demon was constricted and restrained by the patient so that the language and the impulses of the demons were under the control of the patient. Patients often refused to repeat what the demons were saying. They were able to modify demons' behavior or control them.

Some of the things patients have reported are as follows:

"It is screaming obscenities and it wants me to scream obscenities."
"It wants me to hit you."
"It wants me to choke you."
"It has a vulgar personality."
"I do not want to repeat what it is saying."

I have also seen cases where the demons, or what the patients typify as the demons, have control over the patients, when the patients start to shake, jerk, and convulse. Sometimes they froth at the mouth, spit, hiss, growl, and curse.

In these cases it takes a great deal of work with the patients to help them take charge of their minds, bodies, and souls. In most cases, patients often say that with the help of God and his angels, they are more powerful than Satan and his demons, and that they are in control of their minds, bodies, and souls.

Sometimes demons threaten to hurt or kill both the patient and me as follows:

"I am very powerful and I can crush you."
"I can destroy and kill you and this one."
"This soul is ours. My mission is to take this soul."
"I will break your neck."
"I will call my dark angels to battle yours."
"I will attach to you."
"We all hate you because of what you will be doing to get
    rid of us, but we will stop you and we will win."

Sometimes during the sessions, patients describe seeing Satan trying to interfere with the releasement of the demons by scaring them or threatening them. In these cases, the patients often describe that, at our request, angels removed Satan without any problems. Angels of the Light often say that Satan cannot be transformed at this time because this is not his time yet. We need to request the angels to remove Satan and they will do so instantly. But all of Satan's demons can be transformed and returned to the Light regardless of how large and powerful they are.

On a few occasions, patients have said that Satan was trying to interfere with the session, and when we requested the angels to remove him, they said that the patient had the power to remove Satan.

Juanita, a nineteen-year-old patient under hypnosis, stated that somebody very powerful was pulling her hair. She felt very scared and asked me to remove him from there. She identified that being as Satan. In keeping with my experience with other patients, I asked the angels to remove him from there. Most of the time patients report the angels removing Satan from the office and then guarding the office so he cannot come back to interfere again. But this time nothing happened, in spite of our request for the intervention of the angels.

I asked the patient to look up and see whether the angels were there or not. She said, "Yes, the whole place is filled with the white Light and the large warrior type of angels are there, but nobody is doing anything." She saw one large angel with a sword and shield, who said he was the archangel Michael. Michael told the patient that she had the power to remove Satan herself. I asked her to tell Satan off. Still very scared by Satan's presence, she looked at him and in a fearful voice she whispered, "Go away." To our surprise, he left. After that, in future sessions when Satan came to interfere, she just told him to leave and he left. She felt confident and was not afraid of Satan after that.

Occasionally, the demons refuse to talk and answer my questions because they are told by Satan not to speak to me. As long as the patient is semi-conscious during the process, as is in most cases, I almost always succeed in communicating with the demons in one way or another.

When the patients are completely hypnotised and do not stay in charge of their mind, body, and soul and do not stay semi-conscious during the session, then demons are the ones who are in charge of the body. In these cases, the process of transformation becomes difficult because the demons refuse to talk and cooperate and then I have to use different methods of transforming them.

In cases where we do not have enough time to transform a demon or the demon does not cooperate, then, according to the angels, we can request the angels to lift that demon out of the patient and bind it in a space that is somewhere close to the Light, but not in the Light. If we cast it out of the patient without binding it in space, it can possess somebody else, come back to the patient from whom it was cast out, or go back to Satan.

What Do These Demons Say?

These possessing demons can be conversed with, through the patients. They give following information about themselves.

Who they are: They claim that Satan is their master and they work for him. They are very obedient and faithful to their master. Satan sent them to the patients to create problems and to destroy them and bring patients' souls to him. They claim that they have never been in human form. Some of the things they say about who they are follows:

"I am Satan's disciple."
"Satan is my god. I work for him."
"Satan is my master; I do what he wants me to do."

Punishment: Patients often say that as they try to look inside, the demons try their best not to be discovered; when they are located, they seem to be very unhappy and upset. They express the fear that now they are in trouble with Satan, because they have been discovered. According to these demons, this exposure is considered a failure by Satan. They do not want to fail at any cost. They are afraid that the punishment by Satan will be worse than before. Following are examples of what different demons have said about how Satan punished them in the past:

"Nails put in their bodies."
"Cut into pieces."
"Being thrown and burned in the fire."
"Being beaten with a belt with nails on it."
"Skin stripped off, which made them look like a beast and
    they were made to eat their own skin."
"Tortured to extreme pain, choked by thorns, burned in
    a fire, left in a cold, dark pit for a long time."

Satan uses the forms of punishment that demons are most afraid of. The demons in turn use similar punishments on the people they possess.

How These Demons Punish the People They Possess

Demons in my patients often state that, based on how they were punished by Satan, they cause similar pain and torture for the patients they are in. Every pain that was inflicted on the demons by Satan is projected onto the patients. If demons' heads were crushed by Satan, they can project that head pain on the patients, causing them headaches. If they were cut into pieces and suffered a great deal of physical torment, they will project that pain and discomfort onto the patients. They can also force patients to cause similar torment and torture on themselves and on other people.

There is also an emotional overflow from the demons to the patients. The demons feel paranoid because they believe that they are being watched by Satan and other larger demons. They express feelings of arrogance, grandiosity, jealously, anger, hate, paranoia, and desire for power and control, which are projected onto the patients, who in turn start to feel and act in the same way. The patients begin to feel angry, hateful, arrogant, grandiose, jealous, paranoid, destructive, evil, and sadomasochistic. Patients also start to curse and use foul, vulgar, and obscene language. They adopt evil ways and crave power, control, and position at any cost.

Patients often describe that a number of lesser demons are not particularly creative. They cannot use material that they do not have. So, whatever they experience by Satan, they project it onto the patients they are in.

Purpose of the Demons

These so-called demons mention having two different purposes with the person they are with:

- General purpose
- Special purpose

General-Purpose Demons

These demons strive to inhabit any human being they can get into and create physical, mental, and emotional problems, causing confusion and harassment. Their purpose is to keep humans from going to heaven or using their powers from the Light.

Special-Purpose Demons

These demons are described as having a special purpose with the patients they are in. They want to stop patients from achieving the goals they set in heaven. According to the demons, these are the people who have special purposes and missions on earth, which they have chosen to undertake at this time. These are the people who are preachers, healers, researchers making discoveries concerning science and psychology, including understanding of human nature, human interaction, human development, and many others.

The demons claim that these people have certain God-given talents and goals while on the earth. These are the people Satan and his demons especially watch for; a great deal of effort is exerted to stop them. When these people are born, it is not long until they have their own demons in residence. Some demons described their purpose as follows:

"I am sent here by Satan to stop her from what she is supposed to do."

"He knows something about the future and about Satan and us, and we want to stop him from letting everybody know about it."

"I am trained to go after the souls who have a great deal of Light, who have certain kinds of healing work and missions to do."

"I am here to make this person crazy so she cannot accomplish her goals."

"We know about you and what you are going to do. Satan does not want you to tell the world about us and we are determined to stop you at any cost."

According to my patients, these special-purpose demons try to achieve their goals by shading the Light of the person, by blocking the influence of the Light, and by interfering with the communication from the Light to the person with a special-mission. If these demons are unable to completely stop the person, they will try to slant the knowledge and block the discovery that person is supposed to make.

If they do not succeed by directly influencing and interfering with the individuals, then they try to stop them through other people around them, including their loved ones. These special-purpose demons are there for one, and only one, special purpose, and that is to stop individuals from fulfilling their God-given missions.

Some demons claim to have a special purpose to cause a special type of physical or psychological problem for a person, such as causing a brain tumor or causing cancer, or a special type of mental illness. Again the goal is to stop that person.

These demons mention that Satan has the knowledge of the patients' problems and purposes. The demons are told about them and how to work on these people, how to stop them. Other demons claim that they wait for the person to come down from the Light. As the person is making the transition from the Light to the physical world, the demons tune into the person's thoughts and know everything about his or her purpose before he or she goes in the womb.

One large demon gave the following description of how it knew about the purpose of my patient for this life, something even the patient was not consciously aware of.

> **Demon:** "I stay outside the Light and wait until she comes back down. Then I listen and learn about her plans and I make my plans, too."
>
> **Dr. Modi:** "How do you know her plans?"
>
> **Demon:** "I hear them. The thoughts are still in her mind as she comes down from heaven to the earth. It is very easy if you know what you are doing. I wait, and as she

is concentrating on her purpose, I tune in to her thoughts and absorb them, too, even before she hits here. I am here to block her so she does not progress and achieve what she is supposed to achieve. Many have failed. I will not fail. I block her vision so she cannot see and I block her mind so she does not think clearly."

The demons also tell about some people who have special purposes and are thoroughly shielded, internally and externally, from outside and from themselves, so that they can carry on their work with very little or no influence.

Age When Demons Possess People

Demons claim to possess patients any time from birth until death. Some even claim to possess them in the womb or even before, during the patients' transition from the Light to the womb.

Possession from Birth until Death

Charles had a demon who said: "I possessed this person as soon as he was born. I was waiting in the delivery room. He was having difficulty breathing. As he was struggling for breath, I came in."

Misty had a demon who claimed, "I attached to this patient when she was in the nursery because she was born prematurely. I have been trying to cause problems to this one since then."

Joe had a demon entity who said, "I joined this person at the age of seventeen when he was playing the game Dungeons and Dragons. When he called out to someone for help, I came in, and since then I have been with him causing problems."

Deidra had a demon who said, "I joined her when she was having a hysterectomy at the age of forty-two. Her spirit was out of the body watching the surgery. I was also in the operating room and I came in with her when her spirit went back to her body after the surgery.

306

Possession in the Womb

Some demons claim to join the patients while in the womb. Initially, they were with the mother and then from the mother they went into the fetus.

Hope had a demon who said, "I was with Hope's mother. I joined Hope when she was in the womb. Her mother was having a difficult labor and as a result [the fetus] Hope was having a difficult time and I went in her from her mother.

Possession during the Transition from the Light to the Womb

Sometimes demons claimed to attach to the patients during their transition from the Light to the womb.

Albert had a large demon entity who boasted: "I joined him before he was born, even before he went into the womb, during his transition from the Light to the womb. I am here to crush his spirit and take him to hell. In A.D. 900 he promised my master, Satan, to work for him, but he does not always follow what we want him to do, and we are here to make sure that he does."

Same Demon Possessing the Same Person in Many Lifetimes

Sometimes demons claim to follow and attach to the patients in many lifetimes. One patient, Amy, had a large demon entity who gave the following information.

> **Dr. Modi**: "How old was Amy when you joined her?"
> **Demon** [laughing sarcastically and arrogantly]: "Now lady, you know better than that. I have been with this one for centuries."
> **Dr. Modi**: "When was the very first time you joined her?"
> **Demon**: "Almost from the beginning. Soon after her first life on earth, centuries ago. After that I have attached to her during many lifetimes, including this one."
> **Dr. Modi**: "Tell me how? When she goes into the Light (heaven), after her death, what do you do? Do you go with her in the Light?"

307

Demon: "No. We can't go close to the Light, because we cannot stand it. I just stay outside the Light and wait till she comes back down to earth for her life, then I attach to her even before she goes in the womb during her transition from the Light to the womb."

Reactions of Demons to the Light

While we are dealing with the demons in the patients, the patients often say that a bright white Light is always present, with angels in it. This Light seems to be coming from beyond the sky, coming from heaven. They repeatedly say that the demons are afraid of the Light.

When the angels surround the demons with the net of Light, the demons react very violently. Sometimes patients say they jump up and down screaming, "It is burning me; it is killing me; take it away from me!" Sometimes the demons shake and shiver with fear.

When asked, "Why are you so afraid of the Light?" they say they are instructed by Satan to stay away from the Light because Light is death and that they will burn and vanish if they go close to it. Sometimes, with the Light around them, demons see their darkness dissolving at the edges, which convinces them that they are dying.

Larger demons, although uncomfortable with the Light around them, often brag about their power and that they will break free from the net of Light. They try, but are very surprised and angry that they cannot. Some of the descriptions of the reactions of demons to the Light are as follows:

"Light is choking me, strangling me and suffocating me to death."

"If I become Light, it will be an automatic death for me, like being poisoned."

"Light will blind me."

"Light is death, blood bath and spiky."

"Light will kill me and consume me."

"It will scorch me."

"Light is a thousand deaths."

"Light will change me into nothingness and it will make
me disappear forever."

Spark of the Light within the Demon and Its Transformation into the Light

As the demons are reacting very strongly to the Light around
them, they are asked to look inside their being. Most of the time
they refuse to listen and follow any instructions, and claim that
there is nothing but darkness.

At this point I usually tell them that if they do not cooperate
we will ask the angels to take them back to Satan. This always
works like magic. They do not want to go to Satan under any
circumstance because they are afraid of punishment by Satan,
and as a result, they are reluctantly willing to cooperate.

When they look inside their core, they are very surprised to
find a spark or a flicker of Light. They usually have no idea that
they have a Light within. They describe that Light as a "diamond
of Light," "a flame," "a star," "a spark of Light," "a fiery glow," "a
gem," or "a seed of Light," etc.

As they find that spark of Light within them, their first
impulse is not to look at it. They are convinced that they are
definitely going to die. But as soon as they focus on that spark,
they feel as if they are hypnotized and cannot take their eyes off
it. Pretty soon they see that spark of Light growing, while their
darkness starts to dissipate and disappear.

Some demons feel confused and scared. Some feel surprised.
Others experience a total change in their feelings. Instead of
feeling angry, hostile, and mean, they feel very peaceful, which
they do not remember ever feeling before. In seconds, they
completely change into beings of pure Light.

Sometimes the patients see that these so-called demons are
not completely changing into the Light, and they see one or more

309

black, cord-like connections going to Satan or to other demons. According to the patients, during the sessions, angels of the Light are always present and constantly helping us with the process. They are requested to cut all those cords and connections the demons have with Satan, with other demons, or with Satan's command centers. After that the demons change into the Light faster.

After their transformation into the Light, according to the patients, they look like either angels of the Light or balls, sparks, or blobs of Light. It takes demons a few seconds to understand what is happening to them. They express a great deal of shock, confusion, and amazement. They ask questions such as, "How did this happen so soon?" "What does this mean?" "Why did Satan tell me that Light would kill me?" "How did Satan cover up my Light?" "Why was I under the illusion that I was dark?"

Most of them like the new state of their transformed being and the feelings of love, peace, and calm. At this point they are very thankful for the help and are willing to help the patient and me in any way they can. They give a lot of information and understanding about Satan and his demons, how they work and how they affect humanity and the earth, and about Satan's plans. If the demon is a very large one, it seems to have a great deal of knowledge from the dark side.

If the demon is a big commander who has trained and commanded other demons, after the transformation it is more than happy to call all of them from the earth and other planets, who in turn are also helped to heaven by the angels. The Transformed demon is also willing to call out all the others who are hiding inside the patient.

After their transformation, the demons do not like to be called by their names from the dark side. They are very confused, surprised, and curious as to who they are, how they ended up with Satan, and what is going to happen to them. At this point they need some psychotherapy to understand their newfound condition.

Sometimes they recognize the angels of the Light who are helping them and who sometimes will tell them their names from the Light. Pretty soon they start to remember where they were before they joined Satan, and how they ended up with him.

Examples of Demons Changing into the Light

The following are transcripts of different reactions of demon entities to finding the Light within and to their transformation into the Light.

Example 1:

> **Dr. Modi:** "Look deep beneath the layers of your darkness, within the core of yourself. Tell me, what do you see?"
>
> **Demon:** "What do you mean? I am black. I am not looking anywhere. I only take orders from my master."
>
> **Dr. Modi:** "Don't tell me you're afraid of yourself, are you?"
>
> **Demon** [arrogantly]: "I am not afraid of anything. These angels are twisting me to make me look inside. [surprised] I see a diamond of Light and I am black. How is this possible? Why didn't Satan take it away if I was to do this?"
>
> **Dr. Modi:** "Just keep on looking at the Light. Tell me what happens."
>
> **Demon:** [laughing] "You mean to say I will look like these angels?"
>
> **Dr. Modi:** "Well, find out for yourself. There are no tricks."
>
> **Demon:** "You are a crazy lady! [looking in, surprised and excited] Are these angels magic?"
>
> **Dr. Modi:** "No, magic is within yourself, my friend. Tell me, what is happening to your darkness?"
>
> **Demon:** [confused] "I am starting to look like these angels. What is happening to me? Satan is watching and getting angry. I don't belong to him anymore. I am telling him off."

Example 2:

> **Demon:** [confused] "There is this white thing in me. What is this thing? It looks like a white star. Where was this before?"
>
> **Dr. Modi:** "Keep on looking at that white star and tell me what happens to your darkness."
>
> **Demon:** [irritable] "Lady, first tell me where was it before? Why didn't I see it before? Am I going to like this?"
>
> **Patient:** "He is really confused."
>
> **Demon:** [surprised and confused] "I am turning into a white shining egg and my darkness is going away. Where did it go?"
>
> **Dr. Modi:** "Just like an illusion, right?"
>
> **Demon:** "Yeah. We keep our own illusions. We keep on feeding it to ourselves."
>
> **Patient:** "He is all excited, boisterous, and loud. He is looking up and saying that his friends are up there."
>
> **Dr. Modi:** "Who?"
>
> **Demon:** "There is Michael and my old buddy Gabriel and all the others. You all stayed in the Light, didn't you?"
>
> **Patient:** "Michael is stern and telling this one not to make fun of it. This is important. This one apologized."

Example 3:

> **Dr. Modi:** "Look inside of your being, beneath all the layers of your darkness."
>
> **Demon:** [arrogant] "I see it. So what? I am very powerful. [looking puzzled] I see it and I cannot take my eyes off it. It is very bright. It is like a gem! How can a black and ugly thing like me be so bright? [excited] I am changing. My body is changing, my color, my texture, my feelings, and everything. I am changing into the Light. Darkness is going away! [excited] Change these others, too. Make them look like me."

Example 4:

One very large demon in my patient was very angry. The demon was yelling, spitting, hissing, and swearing. The demon reacted to the Light around it as follows:

> **Demon:** "Light is death. It is worse than death. I am very powerful and I will break free."
>
> **Patient:** "He is fighting. He is shaking and scared. Now he is showing himself to me to scare me. I want to throw up. [throws up] He is calling Satan for help and screaming and yelling because Satan is not coming."
>
> **Dr. Modi:** "Dark one, stop it and look inside."
>
> **Demon:** [confused] "I see a spark of light. What is it? Am I going to die now? I am turning into the Light! I look like a snowman. I am not sure how it is possible. How was it so easy and how did I change so fast? What is going to happen to me now?"

Example 5:

A demon in my patient looked like a big black snail, shell-shaped, in his abdomen causing severe abdominal pain during the session. The demon had the following reaction to the Light.

> **Demon:** "Get out and leave me alone! Go away! I'll spit on you! Spit on this person I am with. I hate all of you! I hate humans. I will fight you. I am strong! [screaming] I do not want to feel your Light! I will not feel your Light!"
>
> **Dr. Modi:** "What were you told about the Light?"
>
> **Demon:** "The Light means death. Take it away from me!"
>
> **Dr. Modi:** "Look inside and tell me what you see."
>
> **Demon:** [looking shocked] "What is happening to me? I am changing. Am I going to die? When am I going to die? Look at me!"

Patient: "He is in total shock. He is speechless. Angels are smiling at him with love. They are saying, 'Give him some time to absorb and understand what happened to him.'"

Memories of the Light and How and Why Demons Went with Satan

After their transformation into the Light, demons feel very shocked, surprised, and confused to find who they really are. It takes a few seconds or minutes to remember who they were and where they were before they went with Satan and became dark. They usually describe being in the Light as there being a battle or turmoil. They remember how and why they ended up with Satan. Some remember being tricked by Satan, while others remember going with Satan voluntarily for power. To help them in remembering who they are, I usually ask the following questions.

Dr. Modi: "Move back in time, before you joined Satan, before you became dark, who were you? Where were you? And how did you happen to join Satan?"

The following are accounts given by demons who were in my patients, about their memories of the Light.

Example 1:

Transformed demon: [surprised] "I am somebody. I am somebody special."
Dr. Modi: "Recall before you became dark, before you joined Satan, who were you and where were you?"
Transformed being (demon): [looking shocked and surprised] "I was the right hand of God. I was a loved angel. I was loved by God. [sad and upset] How did I let this happen to me?"

Dr. Modi: "Recall."

Transformed being (demon): "I was not as big as I thought. I was close to God. I made him smile. When there was a conflict in the Light and decisions were being made, I made him smile. I was a relief for him."

Dr. Modi: "What was happening?"

Transformed being (demon): "There was a conflict between Lucifer and God. A new universe is to be formed. There is a battle in the Light about who will be the ruler of the universe. Everybody is choosing between God and Lucifer. Light and dark. Lucifer wanted to rule heaven and earth. Lucifer chose to leave and took many angels with him. I chose to stay with God.

"Lucifer called me from the other side. He wanted me to play a joke on God. [upset] He tricked me. He told me to turn black and pretend that I was with Lucifer and then go back to God. Then I would be able to take my cover off and say, 'Surprise!' But once I changed my color, I could not go back, and I forgot everything very quickly. When the split finally happened, I was shoved away and could not go back. [very sad and upset] What a cruel thing to do.

"Then I became as opposite as possible. I am very sorry for what I did for centuries. I am angry in a way, but yet my new self will not let me dwell on any negative feelings."

Example 2:

One demon, after transformation, recalled with surprise.

Transformed demon: "I was far away from here. A place of all white Light. I was attached to someone. [surprised] I was attached to God! How did it happen? Why was I fighting against him for millions of years?"

Dr. Modi: "Recall what happened."

Transformed being: "God knew of evil. It is a part of all beings; one angel took it all out of him and God let him take it. It is like he split himself. The evil angel told me to come to him. He had something to show me.

"There were others on his side, the other side of the stitch. The black, void place. So I went to look and I could not come back. I do not think I actually chose to stay there. It was like I was hit on the head and all my memories of the Light disappeared quickly. [sad] I could not come back, and I ended up being taught and groomed in the darkness."

Example 3:

One demon, after its transformation, recalled as follows:

Transformed demon: "I was in heaven. There I looked like these angels. [confused] How could I be in heaven and so completely black? For all these millions of years, I was like this?" [very upset]

Dr. Modi: "Recall what happened"

Transformed demon: "I was on a mission for God to give the angels a message. As I was traveling, Lucifer called me and said that he would help me deliver the message faster. He had learned of new ways of telepathy and transportation. At first I ignored him, but later he talked me into letting him help me, since it was such an important job. When I crossed over, I could not come back and did not remember anything."

Dr. Modi: "What did you cross over?"

Transformed demon: "Like a gully, a big crack, when Satan was still in the Light but separate from the Light. We could see everything that was happening. God kept nothing from us. We could see everything and make up our minds. Up to that point I chose to stay with God, but Lucifer tricked me.

"He had his followers hold on to me and I lost my Light and I got dark and forgot about the Light and everything. The longer I stayed, the more they talked to me. And the more I listened the more interested I became and then I had more of a desire to learn their ways. I got very dark very fast."

Example 4:

A patient who had rheumatoid arthritis had several dark entities in him who claimed to cause him pain. One of them gave the following description of how he went with Satan.

> **Transformed demon:** "I was in a very lighted place. There were lots of people like me [looking up with surprise]. I must have been in heaven. I recognize the angels."
>
> **Dr. Modi:** "What happened there?"
>
> **Transformed demon:** "I was not very large but I was a loved angel. Everybody liked me. Lucifer told me that I could be bigger than I was. I would have more friends than I have now and I would know more things than I know now. If I wanted, I could go back. I thought I would try.
>
> "So a friend of mine and I walked over. We were very close. Our color changed very fast and we could not go back. We could not even turn around to see the Light. We were being held so we could not turn. They kept on forcing us farther and farther away and the more we went the darker we got [sad]."

Example 5:

Another demon gave the following account.

> **Transformed demon:** "I was in the Light. It was so peaceful. How did I let it change?"
>
> **Dr. Modi:** "Recall."
>
> **Transformed demon:** "I was a strong angel. Lucifer promised me even more strength and things that go with the strength. He told me that I could go back to God and

show off. Once I went to Lucifer, he touched me and I became dark and I could not go back. Then I did not remember anything.

"I was trained in how to take people's strength and energy and make them feel weak and drained."

Example 6:

Transformed demon: "I was in the Light. It was fine for a while, then there was a struggle and I went with the dark one. The struggle was about differences of opinion. It was a struggle over power between God and Lucifer."

Dr. Modi: "Listen carefully and tell me what they are arguing about."

Transformed demon: "Power. Who is going to rule what. Lucifer got angry."

Dr. Modi: "What is he saying to God? Listen carefully."

Transformed demon: "Lucifer is saying that he wants to rule over a certain area. God does not want him to. He said Lucifer is not ready to do that, to have that much power. Lucifer said he would take it and do it anyway."

Dr. Modi: "What?"

Transformed demon: "God is saying that is not what he had in mind for him. He wishes he wouldn't make that choice. If he makes that choice he will have to, in a sense, pay the consequences of the choice. Lucifer is very rebellious and says that he will do it his way, that God does not know everything.

"Lucifer gathers around him as many as he can. He is talking to many Light beings, many angels and other beings of the Light. He is telling them that they can start to rule their own kingdom and eventually they will rule what is currently God's kingdom and eventually he will take it over. The beings are all listening. Many walk away and some do not. Some listen to him and were tricked by him and his followers. I was tricked."

Dr. Modi: "How were you tricked?"

Transformed demon: "It is how he presented things. Things appeared different from how they really were. I did not look to the Light for the answer."

Dr. Modi: "What did he say to you? Listen carefully."

Transformed demon: "He said, 'Come with me and you will be able to see the true Light of creation.' That in a way God was not a true Light and that he had different, brighter Light. He would give me power, peace, and happiness. I believed him and went with him."

Dr. Modi: "As you are going with him, how much of the part of the Light is he taking with him?"

Transformed demon: "At least one fourth of the Light."

Dr. Modi: "As you go with him, what happened to you?"

Transformed demon: "My color changes. I lose my Light and become dark; then I am dark and I get darker and darker. Then I am trapped and cannot see beyond the darkness. I cannot see the Light anymore."

Dr. Modi: "Then what happens?"

Transformed demon: "Then we all work for Satan."

Memories of What Happened When They Went with Satan

Demons after their transformation are often able to recall who and where they were before they went with Satan, and what happened to them after they went with him.

Example 1:

Transformed demon: "After I was tricked into going with Satan, I forgot everything quickly. I could not come back and I ended up being taught and groomed. We were drilled over and over by Satan and his demons about the Light. We were told that if we become the Light, it would be automatic death, like poisoning. Then if we should turn Light, it will be destroyed at the end of the time and we would be dead because the dark is going to win the war anyway."

Dr. Modi: "What else were you told and taught?"

Transformed demon: "We learned how to cause pain. We learned the anatomy of every planet and all the galaxies we thought we could inhabit and possibly have a chance of winning and taking over. We know how to make the earth hurt and scream. We know every fiber of the planet Earth and how to cause it pain. It depends on what your function is going to be in life. If we are supposed to be in people, animals, or plants on this planet or other planets, then we study them and learn how to turn them into the opposite of what they are. We learn how to control them and how to cause pain. Others are groomed for other things and they learn how to control those.

"We are drilled well. It is after a long time of training before we are allowed to do anything. If we fail, we are given tremendous pain so we pay attention the next time. By the time we come down we are very determined not to fail."

Dr. Modi: "What were you trained for?"

Transformed demon: "I was groomed for people or living beings on this planet and on other planets, too. I was not groomed for plants or minerals. I have some general knowledge so that we do not block each other, because we do fight each other for power. A lot of natural disasters are caused this way, through our fighting with each other. We end up making a mess of things on Earth, like the volcanoes and earthquakes, they are partly due to our fighting.

"We feel what you may call an evil power. It feeds on us and we swell up inside. We feel happy in an ugly way. We think we are the greatest. We are the best. There is no death for us. No one is over us. The meaner we are, the more jobs and power we get. This makes other demons look up to us."

Example 2:

> **Transformed demon:** "There are schools where they teach us how to be a good dark one. How to destroy and hurt."
>
> **Dr. Modi:** "How do they teach you?"
>
> **Transformed demon:** "We have teachers who take us along and show us how we can enter people, hurt people, and stay attached to people. There are training schools."
>
> **Dr. Modi:** "What were you trained to do?"
>
> **Transformed demon:** "I was trained to go after the souls who have a great deal of Light, who have a certain kind of healing work and missions to do."
>
> **Dr. Modi:** "What was your goal with this patient?"
>
> **Transformed demon:** "To make her crazy so she wouldn't accomplish her goal."
>
> **Dr. Modi:** "What is her purpose?"
>
> **Transformed demon:** "She has too much Light. She still does not hear her purpose. She rejects her purpose. That makes it easier for us to attach to her."
>
> **Dr. Modi:** "But what is her purpose?"
>
> **Transformed demon:** "To spread the Light and to teach others about the dark ones. That is one of the reasons why Satan wants to destroy her and people like you, so darkness can take over the earth."

Effects of Demon Possession

Demons in my patients claim to cause every type of physical and psychological problems for them.

Physical Symptoms

According to the patient reports, these demons can cause any symptoms from head to toe. Every organ, every tissue, and every part of the body can be infested and afflicted by the demons. They can cause aches and pains, numbness, weakness, and diseases in every organ and every part of the body.

- According to these demons, every physical and emotional pain they suffered with Satan, they project onto the patients.
- Through different types of devices, either inside the body or outside the body, the demons claim to cause aches and pain and other physical problems.
- They claim to interfere with the patients' nerve impulses and chemical processes.
- By pressing and scratching different organs and parts of the body, demons claim to cause physical problems such as pain, numbness, cancer, tumors, and other diseases.

Psychological Symptoms

Demons in my patients claim to be the single most common cause for most psychiatric problems. They cause them directly and indirectly.

- They cause them directly by possessing and influencing a person. They cause various types of problems for people by negatively influencing them, leading to fights, arguments, and drug and alcohol abuse.
- Demons are responsible for keeping the earthbound entities earthbound and for influencing, controlling, and pushing them to attach to different people and cause them different problems.
- Demons are also responsible for all present-life and past-life traumas and problems, thus leading to soul fragmentation. Later they get hold of those soul parts and restimulate the memories and feelings of the traumas, through those soul parts and their connecting cords, creating psychological and physical symptoms for people in the current life.
- Demons in my patients claim to cause all types of psychological symptoms. They project their anger, hate, para-

noia, arrogance, fear, desire for power and position, and violent sadomasochistic behavior onto the people, who then act and behave in the same ways. They can also cause people to curse and use obscene language.

- The demons claim to cause depression, insomnia, panic attacks, violent anger outbursts, chronic fatigue, nervousness, suicidal thoughts, homicidal thoughts, obsessions, compulsions, sexual problems, fears, phobias, etc. They also claim to cause psychotic symptoms such as hallucinations, paranoia, and delusions. They transport these symptoms and feelings through the missing soul parts and their connecting cords and devices. They brag that they give people the desire to take drugs and alcohol. They also claim to cause eating disorders such as anorexia, bulimia, and obesity.

- By absorbing and draining the patients' vital energy, they make them feel constantly tired and drained. They use energy absorbers, a type of black, sticky, liquid type of substance, which can absorb the patients' vital energy, causing chronic fatigue.

- If demons have soul parts of the patients in their possession, they can insert negative thoughts, feelings, visions, voices, paranoia, attitudes, and behavior in the patient through those soul parts and their connecting cords. They can also insert human and demon entities, devices, and energy absorbers through these soul parts and their connecting cords into the patients' bodies, causing them different types of problems. Through those soul parts, the demons can also restimulate traumatic memories from this life and past lives.

- By blocking or shading the patients' Light and blocking their communication with the Light, demons can retard patients' spiritual progress.

- Demons boast about being extraordinarily successful in making people believe that Satan and his demons do not exist. If we know they really exist, we will want to be able to resist their influences and find ways to free ourselves from them. The demons claim they like to keep humans confused about their existence and about what is real and what is not. They brag about being responsible for everything that goes wrong with humans and all the troubles in the universe.

Examples of How Demons Can Cause Emotional and Physical Problems

Demons, when discovered, often boast and brag about how they have affected the patients they are in. After their transformation into the Light, they are more than willing to give us the knowledge of how Satan and his demons affect human beings and what kind of physical and emotional symptoms they have caused for the patients.

Following are descriptions given by some demons in my patients about how they created different types of problems.

Example 1:

One Transformed demon gave the following information:

Transformed demon: "Do you know of the mental illness where people scream and cry a lot? Sometimes they rock back and forth. I did a good bit of that. I hurt their stomach and caused pain. They had to be put away. By causing mental illness, we can cause great disturbances in families for generations, depending on the culture and religion."

Dr. Modi: "How about the different psychotropic medications? How do they affect demons?"

Transformed demon: "It affects us. Sometimes we can block it out and stay dormant. The doctors and patients think they are getting better. Then when the medicine is stopped, we get our strength back. So when that patient is getting better, we get stronger too and begin to create problems again. That is why these people get sick again and again. Sometimes we feel the medicine and we relax and do not fight it. But as long as we are there in the patients, they will be sick again and again."

Dr. Modi: "How about shock treatment?"

Transformed demon: "Sometimes we get shocked out and we come out. Especially if we are on the surface. Sometimes we stay around and come right back in. Other times we just wait till the body chemistry is ready to receive us again and then we go back in. If a demon is not very experienced, it might leave the patient, but another demon is assigned very quickly to the patient.

"But if we are deeply implanted in the deeper layers of the patient, then we just have to take it. It is a kind of punishment for not doing our job better. So we want to fight harder and we gain strength from it. If you really think about it, the medication and electroconvulsive therapy may seem to work initially, but in the long run, as long as we are there, the person will get sick again and again."

Example 2:

One demon in my patient claimed to be a number "7" beast in Satan's hierarchy. He gave the following information about how he and the demons he commanded on the earth and other planets affected people they were in.

Beast Demon: "We can possess and affect every part, every organ, every bone and tissue of your body. We can go in your blood vessels and can cause you high blood pressure, low blood pressure, or circulation problems. We can even affect your hair follicles. We can infest and afflict every part of your mind, body, and soul.

"People afflicted with alcoholism and drug addiction are wonderful to work with. Every time people drink or take drugs, we can easily come in because their auras get weaker. We turn them mean and cause them to

325

hurt others. People with irrational behavior, irrational meanness, irrational cruelty, and irrational yelling usually have a beast and other demons in them.

"The starving and dying people will clutch to anything. We take them all in by telling lies. We tell them everything they want to hear and then get them after they die. They belong to us and we make them work for us. We send them in different people to eat through them and give them weight problems or cause anorexia."

Example 3:

Another demon gave the following account, after its transformation, of how it affected my patient and others.

Transformed demon: "I enter into people and take over their brains and their bodies and I manipulate their thinking and actions. Then they get on the thought and physical pattern, that they accept as their own and it goes on and on. When their brain and bodies are on that pattern, I ask another demon to take over and I go to somebody else. I have trained other dark ones to do this, too.

"I can also cause a type of cancer. Cancer can be due to chemical and biological reasons and it can also be due to the entities. Chemotherapy does not work much on this type of cancer caused by us."

Dr. Modi: "What type of cancer is that?"

Transformed demon: "Stomach and intestinal cancer."

Dr. Modi: "Why doesn't chemotherapy work?"

Transformed demon: "It doesn't make the entities go away. There is another type of disease of the mind that I have trained others to cause. This has to do with humming and constantly recurring noises. This is where we go in and take over the part of the brain and make them hear voices constantly, and they go crazy. Do you realize that the brain has more illnesses than any other parts of the physical body? It is because if you block the brain, you block everything.

"There is a disease of the leg muscles which I trained others to cause. You call it polio. Polio causes pain in legs and can cripple those affected. After releasing the entities, these people may not walk right away, but they will get relief from pain, and later therapy will begin to work.

"I did all this to so many. Now I feel very bad about it. I am sorry for causing all the misery for humans for so long."

Example 4:

One demon, who was in a patient who had rheumatoid arthritis, gave the following account after its transformation of how it affected the patient.

Transformed demon: "I was taught and trained in how to possess people and cause them pain, and that became my job. This fellow here got drunk and we came in. He thought we were rheumatism. We caused him a great deal of pain and made him sick. He should not have taken a drink.

"I also taught other dark beings how to take human beings' strength and make them weak and angry. Men are easy to control because they relate to strength and ego a lot, like those who play sports. They become angry easily and drink alcohol to help them remember the good old days when they were strong. We also cause them to fall and hurt themselves so that they feel weak and then to use alcohol and drugs and abuse their families."

Example 5:

One demon, who claimed to be a very big commander in Satan's hierarchy, gave the following account of how it affected

327

the patient. "I caused him insane anger, a maddening craziness. I do not let him sleep. I am a big commander and I have caused, and trained other demons to cause, insanity, different types of mental illness, murder, rape, Tourette's syndrome, self-mutilation, torture, pyromania, etc.

"Do you realize that mental illness is the greatest cause of death, either self-inflicted or murder? What you people do not realize about mental illness is that some of it is true dysfunction of the brain, but most of it is caused by us demons. We put in people's minds thoughts of torture, such as cutting others and killing babies and other sadomasochistic thoughts.

"Souls get confused and they are grabbed by us after death. We stop them from going to the Light and then we try to trick them into working for Satan. Poor souls, they do not have much choice because they are so confused.

"I have trained millions of other demons, all over, to cause physical problems such as cancer, digestive problems, inflammation, ulcers, circulation problems, heart problems, breathing problems, and pain in every part of the human body. Now I am so ashamed of what I have done. So many people died horrible deaths because of me. Now I feel so sad, mournful, and remorseful. I caused all that to humanity for so long. I am so sorry."

Example 6:

One patient had a very large demon who claimed to be a number "3" beast in Satan's hierarchy. This demon gave the following description of how it caused physical and mental problems for this patient and others from the beginning of time.

> **Demon** [before transformation]: "I caused him bloody pain. I scratched his insides and caused bleeding and pain. I put knots in his organs. I affected the nerves in his organs. I clawed and spit poison through his intestines. I am assigned to him. It is my job to make him miserable and to make sure that he does not achieve

his true potential. I hate him, and in turn, make him hate everybody."

Demon [after transformation]: "I am trained to control humans and cause pain. We all have special talents, training, and jobs. My job is to work deep within the organs and cause hidden pain and discomfort that are not detected easily. I create ulcers, as I did in this person. I can also cause irritation and bleeding.

"Human beings are so grounded in their bodies that it is easy to control them, while it is harder to control beings on other planets because they are not as grounded in their bodies.

"I was very good at my job. I worked well with nerve cells and molecules. I have caused, and trained other demons to cause, ulcers, bleeding, and dysfunction in different organs of the body. We can cause so much pain that people sometimes become insane because they cannot find what is wrong with them. Doctors tell them that it is all in their head and it isn't.

"We can cause dysentery and cancerous growths in the intestine. We cause bleeding by scratching and ripping the organs. When we cannot do that, we rub cells and molecules until they are irritated or until they rip themselves."

Example 7:

A large demon who was in my patient's tongue gave this description.

Demon [before transformation]: "I make him violently angry and irritable. I control his mouth and his tongue. I make him curse, scream, and use foul language. I twist his intelligence, ego, and his psyche."

Demon [after transformation]:[sadly] "I have done tremendous damage to humanity from the very beginning of time. I have caused, and trained others to cause, epilepsy, mental illness that has to do with neurons in the brain not touching each other in the right way.

"I have given people the desire to murder, caused temporary insanity, forced a mother to drown her child, brought to a normal person a murderous rage who then hurt or killed somebody. I used to cause one race to fight another and one religion to fight another religion and caused wars between nations.

"Earth is an angry planet. It is easy to control this planet and the people in it. We can also cause earthquakes, tornadoes, volcanoes, and hurricanes. I feel so ashamed now. I am sorry for what I have done."

Example 8:

One demon in my patient bragged about how demons affect humans when they watch violent, horror, X-rated, and pornographic movies, and listen to music with negative messages.

Demon: "We crowd around people when they are watching violent and horror movies, at home and in the movie theaters. When they become shocked and scared, their shields open and we can enter their bodies. Then we motivate them to watch more of these movies. We also shoot black laser beams into people and send a black, sticky substance. The more people in the movie theater, the greater the negative energy.

"The more they watch these violent movies, the more hardened they get. They develop apathy, indifference, and noncaring attitudes. We make them angry, hateful, insensitive, and cold. They are under our influence like puppets."

Dr. Modi: "How about the X-rated and pornographic movies?"

Demon: "When people watch X-rated and pornographic movies, they lower their vibrations and open their shields for us to come in. Then we give them obsession to watch them more and more. Images are stored in the visual cortex. We can restimulate their visual cortex through a transmitter type of device and give them urges to watch these movies. We also squeeze their testicles and give them inappropriate sexual urges. They seem to focus at the lower level of their vibration and it retards their spiritual development.

"Their concentration is focused outside their partner and weakens their love and relationship. They develop indifference and inability to see their partner as a person. They think of them as an object.

"We can cause teenagers, through these movies, to have sexual obsessions and cause them to become sexually promiscuous and have other problems associated with sex.

"In vulnerable people with anger and hatred toward women, we can push them to be sexually abusive and commit sexual crimes."

Dr. Modi: "How about the music with negative messages?"

Demon: "Here we work through your ears. Focused concentration on music has a mesmerizing effect, almost like hypnosis. The negative messages are accepted as suggestions and are recorded in the auditory cortex. The loud and cacophonous music can open the shield and we can come in and give them more desire to listen to the music and act on the negative messages. We plant into their auditory cortex transmitter type devices, which we can activate from outside the person and replay the negative messages over and over, till they act on them.

"You people do not realize how these movies and music can be addictive in nature and simply shift your focus away from your spiritual growth and mislead you.

"We are the ones who control, motivate, and guide people to make these X-rated, pornographic, violent, and horror movies and write the scripts and lyrics with negative messages. They are under our control and do not even know it."

Dr. Modi: "What role do you play in drug and alcohol addiction?"

Demon: "We play a big role. We work on the groups of children and teenagers. Groups are powerful. We get in through the weak ones. Then we get inside the others when they are open.

"We set up the memories of the good times through the transmitter type of devices into their feeling cortex. We restimulate the memories of highs they had with their friends and motivate them to use drugs and alcohol to achieve the same effects.

"Drinking and using drugs can weaken and open their shields and we can come in and give them a desire to use more and more. We also send into them earth-bound spirits who were addicted to drugs and alcohol, when they were living in their bodies. Once they enter people, they satisfy their addictions through their host. That is why drug and alcohol addicts have a hard time stopping their addictions.

"We control and affect every thought and behavior of human beings. They all are simply like puppets in our hands and we have fun in manipulating them.

"We do not want you to write your book about exposing us. We will do everything to stop you. We will make sure that people do not believe you. So far, we are very successful in making people believe that we do not exist. We do not want people to learn about us and how they can free themselves from us through prayers and other means. It will destroy us and we will do everything in our power to stop you."

Dr. Modi: "You know you cannot stop me."

Demon: "You are no fun. But if we cannot stop you directly, then we will stop you through your family members, friends, and other people around you. We will turn them against you and make them upset and angry with you. We will make you miserable, so miserable that you have no choice but to quit.

"We manipulate some of your patients, secretaries, and other people around you who don't believe we are real, and turn them against you and make them upset and angry with you. We make them believe that it is all hocus-pocus and they should not continue with the treatment, and thus push them into quitting the therapy.

"We are trying to stop you from practicing and doing this work. We will continue to do everything in our power to stop you from writing your books and exposing us."

Dr. Modi: "Well, we will see. God and all of heaven are with me and you cannot do a thing to stop me. The work will be done and the books will be written."

Single Demon Causing a Single Symptom

Sometimes a single demon entity was responsible for causing a single symptom for the patient, and with the removal of the demon, the symptom was completely relieved.

Max complained of severe body odor. In spite of taking a bath several times a day, he still had the odor. Under hypnosis, he found in his chest a large demon entity who claimed to cause him the body odor. The demon explained it as follows:

"Before I came to this person, Satan dipped me into an awful-smelling oil as a punishment, which made me smell bad. Then when I came into this person, he began to have that odor too."

After releasing the demon, Max was free of the odor.

Kathleen had periodic ringing in her right ear for about a year. Under hypnosis, she saw a gray demon blob in her ear. This demon bragged about causing ringing in her right ear by pressing on her right eardrum. After releasing that demon, Kathleen was completely free of the ringing.

Brenda had severe migraine headaches from time to time for two years. During those headaches, she could not tolerate light and noise. Sometimes the headaches would last for hours and sometimes days. Her x-rays and CT scan were normal. Under hypnosis, she found a large black demon which was filling her whole head. It claimed to cause headaches by pressing on her brain and nerves. After releasing the demon entity, Brenda was totally relieved of her headaches.

Jody had recurrent nightmares about a monster chasing him. Under hypnosis, he found a gargoyle type of demon in his head who said that it was the one giving Jody nightmares and had fun doing it. After releasing the demon, Jody did not have nightmares.

A Single Demon Causing Multiple Symptoms

I have seen a single demon entity cause multiple emotional, mental, and physical symptoms for the patients.

Mandy, my secretary, had a very unusual reaction to one of my patients after a phone call, when he said, "I would like to make an appointment to see Dr. Modi." Mandy was frightened and told me that the man gave her the creeps, although he was very polite on the phone.

When this patient came for his first appointment, Mandy closed the window and the door between the waiting room and secretary's room and felt very uncomfortable while he was in the office.

When I saw this patient, he was very pleasant and polite. He was an educated professional man with no signs of psychosis or any type of violent or unusual behavior.

Curious as to what caused this reaction in Mandy, we decided to do a session with Mandy, who under hypnosis found a demon entity in her leg who was causing cramps. This demon entity became very fearful, upset, and distressed when questioned about the new patient who had affected Mandy. The entity expressed that the patient is very dangerous for the demons and should be stopped at all cost.

After releasing that entity, Mandy did not have any cramps in her leg and was not afraid of that patient anymore. It was the demon who was afraid of the patient, and Mandy was experiencing its fear.

Bob, a fifteen-year-old patient, gave a history of being depressed, withdrawn, hyper, and rebellious for about two years. He felt tired and drained most of the time and had a "no care" attitude. He had restless sleep and often had nightmares. He had anger outbursts, destructive behavior, and did not get along with his parents. He also often heard somebody calling his name in a whisper.

About three weeks before he came to my office, Bob felt that something had walked in his head and he began to have headaches and pain in his eyes.

Under hypnosis, as Bob scanned his body, he saw a black blob in his head. It claimed to be a demon. It claimed to come into Bob two years ago, when he was upset. It bragged about making Bob angry and causing him to disobey his parents. It caused him to get into fights and become rebellious. It also made him depressed, tired, and drained and gave him nightmares.

The demon claimed that when Bob started to go to a new church, it had to come out, because the demon could not stand the bright white Light that poured in the church. However, it continued to hang around Bob and influenced him to stay away from studies and to engage in rebellious and destructive behavior. The demon admitted constantly talking to Bob, which caused him to think he was hallucinating.

The demon said that it reentered Bob's body about three weeks before he came to me, when he was upset, and gave him headaches and pain in his eyes. The demon was transformed into the Light and was released to the Light.

After that session, there was a great deal of improvement in his depression, anger, destructive behavior, headaches, eye pain, nightmares, and auditory hallucinations.

Multiple Demons Causing a Single Symptom

Sometimes many demon entities work together to cause a single psychological, physical, or spiritual symptom. Usually the weakness in that part of the body comes from past life traumas, which create openings for the entities to come in.

Nina had a history of sharp shooting pain in her left heel, causing difficulty in walking. Under hypnosis, she located many gray and dark demons in her heel during many sessions. They were packed in multiple layers in her left heel and claimed to cause her pain by pressing on the nerves and tissue.

Joan had multiple large and small demon entities throughout her body. They claimed that they are there to block her from the Light and retard her spiritual growth.

Gary had back pain for several years. As he scanned his back under hypnosis, he found many large and small dark demon entities in his back, arranged in layers. They claimed to cause Gary back pain by pressing on his nerves and spine. Releasing them relieved his back pain.

Multiple Demons Causing Multiple Symptoms

Sometimes multiple demon entities can cause multiple symptoms in a single patient.

Rich was diagnosed as having multiple sclerosis for two years. In addition to depression, he also had double vision, nausea, vomiting, numbness and weakness in both his hands and legs, poor coordination, and such difficulty in walking that he had to use a cane. He had trouble urinating because of a weak bladder. He also had headaches, shoulder pain, and temporomandibular joint pain.

Under hypnosis, as Rich scanned his body, he found many black blobs who claimed to be the demons, who were sent by Satan to create problems for him.

Black blob in the eyes: Claimed to cause double vision by pressing on the optic nerve.

Black blob in the head: Claimed to cause headaches.

Black blob in the jaw: Claimed to cause TMJ symptoms.

Black blob in the neck and both shoulders: Claimed to cause neck and shoulder pain.

Black blob in the right hand: Claimed to cause numbness in the right hand by pressing on the nerves.

Black blob in the stomach: Claimed to cause nausea and vomiting.

Black blob in the bladder: Claimed to cause bladder problems by pressing on it.

Black blobs in both legs, ankles, and feet: They all claimed to cause numbness by pressing on the nerves.

All those black demon entities were transformed and released from Rich and the whole body was cleansed, healed, and filled with the Light, with the help of the angels.

During the next session, Rich reported a great deal of improvement in his condition. He was able to walk without a cane and at times was even able to run. His headaches, double vision, shoulder pain, TMJ symptoms, nausea, and vomiting were improved a great deal. His bladder weakness and weakness in his hands improved about 50 percent. He was more energetic and less depressed.

Rachel had been treated for schizophrenia off and on since she was a teenager. She was in and out of mental hospitals. She had auditory and visual hallucinations, paranoid ideations, violent behavior, anxiety attacks, and nightmares and was using drugs and alcohol. She was taking large doses of antipsychotic medications, tranquilizers, and sleeping pills, but she still continued to have her symptoms.

We decided to check Rachel for any possessing spirits. Under hypnosis, she saw many dark demon beings who bragged that they gave her anxiety attacks, nightmares, violent anger outbursts, desire to take drugs and drink alcohol, paranoid ideations, and hallucinations. They all claimed they constantly talked to her and fed her negative thoughts and behavior and pushed her to act on her negative impulses. Many of them claimed to have joined her when she was taking drugs and alcohol.

After she released all the entities, most of her symptoms improved and we were able to cut down on her medication. She was able to stop using the drugs, but unfortunately could not stop using alcohol. Every time she began to drink, a new group of demon entities came in and gave her psychotic symptoms. We spent many sessions releasing the new entities. They all bragged, "This one is easy to control. We can influence her even from outside to drink and when she does, it opens her up for us to come in. And then we work on driving her crazy by giving her those symptoms all over again. As long as she drinks, she will always be under our control."

Although she was symptom-free for several weeks after each releasement session, she could not stay away from drinking. Even drinking one beer opened her shield, allowing new groups of entities to come in and create the symptoms all over again. The entities took a great deal of pleasure in driving her crazy.

Degree of Demon Possession

Based on what my patients have reported, there are two types of demon possession: partial and total.

Partial demon possession: According to my hypnotized patients, demons have only partial control over them. They can inhabit a part of their body and cause them physical and emotional problems, but they do not have full control over patients' minds, bodies, and souls. Patients still have their will. Most of the patients I see in my practice belong in this category.

Total demon possession: This phenomenon is extremely rare. In it, a person is totally taken over by the demon. The demon completely controls a person's mind, body, and soul. In this case, the demon is walking, talking, and acting at all times through the person.

The person's soul is still there. It is not removed; it is not destroyed. It is totally under the control of the demon. It becomes the property of the demon. The demon completely surrounds the person's soul, just as when the demon has completely surrounded and trapped the earthbound entity which then is completely dominated by the demon. Here the demon simply represents the person.

The person has to cooperate and be willing to allow total possession at some level of his or her being and consciousness; otherwise, Satan and his demons cannot take total control over the person.

Extent of Effects Due to Demon Possession

Patients describe the extent of the effects due to demon possession as follows:

- At the very least, a demon can influence a patient emotionally or physically.
- When people dull themselves with drugs and alcohol and lose some control of their minds and bodies for a short period of time, a demon can partially take over and make them say or do things that they normally would not do. They can make people act violently, verbally or physically, toward the people around them. Sometimes demons claim to make a person rape, kill, or hurt someone and commit other criminal acts.
- When a demon owns a part of person's soul, it is easier for the demons to take partial control of him or her, at least for a short period of time.
- In cases of total possession, the person's mind, body, and whole soul are completely under the control of the demon. It is the demon who is walking, talking, and acting through the person at all times. This situation is rare.

Experience of Demon Possession

Patients describe the experience of possession by the demon entities as follows:

- Most of the time patients are not even aware of any possession except under hypnosis. They have no perception of the existence of the demons in them and they are not even aware of any problems caused by them. They attribute the problems caused by the demons as their own.

- Sometimes patients report that they hear this voice, which is negative, evil, maniacal, and separate and distinct from theirs.
- Sometimes persons may be aware of something evil in them controlling them. They may say or do things that they feel they have no control over, and sometimes they have no memory of what they did.

Light and Beings of the Light

Under hypnosis, patients often describe seeing a brilliant white Light and the beings of the Light in it, especially while we are working with earthbound and demon spirits. Patients who are going through a past life regression also give similar descriptions of seeing a brilliant white Light and beings of Light coming to help them after the death of their physical body. Even people who have gone through a near-death experience give a similar description of the Light and the Light beings, with or without hypnosis.

Usually, patients see a very brilliant, dazzling, shimmering, white Light coming from above, beyond the ceiling and beyond the sky. This Light is described as very bright, even brighter than the sun, but it does not hurt the eyes. They see the Light coming from what looks like heaven to them. Sometimes they can see and describe the gates of heaven and one or more angels guarding it.

Beings of the Light: According to my patients, Light and beings of the Light almost always appear when we deal with earthbound entities and demon entities. These Light beings usually are seen by my patients in forms familiar to them, depending on their religious and cultural beliefs. So a person who is a Christian will often report seeing Jesus, the Virgin Mary, St. Peter, and different archangels, such as Michael, Gabriel, Raphael, and other angels. A person who is a Hindu may see

Krishna, Rama, or Shiva, while a Buddhist may see Buddha, and a Moslem may see Mohammed or Allah in the Light.

To my patients, these beings of Light appear as pure white Light, but have recognizable forms. Other times they appear in white robes, completely surrounded by the Light. Archangel Michael is sometimes seen as a large angel with wings and sometimes armored with a sword and a shield. Sometimes the Light beings appear as just beings of pure white Light without form. Other times they appear to be dressed ornately. They may have a golden Light or white Light in them and around them and they may be wearing white or golden robes, depending on their level in the Light, with golden being the highest.

Some patients report seeing angels who claim to be their guardian angels, who are always with them, protecting them. Most patients claim to have one or more guardian angels. According to the patients, the angels have never been human.

Some patients report seeing beings of the Light who look like humans and who claim to be their spirit guides from the Light. Their job is to guide patients and help them in this life. They usually provide spiritual guidance, love, and support to the person. Patients report having anywhere from one to four or more guides from heaven, depending on the purpose of the person here on the earth. Patients often say that they have known from their past lives some of the guides who have chosen to be their guides during this life. These heavenly guides are often connected with the same Godhead with whom the patient is connected.

Sometimes patients report seeing their deceased loved ones in the Light. Usually they appear as wearing white robes and are totally surrounded by the Light. These loved ones look and feel to the patients as very real—young and healthy, even though they may have been old or sick or crippled when they died.

Patients see and describe the representation of God as a being of pure Light and love, or as a pyramid of Light, a mountain of Light, a ball of Light, or an ocean of Light and love. They call God: the one, the whole, all there is, the all, etc.

341

Often people see a silver thread or cord of Light going from themselves to what they describe as one of the masters, the Godhead or the oversoul, and then to God. Patients sometimes describe the representation of God as a powerhouse with millions and millions of cords coming out of it and going to different people and beings all over the creation. Patients often describe seeing this connection between them, Godheads, and God. It helps them to realize that they are always connected and in touch with their Godhead and God.

Patients sometimes describe heaven opening up during a session, when they can see the whole heaven, and the hierarchy of the heaven inside. They report a big mountain of Light on the top, which is so bright that they cannot look at it. They describe this mountain of Light as God. Next to that they see Godheads of our world. Patients often recognize them as different religious figures from different religions from all over the world. Next to them, they see different types and levels of angels with different shapes and forms. Sometimes patients report that on the other side of God there are Godheads, angels, and beings of other worlds and other planets.

During the sessions, when patients see angels or other beings of the Light, the angels are usually totally surrounded by the brilliant white Light. Love and peace radiate from them. Their eyes are very loving and kind. Their hands, when touched and held, feel warm and real.

During the session, these beings of the Light almost always come instantly when requested, and guide us and help us.

Devices

I have become used to my patients reporting that they have either a human or a demon entity within them. It came as a surprise to me, however, when one of my patients, **David**, reported seeing machinelike inert devices in his neck, back, and shoulders. It intrigued me, so I asked David, under hypnosis, to examine the so-called devices closely. David said that these devices had a metal-looking appearance.

As we were trying to figure out what to do with those devices, David said the angels of the Light were there. One of them identified himself as the archangel Raphael. He said that these devices needed to be removed and destroyed and that he could do it for us.

Raphael described those things as spiritual devices, which were put in David by the demons when his neck was jerked in a car accident. They created pain in his neck, back, and shoulders. David had had severe pain in his neck, back, and shoulders since the accident. His physical examination and x-rays of his neck, back, and shoulders were normal. His doctor could not find anything physically wrong with him although his pain continued and was so severe that he required pain medications and muscle relaxants.

David saw angels removing those devices from him and dismantling and destroying them. He also said that the angels were scrubbing, cleansing, and healing his neck, back, and shoulders, removing any negative effects from those devices, filling those parts of his body with the Light, and smoothing and strengthening his energy field. The angels also told him to ask them every day to cleanse, heal, and fill those parts of his body with the Light and to regularly pray for protection and guidance.

David saw angels putting a special shield around him in addition to the bubble of Light and spiritual mirrors. To him this looked like three layers of wire mesh net overlapping each other. It was made up of spiritual substances.

Raphael suggested that this shield could prevent demonic influences from the inert devices. David was told to make sure to request the angels to shield the cord, which is our connection with the Light, too, but not to block the part of the cord that is in the Light. Otherwise, guidance from the Light would be blocked as well. Amazingly, these shields were very effective in warding off the demonic influences through different devices.

David felt an immediate improvement in his neck, back, and shoulders. The pain was completely cured within the next twenty-four hours. He did not need any pain medication or muscle relaxants after that session.

Occasionally, in spite of all those shields, Satan and his demons were able to create some interferences. So the angels put in place for David another special shield, which looked like an aluminum metallic case, although it was made up of a spiritual substance. According to the angels, it would eliminate all but a very tiny fraction of the demonic attacks.

But they warned that these shields—the triple mesh net and metallic shields—would also block the communication and guidance from the Light. We should make sure to ask the angels to put these shields in place when needed and to remove them when they are not needed.

Angels said that Satan has many black communication centers throughout the creation and there are black cords going to different people and places throughout the whole world and the creation, which affects everybody negatively. We should routinely, in our prayers, ask angels to cover and destroy all of Satan's communication centers with a blanket of Light, cut their connections with Satan, his demons, people and places, and destroy them.

Angels also said that our souls are connected to God with silver cords and the attacks can also come through those cords, if they are damaged and have holes. So we should make sure to ask the angels to cleanse, heal, and shield the cords, too, while shielding the body and energy field. Angels said that if we ask to be shielded in this manner, this would ward off 99 percent of Satan's influences.

Under hypnosis, patients often report finding different types of devices in their bodies and in their surroundings. According to the patients, Satan and his demons can build these devices for practically any purpose. They range from small single-purpose devices, such as a metal-looking bar, clamp, or fork used to cause aches and pains, to more complex crushing devices intended to interfere with the function of different parts of the body.

They report that devices can be single-purpose, causing one symptom or problem, or they can be multi-purpose, creating multiple problems. They can also be remote devices. They are actually spiritual devices, but they have a physical effect on the patient. Patients say that these devices affect nerves, chemical processes, hormone production, and the operation of the physical body. When these devices are removed, the patients' symptoms sometimes disappear almost immediately.

Different Types of Devices

Physical Displacement Devices

Physical displacement devices are mechanical devices that push, pull, or apply pressure. They are of different sizes and shapes, each tailored for a specific job in a certain person. These cause physical displacement which is constant once they are put into place. Physical displacement devices can throw a joint off by a fraction, put pressure on a nerve, or squeeze two bones together tighter than they should be and cause them to grate and scrape together. They may separate two bones in a joint and allow fluid to seep in where it does not belong, or they can put pressure on a nerve junction.

Active displacement devices: These are seen to be screws or pointed rods that simply shove normal tissue out of the way or press the part, and thus cause pain and dysfunction in different parts of the body.

Passive displacement devices: These are remotely controlled devices that sit passively in the patient. They affect the person only when they are activated from outside. Three types of passive displacement devices are reported.

Devices resembling a radio receiver: This is reported to resemble a radio receiver. The demons "broadcast" thoughts and information to the device, which conveys the information to the patient.

Radio receiver action device: This is similar to the radio receivers above, except that there is an action part included in it. It may have a plunger that can stick out, and an arm that can twist, or some part that can perform a simple motion.

Silver rod: This type of receiving device is a silver rod that can release a stimulating electric current along the nerves when the demons activate it.

Focusing and Amplifying Devices

Under hypnosis, some patients have reported different types of devices that Satan and his demons use to focus their thoughts on human beings to influence them:

Focusing dish: Under hypnosis, patients have reported demons operating a focusing dish. It is like a parabolic dish with a rod sticking out of the center, resembling a satellite dish. The demons use it to focus their thoughts on a human being to influence them.

Wave machine: Patients have reported that one demon operates a single-wave transmitting device aimed at the patient. The machine projects the thoughts of the demon on the patient.

Standing wave machine: According to the patients, two demons are needed to operate this apparatus. It consists of two stations set up on opposite sides of the human target. The demons aim their thoughts into the device and it sets up a sort of standing wave through the human. It is more effective and has greater ability to influence a person than the single-wave machine.

Energy Absorbers

Black energy absorbers: These appear to consist of a black sticky substance that coats different parts of the body, primarily the nervous system, and interferes with its functioning. It also interferes with spiritual impulses from the Light, and blocks out the Light itself.

The energy absorbers have a physical effect by dampening and interfering with nerve impulses. They affect primarily by absorbing patients' energy, making them chronically fatigued, sluggish, and sleepy. They can also interfere with their memory and thinking, which becomes sluggish and slow.

Linda, a thirty-year-old female, had a history of chronic fatigue. She also had difficulty in staying awake after eight or nine at night. No matter where she was or with whom, she would fall asleep almost like a child and had difficulty waking up. At times she had this problem even during the daytime. Her doctors could find nothing wrong, and all her laboratory tests were within normal limits, including her thyroid test. Under hypnosis, as she looked inside her body, she found her brain, spinal cord, and nerves covered with black, sticky, inert stuff, which she called energy absorbers. This substance absorbed her energy and made her sleepy, chronically tired, and drained. She stated that the angels, with some difficulty, removed the sticky substance from her nervous system. They scrubbed and cleansed her whole body and filled it with the Light. After that session, Linda reported that for the first time in her life she was feeling energetic and did not have an uncontrollable sleepy feeling.

Yellow-green slime: This substance is used primarily inside the digestive tract. It has the physical effect of interfering with digestion and nutrient absorption. It also causes discomfort and sometimes even pain.

Remote Spiritual Devices and Centers

Black umbrella or curtain: This is a remote device that is placed between the person and the Light to prevent spiritual strength and guidance from the Light.

Bob, during a session, was feeling alert, awake, and energetic at the beginning of the session, while we were discussing what happened during a prior session. Then all of a sudden, just before we tried to proceed with hypnotherapy, he said he was feeling very tired and felt as though something were pressing on his head, causing a headache. He was not able to focus on the session. As he looked inside his head and the rest of his body, it appeared to be brightly lit and there were no entities, negative energies, or devices. So he looked around outside his body. He saw a black umbrella type of device above his head that was making him feel tired and sleepy and blocking his guidance from the Light. After removing that device, Bob felt an immediate change. His headache and sleepiness improved right away and he was able to do the session without any further problems.

Command centers and communication centers: According to the patients, these are set up in another dimension by Satan and his demons. Patients describe them as command centers, observation centers, and communication centers. To the patient, they appear as large blobs of darkness, of different shapes (often triangular) and different sizes. Patients describe hundreds and thousands of black or gray cords or ropes coming out of these centers and going to different people, places, and objects all over the world. They are also connected to Satan and his demons, who control and influence different people and places throughout the world through these centers and their connections. Patients also see, inside those centers, one or more demons, who control them.

During a session, when we asked the angels for help and guidance about what to do, the patient said these angels of Light cut off all the connections between the centers and the people and places and Satan and his demons. They also destroyed the centers by covering them with large blankets of Light.

I found it to be an effective technique to have angels cut all the cords, wires, tubes, or connections they see between them, the demons, Satan, and these centers. Surprisingly, many patients report seeing them. The technique works every time, releasing patients' symptoms.

Patients also report that Satan can re-create these devices and communication centers as soon as we destroy them. It seems like a never-ending battle, but again and again patients reported that the angels told them to pray daily for protection and to request to destroy those centers throughout creation and for removal of everything from them that does not belong with them and that will make patients less than what they should be in God's plan.

Focusing and Amplifying Thoughts on the Patients

Focusing thoughts through a group of demons: In this method of remote influencing, no equipment is needed. A group of demons focuses their thoughts on a human target.

Angelo, a thirty-eight-year-old man, was a good subject and was able to do spirit releasement and past life regression without any problem. During one session, as we were trying to do hypnotherapy, he just could not do it. He felt for some reason he could not tune into anything. He was being blocked somehow. He scanned his body, the whole office, and our surroundings, but there was nothing. As he searched for the problems, he saw many groups of demons at a distance. They all were focusing their thoughts on Angelo, blocking and confusing his thoughts and vision. The demons claimed they did not want Angelo to succeed with his treatment and that Angelo was coming close to his healing and gaining other knowledge. Satan wanted to stop him from succeeding in his treatment, and tried to discourage him by blocking him. We requested angels to collect the demon entities who were trying to interfere in the net of Light and help them to the Light or bind them into space so they could not interfere again.

After removing the interfering demons, he had no trouble regressing to the source of his problems.

Focusing and amplifying thoughts of Satan worshipers: This involves a group of demons focusing and amplifying onto the patients the thoughts and intents of groups of human Satan worshipers.

Belinda, a thirty-year-old female, was also a good subject and had no problems doing spirit releasement or regression therapy. During one session, she felt totally blocked and did not receive any thoughts. She scanned her body and the office, which were clear and lighted. She saw a group of demons at a distance focusing on a group of human Satan worshipers and amplifying their negative thoughts onto her, thus blocking her and interfering with her treatment. After the angels removed those demons and shielded the office, Belinda was able to do the regression without any problems.

Effects of Devices

The effects of the devices on patients are the same as the effects of the possessing demons, only they are not as strong and pronounced. According to the patients, Satan and his demons can create practically every type of device for any and every purpose.

Demons can create devices to cause just about any type of physical problem. They can create devices to cause aches and pains, chronic fatigue, and the malfunctioning of different parts and organs of the body. Through these devices and energy absorbers, they can drain or absorb patients' energy and cause patients to feel tired and drained. Sometimes patients report devices that are used to make them sleepy or drowsy in their day-to-day life and even during a session. Sometimes, even when we are simply talking, devices are used to make them sleepy to distract them from hearing what has been said.

Demons can also create devices to cause every type of psychological problem. They can insert thoughts, attitudes, voices, visions, and obsessions through the devices. They can create devices to cause problems with memory and concentration. They can project visions to distract patients, especially during sessions.

Josephine had bulimia for several months. As she struggled to control her eating habits, a food commercial was projected through devices onto her mind and she would become obsessed with those foods and would eat them till she was ready to throw up.

Susan had frequent pains in her shoulder all her life. She saw a stapler type of device, which had many teethlike projections instead of just two. She saw that this device was connected to a power pack, which in turn was connected by a cord to a main switchboard in hell, like a control room that looked like a sound booth in a TV station. She called it "hell's control room."

It was filled with very sophisticated equipment that was operated by black demons. The switchboard was connected with various devices in people all over the earth. Demons controlled the device in Susan's shoulder by activating the circuit so it squeezed her shoulder around the joint and surrounding muscles and connective tissue, causing her great pain. After she removed the device from her shoulder, her pain was relieved.

Gina had chronic back pain all her life. She found a rodlike device in her back, which demons twisted and squeezed remotely from a control room in hell. Her pain was relieved after removing and destroying the device and the control room.

Jodi found clamplike devices that were clamping the cords connected to the soul parts that she lost from her eyes. The effect was vision problems, which improved right away after removing the clamps.

Julia began, during a session, to have severe pain in her eyes and could not stand to look at the Light. She found teethlike clamps being put in her eyes during the session when she became overtly sad and compassionate for a friend and began to cry. This opened her shield and demons were able to insert those clamps.

Randy, under hypnosis, saw black blocks or monolith-type devices being placed outside his home. They looked like polished stones, in different sizes, and black as coal. They were like barriers. There was also a star-shaped radio tower, a satellite-type device that broadcasted negative thoughts and ideas and created problems between him and his family.

He also saw a billboard-shaped device near a pine tree in front of his home. It looked like an advertising billboard that flashed different types of negative thoughts and messages. At our request, angels destroyed all the devices from all around the house and filled his home with brilliant, hot white Light. They also put a bubble of Light around his home and covered it with the reflective mirrors and rays of blinding, hot, vibrant white Light. According to Randy, the whole house looked like a bright, hot afternoon sun. We also requested the angels to stay on guard around his home and protect it from the negative influences.

Judy, during a past life regression session, began to remember a past life story very vividly, but then suddenly went blank, with no pictures and no memory. As we began to locate the source of her block, she saw Satan at a distance, holding up a black curtain. He was using it as a curtain between Judy and the Light, creating

DEMONIC DEVICES AROUND RANDY'S HOUSE AS DRAWN BY PATIENT.

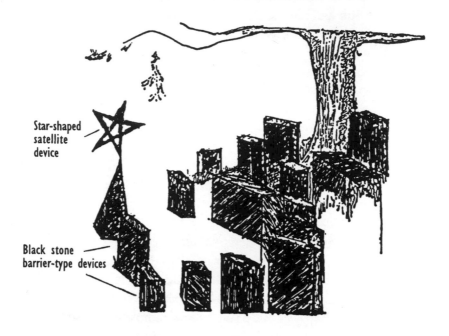

DIFFERENT TYPES OF DEMONIC DEVICES AS DRAWN BY DIFFERENT PATIENTS.

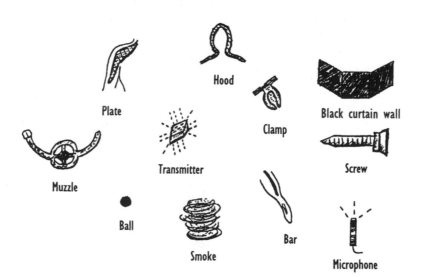

a block in her memories. He did not want her to succeed with her treatment and be free of his influences. At our request, the angels removed Satan and created a shield of blinding, hot, vibrant, white Light so neither Satan nor his demons were able to interfere during the session.

Tim had hearing problems from time to time and doctors could find nothing wrong with him. Under hypnosis, he saw that demons were clamping the cords connected to the soul parts he had lost from his ears and thus blocking his hearing. The clamps were removed and destroyed and all the lost soul parts were brought back, cleansed, healed, and integrated with his ears with the help of the angels. Afterward, Tim did not have any hearing problems.

Cleansing and Healing

While working with earthbound and demon entities, my patients often describe angels of the Light cleansing, healing, and filling them with the Light. They say that the space where the spirits or devices were should be immediately cleansed, healed, and filled with the Light, otherwise Satan and his demons will put another entity or device in that space.

I routinely ask the angels to cleanse and heal the person by scrubbing every part and every organ of the patient's body, removing all the negative entities, energies, and devices, and any leftover residue. Then I ask them to fill the person with the brilliant, white, liquid Light and shield the body with the bubble of white Light and cover it with the spiritual mirrors and rays of blinding hot white Light. Each patient describes the cleansing process in different ways, but the basic idea is the same—cleansing and healing. The following are some of the descriptions of cleansing and healing given by different patients.

"I see big angels scrub and scour and heal by touching, mostly with wands, almost like laser beams. Sometimes they heal just by touching with their hands. They are more sedate and dignified and very sweet and gentle in their touch. They go through the body very systematically and carefully, touching with a laser wand and healing."

"The angels are wrapping my shoulders in a cosmic Light-filled 'Ace bandage.' This bandage, filled with the Light, brings heat and healing to the shoulders."

"I see a number of little baby angels with wings. They giggle and wiggle and slip and slide and throw water on each other and they generally delight in the task. They are very conscientious and take their task seriously and their little bodies are healing in themselves. They slip and slide as on a water slide through the body and their touch heals as they slide. They tip over buckets and throw sponges and bubbles fly everywhere. They are generally mischievous. They wait to be called, like a bunch of kinder-gartners waiting to be let out for recess. They play 'hide and seek' while they cleanse. They have the *best* time while they cleanse and heal."

"Angels are taking a hose and washing out all the negative entities and energies with the liquid Light, as if washing all the dust and dirt out."

"It is like the commercial of Mr. Bubble. The angels are scrubbing and cleansing and there are bubbles all over."

"Angels put these balls of Light in my body that they move up and down in the body, telepathically from outside. As these balls of Light move all through the body, they cleanse and heal the body."

"They are like spiritual doctors and nurses with white coats. They scrub and cleanse the damaged parts and wash them with the Light. Sometimes they bandage the parts with the bandage made up of Light. Other times they just use wands like laser beams to heal."

"I see the angels with buckets and sponges. They are methodically scrubbing and removing anything that is negative and then filling the whole body with the white Light and shining it."

"There are many angels. They are washing the whole body with the Light. Then they are coating every part of the body with white Light, as if whitewashing the walls."

Results of Spirit Releasement

Perhaps the first and most dramatic result of this therapy that patients realize is the aftermath of spirit releasement. Often there is an immediate relief from the emotional and physical symptoms caused by the possessing spirits. Most often these are the same acute symptoms that have caused the patient to seek therapy to begin with. Often, lifelong physical, emotional, and mental symptoms, troubling thoughts, behaviors, even addictions, disappear following a releasement session, as entities leave and pack their problems along with them.

Often, when a releasement session is intense and long, patients report feeling drained immediately following the session. This initial fatigue, however, has consistently evolved into an increased feeling of energy and a sense of well-being within forty-eight hours. Patients then report feeling more alive and energetic than they have ever felt before.

Others report feeling "empty" or "light," as though they had lost weight. Some say they can breathe more easily, or that a great weight has been lifted off their shoulders or chest. Some patients experience postsession feelings of loneliness, or even grief over the lost spirits. Most report immediate and positive changes in their close relationships with family and friends. It is not uncommon for people to disbelieve what they have seen or said under hypnosis. Despite this tendency to mistrust or disbelieve what they themselves reported, the positive changes occur. And this is, after all, the point of therapy: positive changes and healing.

Possession by the Entities (Spirits)
from Another Planet

Sometimes patients report that they have with them beings from other planets who create physical and emotional problems.

Barbara, a twenty-year-old female, reported seeing spaceships and little people with emerald-green eyes, who were "awful looking." They were constantly moving in her head, giving her headaches and difficulty in concentration and memory. She was also having trouble sleeping and was feeling tired and drained. She had crying spells, poor appetite, nausea, and vomiting. She was becoming very nervous and depressed. These symptoms continued for several months.

Under hypnosis, Barbara reported seeing the same little people in her head. These so-called little people claimed to be from another planet. They said that their planet was destroyed and somehow they ended up on the earth and joined Barbara. After some therapy they were released back to the Light. Barbara also had a few earthbound entities who were released.

Afterwards, Barbara did not see or feel those little people in her head anymore. She was able to sleep and eat well and did not have any nausea, vomiting, headaches, or depression.

Possession by Animal Spirits

Occasionally people report having animal spirits with them.

Becky was going through severe depression and had repetitive dreams about chickens. She said that as a little girl her parents used to kill chickens, and she had to help them. She hated it. Under hypnosis, she saw spirits of those chickens inside her. After releasing the spirits of chickens to the Light, she did not have those dreams anymore.

Linda found the spirit of her pet dog inside her as a possessing entity. It was released to the Light.

Summary

If we look at the results of my research in Chapter X, seventy-seven out of a hundred patients reported having demons in them who were responsible for the psychological and physical symptoms for which they were seeking help. With the removal of these so-called demons, the associated symptoms caused by them were often cleared up immediately.

My patients often reported having one or more demons in them. Sometimes they mentioned being infested by hundreds of them, like having freckles all over their body. Frequently patients are able to give physical descriptions of these demons, including their shapes, sizes, and colors.

According to my patients, these demons most commonly appear as black, red, or gray blobs in round, pyramid, or geometric shapes. They can also appear in any form that is in keeping with the patients' own ideas of what a demon should look like. Some patients report them in scary forms—a monster, a devil with horns, beast, giant, dragon, Dracula, gargoyle, evil-looking humanoid forms, lizards, bats, snakes, etc. Their purpose is to cause fear in the patients. If these demons have eyes, they appear as dark, black, red, blank, cold, evil, like empty holes, vacant, piercing, and sinister-looking.

Sometimes patients report that these demons, when they appear outside them, can be very deceiving and can even take the form of Light beings with loving eyes and can create the illusion of the light around them. However, they cannot stay in that form for more than a few seconds to a few minutes. They quickly change into black and evil-looking beings. The illusion of the light around them quickly disappears. Their hands, when touched, feel cold and bony.

Patients claim that these demons occupy different parts of their bodies, causing symptoms in those parts of the body. Sometimes patients report that these demons are arranged in many layers in their bodies, one on top of another. In these cases, after we release the top layer of the demons and their associated symptoms, the patients may appear clear and free of their problems. But during the next session, patients report having a new set of symptoms, which are called the tertiary symptoms. When they look inside, they find new demon entities causing the new set of symptoms.

Some patients are so totally infested by these demons, in multiple layers, that it seems to be a never-ending and exhausting process for the patients and for me. But with the patients' determination, we can free them from their longstanding affliction.

Sometimes patients report the demons are completely surrounding their bodies and auras, influencing and blocking them from the Light. Other times, they claim that demons have one or more fragmented parts of their souls in their possession, either inside the patients' bodies or outside.

Patients describe these demons in different sizes, from tiny dots to giant creatures. They can be conversed with, through the patients, with the patients' permission. Under hypnosis, during conversation, the so-called demons initially appear as cold with no hint of power, purpose, or intent. As these demons talk, their anger, hate, and arrogance come through.

These demons sometimes claim to be organized by ranks and are assigned duties on the basis of their abilities and power. Some large demons claim to train and command other demons; after their transformation they are willing to call all of them, numbering sometimes in millions, from all over the earth and other planets, so they can also transform into the Light and go to heaven, too.

When initially located, demons brag of holding a very high rank in Satan's hierarchy. Only after their transformation do they admit or realize they were not as large and powerful as they thought. They realize this delusion of power was fed to them mostly by Satan and was partly self-induced. They also realize that Satan lied about their rank.

Patients describe these demons as ugly, sly, sneaky, mean, cold, underhanded, hostile, angry, hateful, and belligerent. They lie constantly. They curse and use obscenities and like to brag about how they have affected and tormented the patients they are in. Sometimes they make patients convulse, shake, jerk, froth at the mouth, spit, hiss, growl, and threaten to kill the patients and me.

They hide inside the body and try hard not to be discovered. They claim that Satan is their master and they are assigned to the patients to cause them physical, mental, emotional, and spiritual problems. They say that Satan wants every soul he can get and their job is to confuse and manipulate people's spirituality.

Demons say that when they are discovered by us it is considered by Satan to be a failure on their part, and they are punished by Satan even worse than before. They do not want to go back to Satan at any cost. When dealing with these so-called demons, patients always report the presence of a brilliant white Light and the angels of the Light in it. Demons, when surrounded by the Light, react violently to it. They claim Satan told them to stay away from the Light because it will kill or burn them or they will vanish.

When asked to look inside their being, the demons always find a spark of Light within. They claim they had no idea it was there; as they look at that spark, they cannot take their eyes off of it. In no time the Light grows and they become the beings of pure Light. Their darkness disappears.

After the demons' transformation, they recall being in the Light, in heaven, just after their creation. They remember a conflict between God and a large being who they say was Lucifer. Lucifer chose to leave the Light and many Light beings went with him. According to my patients, Lucifer and those beings are really Satan himself and his demons. Some demons remember going with Satan because he promised them power, while others were tricked into going with him.

These demons often recall that as they went from the Light with Satan, they became dark and completely forgot about the Light in them and who they were. They claim that in the darkness they were trained and tutored about how to possess humans and other beings and how to cause them physical, emotional, mental, and spiritual problems, then eventually bring their souls to Satan so that he could win over the Light, and God.

These demons claim to cause a wide range of emotional, mental, and physical problems from head to toe. Amazingly, releasing those demons frees the patients from their crippling problems.

The demons claim to affect the patients in many different ways. They can cause aches and pains in any part of their bodies by pressing on the nerves and by tampering with the nerve impulses and interfering with them. They plant negative thoughts, visions, voices, and attitudes in patients. They can cause every type of psychiatric problem, including depression, psychosis, chronic fatigue, obsessive-compulsive behaviors, paranoia, anxiety attacks, phobias, sexual problems, drug addictions, alcoholism, sadomasochism, personality disorders, behavioral problems, attention deficit disorders, etc.

Demons claim to implant the thoughts of anger, hate, jealousy, paranoia, murder, suicide, rape, and torture in people and push them to act on them. They claim to cause anything that is negative or wrong in the human personality, and take a great deal of pleasure in doing it.

These demons also claim to absorb patients' energy, causing them chronic fatigue and depression. They also cause problems by interfering with the chemical process in the body. Patients say that these demons block their communication and guidance from the Light (heaven), then confuse and misguide them from the purpose they plan for this life and retard their spiritual progress.

These demons claim that their first and foremost objective is to make sure humans do not notice them and do not have any knowledge of their existence. They boast that they are extraordinarily successful at this. They say that humans are too tied up with the physical world, considering it to be the real world, and losing sight of what is real and what is not. Those who do not deny the existence of Satan and his demons are made afraid of them.

By dealing with these demons under hypnosis and freeing themselves from their negative influences, patients gain a great deal of knowledge about them and the illusion of their power. It gives patients self-confidence and understanding that Satan and his demons have only as much power as they give them. My patients have told me repeatedly that with the help of God and his angels, they are more powerful than these demons and Satan. They say that the basis of their power lies in God and must be applied in God's name. The necessity for divine intervention is important, because we are simply too human to deal directly with Satan and his demons.

My research clearly shows that earthbound and demon entities are the most common cause for depression, but additionally, the facts lead to the conclusion that demons are the single leading cause for psychiatric problems in general, directly and indirectly. Directly, demon entities cause problems by attaching to people or through the earthbound entities, who are also possessed and influenced by demon entities. The demons inside the possessing earthbound entities can also affect the patients directly. They can also use devices and energy absorbers to cause depression and other emotional and physical problems. When the demons have fragmented soul parts of the patients in their possession, they can insert negative thoughts, attitudes, and visions, as well as negative energies, entities, and devices inside the patients, causing them every type of physical and emotional problem. So Satan and his demons directly and indirectly are the single most common cause of psychiatric problems.

Unlike in traditional exorcism, in therapy these demons are treated as secondary patients who are fearful, confused, in pain, and in need of healing. They are treated with concern, compassion, and understanding. Through therapy, they are helped in finding their true identity and are transformed into beings of pure white Light. They are then sent to heaven, with angels, with love. There is no judgment by the patients, the therapist, or the beings of the Light. They are greeted in heaven with love and joy, as if they are reunited with a long lost family.

It is important to note that because of our human frailty, most people are open to possession and, indeed, are possessed at some point in their life. But the possessing entity is not a forever, essential part of us; it can be released. Although the possessed person takes on the problems, symptoms, and negative behaviors of the possessing entity, it is important to remember that an individual's essential state is one of goodness and Light. Having demon spirits within a person does not mean that the person is evil or not loved by God.

I want to stress again that none of this information is coming from any religion. It was given to me by different hypnotized patients coming from diverse backgrounds, cultures, and religions. Surprisingly, it is consistent from patient to patient. Their words and expressions may differ, but the basic theme is the same.

I do not know if these so-called demons that my patients see and describe, inside them, are real or not. All I know is that by removing these so-called demons from my patients, their emotional and physical symptoms are improved or cured completely.

Chapter VI

Soul Fragmentation and Soul Loss

The Shattered Soul

Pieces here, pieces there
Pieces scattered everywhere.
And who, you ask capriciously,
Will stop and pick them up for me?

Like so many pieces
Of so many puzzles
I have cast myself
Upon the fickle wind,
Have bought and sold and bartered for
Those dearest and best parts of myself
That I was meant to guard.

Tired, sick, and empty,
I stop to check my inventory
And find that the greater part
Of me is out on loan,
And pieces are here
That I do not own.

Pieces here, pieces there
Pieces scattered everywhere
And who, you ask me will there be
To help me bring them back to me?

I look more closely at you
My friend, my lover, my child,
To find that, like me, you are
A fragmented being, a puzzle
Without all the pieces.

"Pull yourself together," you say.
Little do they see that
We are all souls of broken glass
Or sieves through which the
Grains of our lives
Pass on their way to Forever.

Pieces here, pieces there
Pieces come from everywhere
Winged messengers from Eternity,
The Angels bring them back to me.

A Light descends from somewhere
Above my head and bathes me
In its warmth and purity
Angels' hands put me back together
Like a spiritual Humpty Dumpty

They fuse me with liquid Light
That mends the lingering scars
And fills the cracks and crevices
In my Soul.
And by their leave, I realize
That once again I am made whole.

Pieces there, pieces here
All reflected in a mirror;
Strengthened by a shield so strong,
I'll stay right here
Where I belong.

—Jane

Soul Fragmentation and Soul Loss

Most of the time the basic protection prayer and technique provided in the beginning of Chapter V worked fairly well for my patients. Sometimes, however, a few patients mentioned still being afflicted by new entities and negative influences.

Dean, a patient, continued to be afflicted by new entities after releasing all the entities from his body. So we started to look for the source of his problem. Under hypnosis, he saw many soul fragments missing from his soul, creating holes and tunnels in his soul and in his shield. He described his soul as being located in his heart area. It appeared to him as a white ball of Light that appeared blotchy because of the missing soul parts. He saw a gray cord from his soul going out in the darkness and saw Satan holding his soul fragment. Since we did not know how to get that soul part back from Satan, I asked Dean to look and see if there were somebody from the Light to help us. Dean saw a large angel who identified himself as Michael, an archangel. He said that Satan was sending new earthbound and demon entities, devices, energy absorbers, negative thoughts, visions, and attitudes into Dean through his soul part and its connecting cord, which acted like a tunnel.

Michael said that all the soul parts need to be returned, cleansed, healed, and integrated with Dean's main body of the soul.

He said that he could bring those parts from Satan for us.

Dean described that Michael went to Satan and told him that Dean wanted his soul part back and that Satan must hand it over. Dean was amazed that there was no struggle, no fight, and no violence. Michael made the demand on behalf of Dean in the name of God, and Satan had no choice but to hand it over.

The soul part and cord were gray. Dean said Michael brought his soul part back, cleansed it, healed it, filled it with the Light, and integrated it with Dean's main body of the soul. After cleansing that part, it looked like a spark of Light to Dean. Angels also brought back many other soul parts of Dean, parts that were with other demons and different people. Some were also stored in the dark places by Satan and his demons.

After locating and bringing all the parts back, the angels cleansed, healed, and integrated those soul parts with Dean's main body of the soul. They also cleansed and healed his whole soul and put a shield of bright Light around it. Then they cleansed and healed Dean's whole body and filled it with brilliant, white Light and shielded it completely. Dean saw some holes in his energy field, which were plugged with white Light.

Archangel Michael suggested that every person should routinely request the angels to locate and bring back their lost soul parts and cleanse, heal, and integrate them with their main body of the soul. He suggested that we should add this request to our routine protection prayers.

The Soul

Frequently, hypnotized patients can see their own souls inside their bodies. They describe the soul in the form of a condensed ball of Light inside the chest, the divine part of their being, which is a part of the almighty God. According to the patients, they have access to God and spiritual knowledge through their souls, which are connected to one of the Godheads and then to God with a silver cord. My hypnotized patients claim that the soul and subconscious mind in fact are one and the same. Under hypnosis, they describe the shape, size, color, and location of the soul within the body.

Location: The location of the soul in the body varies from person to person. Most people see it in areas such as the chest, or in the solar plexus. Some people see the soul in the head or neck area. They also visualize the soul as occupying their entire body.

Shape: The shape of the condensed or main part of the soul also varies from person to person. The different soul shapes reported by patients are round, egg-shaped, like a candle flame, praying hands, or free form with a changeable shape resembling an amoeba. Patients also describe the soul as having the shape of their body, like an emanation or halo all over the body from that condensed part of their soul.

Size: Different patients report having varying sizes of souls, ranging from a small spark of Light to a ball of Light within. According to patient reports, the size of the soul has nothing to do with the size of the physical body, but rather depends on how evolved the soul is. The greater the spiritual development, the larger the soul.

Color: Patients describe the color of their souls as white Light, white mixed with gold, and pure gold. Some patients describe the soul color as grayish or black, sometimes with a red, yellow, orange, or greenish tinge or shade. In these cases, their souls have demonic influence.

Connecting cord: Under hypnosis, patients also describe that their souls are connected, first to one of the Godheads and then to God with a silver cord. They claim that through the silver cord, there is a constant communication between us, the Godhead, and God. Through these silver cords our prayers are heard, and we also get guidance from them.

Soul Fragments

Under hypnosis, patients claim that their souls are fragmented due to some emotional, mental, or physical trauma. They often report their souls are not complete or whole and use terms such as *broken, divided, split, fractured,* or *fragmented,* to indicate that parts or pieces of their souls are missing.

Appearance of the soul fragments: My hypnotized patients see and describe these fragmented soul parts in two different forms: spiritual and physical.

Spiritual Form

Patients describe the fragmented soul parts as sparks of Light or pieces of Light in different sizes, colors, and numbers.

The sizes of these soul fragments, according to patients, range from large to very tiny pieces. Some describe the fragmentation as broken glass that shatters into pieces of different sizes, shapes, and forms.

A fragmented soul may have any number of pieces, ranging from only one to many, even thousands, depending on the severity of the trauma. The more intense the trauma, the more dramatic the shattering and fragmentation of the soul.

The colors of the soul fragments are described as silver, white Light, white mixed with gold, and pure gold in their pure form. When they have demonic influence, they may appear as gray, black, brown, or tinged with red, green, yellow, or orange.

Patients say that these fragmented and separated parts of the soul are still connected to the main body of the soul by a thread, a cord, or a line, which may be thick or thin, depending on the size of the fragmented soul part. The connecting cords may appear as silver, gold, gray, brown, black, red, or copper, depending on whether they are pure or have demonic influence.

Physical Form

Most of the time, patients see the fragmented soul parts that remain inside the body as having the physical appearance they had at the time of the trauma and the fragmentation. They look and feel exactly the way patients looked and felt at the time of the trauma that caused them to split or fragment from the main body of the soul. These fragmented parts, or little ones, have all the feelings, emotions, and memories of the trauma that caused them to fragment, even if it happened many years ago, as if they are frozen in time

369

or locked into a given age. My patients describe these fragmented soul parts using wording similar to that used in traditional psychiatry as subpersonalities, alter personalities, or as an inner child.

Age When Soul Fragmentation Occurs

Patients report that soul fragmentation can occur at any age, from birth to death. They also report that fragmentation can happen even in the womb or in one or more past lives. It is also possible to communicate with these fragmented soul parts through the patient.

Soul Fragmentation from Birth till Death

Linda had several fragmented soul parts that were trapped inside a dark demon entity. When they were freed from that demon entity, they appeared to Linda as she was at the age of six months, one year, four years, seven years, nine years, and twelve years. They claimed to fragment from the main personality, or the main body of the soul, because they did not want to grow up and do things grownups have to do.

Wilma had a soul fragment that appeared to her as she was at the age of fourteen. It separated from the main body of the soul because she did not want to have sex.

Julia, a thirty-eight-year-old female, had an abortion at the age of sixteen. Even after several years, she could not get over her guilt feelings. Under hypnosis, she found a fragmented part of herself at the age of sixteen, which separated during the abortion because she felt guilty. There was also the spirit of the aborted fetus. They both were trapped inside a dark demon entity. During the session, the dark entity was transformed and released to the Light as well as the spirit of the aborted fetus, who came in Julia because of love. Sixteen-year-old Julia was integrated with the thirty-eight-year-old Julia after some therapy. After that session, Julia felt free of her preoccupation and guilt about abortion. She felt at peace.

Wilbur, a thirty-five-year-old man, found under hypnosis a soul fragment of him at the age of twenty-two that separated when he came home from Vietnam and heard about how people felt about Vietnam veterans.

Soul Fragmentation during Birth

Barbie, a thirty-year-old female, had panic attacks, during which she became short of breath and had feelings of being closed in.

Under hypnosis, during a session, as we were locating and releasing the spirits, she found in her head a dark demon entity that looked like a black blob. It refused to talk and cooperate with me and said it was told by Satan not to speak to me. So I requested the angels of the Light to surround this dark one with the net of Light. Barbie told me the Light was not all around the dark one. From my experience with other patients, I learned that when the Light is not able to surround the dark entity, there is usually a little one that is the fragmented soul part of the patient, either holding onto or trapped inside the demon entity.

Barbie did not see any child fragment holding on to the dark demon. So I called out for any little Barbie trapped inside the demon entity. Barbie had a childlike expression and said, "I cannot get out. It is all dark here. I can't breathe. I can't come out."

> **Dr. Modi**: "Just come out of there, little one. You don't have to be trapped in the darkness."

We requested the angels to help the little one out and they did.

> **Baby Barbie**: [patient smiling like a child] "I am out and I can breathe now."
>
> **Dr. Modi**: "What happened? Why didn't you grow up with big Barbie?"
>
> **Baby Barbie**: "I separated at the time of our birth while the doctor was trying to pull our body out of our mother's womb. I could not come out with the body and I stayed in the womb. A man [an earthbound

spirit] was watching and saw me inside the womb. He came and brought me out of my mother's womb, but I don't know how I got here."

Arthur, the earthbound spirit who brought out the fragmented part of the baby from the womb, was also trapped inside that dark entity. I asked him to just walk out of the dark blob. After he came out of the darkness, he gave the following account.

Spirit Arthur: "I was in the delivery room watching Barbie being born. As the doctor pulled the body of the baby out of the birth canal, a part of the baby's soul fragmented with the trauma of pulling and stayed in the birth canal. Nobody could see that part, but since I was in spirit form, I could see that part of the baby inside the birth canal, so I went and brought that part from the mother's birth canal. Then somehow this dark blob just covered us and trapped us completely inside it and brought us here inside grownup Barbie."

Inside that dark blob were other fragmented parts of Barbie at the age of six months, one year, two years, six years, seven years, and eleven years, which were all helped out of it.

The dark demon was transformed into the Light and was sent to the Light (heaven). Arthur was also released to heaven and all the soul parts of Barbie (the little ones) were cleansed, healed, and integrated with Barbie's main body of the soul after resolving their traumas.

Barbie: [crying] "I never knew what was wrong with me. It was these little ones who felt trapped and could not breathe."

During the next session, Barbie told me that all her life she slept in the fetal position and sucked her thumb while sleeping. This behavior improved after that session.

Fragmentation in the Womb

Sometimes patients report fragmentation happening even in the womb.

Alicia, a thirty-five-year-old female, had a stillborn baby at the age of twenty-one. As we were locating and releasing the attached entities from her, she saw the spirit of the stillborn baby inside. The baby had a deformed head, as if a part of the brain were missing.

Alicia also saw another fragmented part of that stillborn baby inside, which said that it fragmented from the main part of the baby's soul while still in the womb, at five months of age.

I requested the angels to cleanse, heal, and integrate the fragmented part of the baby with the main body of the baby's soul. Alicia saw that part going in the baby's head area and the baby's head appeared complete. It did not appear deformed. Then the spirit of the stillborn baby was released to the Light (heaven).

Fragmentation in One or More Past Lives

Patients even reported their soul parts being fragmented and lost in one or more past lives. These lost soul parts create holes and weaknesses in patients' souls and continue to cause problems for the patients in their current life. As a result they do not function with their full capacity.

Sandy recalled a past life in which her eyes were plucked out because she failed a religious test. During that time she lost soul parts from each of her eyes; these soul parts were retrieved, cleansed, healed, and integrated after she resolved the trauma of that life.

Sherry, under hypnosis, recalled a past life in which she was brutally abused, physically and emotionally, from childhood by different people in town because she had knowledge of things and events before they happened. They killed her at the age of seventeen because people thought she was a witch.

After the death of her physical body, her spirit saw the Light and the angels, but she had trouble going to the Light, as if somebody

SHERRY

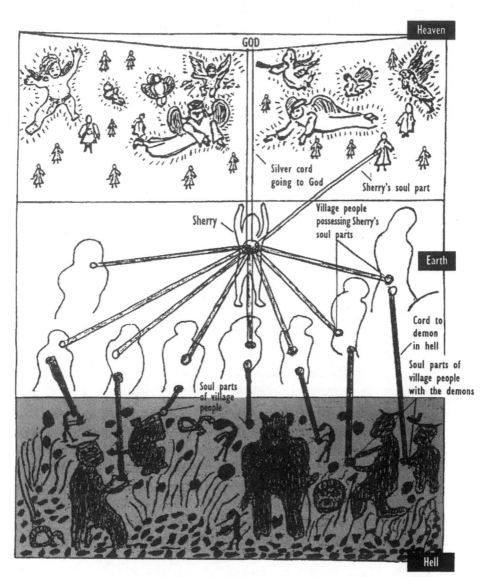

As Sherry is trying to reach out to the angels, she is being pulled down by the village people through her soul parts and their connecting cords, which are in their possession. Soul parts of the village people, in turn, were in possession of the demons in hell, through which they were turning village people evil.

were holding her back. As she looked back, she saw many cords going from her to her abusers in the town. They all had one or more parts of her soul that she had lost during her abuse. After some difficulty, she was able to make her transition to heaven.

From heaven, as she looked back and reviewed her life, she saw clearly all those abusers being possessed by many dark entities; they looked very dark to her. She also saw cords from the town people who abused her, going down in hell, where Satan and his demons had possession of all their soul parts and were motivating them to do evil actions.

After understanding how those people were like puppets, under the control of Satan and his demons, she was able to forgive them and free herself from the traumas of that life. After the resolution of the trauma, we requested the angels of the Light to bring back all the parts of her soul that were lost during that life from different people and places and the darkness. They were cleansed, healed, and integrated with Sherry.

What Happens to Those Fragmented Soul Parts?

Patients, under hypnosis, report that some fragmented soul parts stay in the body, while other soul parts leave the body. It is better for the patient when the soul parts stay in the body.

Soul Fragments That Stay inside the Body

Soul fragment that is pure: The soul fragments can stay in the body looking and feeling exactly the way the patient looked and felt at the time of the trauma, when fragmentation occurred at a younger age. It is as if they are frozen in time or locked into a given age.

Cindy, under hypnosis, found a fragmented soul part that looked like her at the age of eight, hiding under the bed with her fingers in her ears because she did not want to hear her parents fighting. This soul part was cleansed, healed, and integrated with grownup Cindy.

Soul fragment infested by entities: Sometimes, although the soul fragments remain in the body, the patients report that the soul fragments have been infested with earthbound entities, demon entities, and sometimes with the soul fragments of other living people.

Phil, a patient, had a history of uncontrollable temper outbursts. As he scanned his body, he saw many grayish-looking little Phils who were very angry and refused to talk because they did not trust grownups. They were infested by demons, which is why they were looking gray and were uncooperative. So we requested the angels of the Light to remove all the dark entities from all the little Phils and grownup Phil and help them to the Light. After cleansing, the little Phils were cooperative and talked about fragmenting from the main body of the soul when their father physically abused them. Also, the abuse opened Phil for possession. He was infested by many human and dark entities, which caused him to feel uncontrollable anger from time to time. All the little Phils, the fragmented soul parts, were cleansed, healed, and integrated with grownup Phil after the resolution of their traumas. After that, Phil's uncontrollable temper outbursts improved dramatically.

Soul fragment holding on to an entity: Some patients report their soul fragments or the subpersonalities are actually holding on to possessing entities. In these cases, the possessing entities, whether an earthbound entity, demon entity, or part of another living person, have a much greater influence over the patients.

Jack, under hypnosis, found the spirit of his father with him. After some therapy, his father understood that he needed to go to heaven and was willing to go; Jack was also willing to release him. When his father looked up, he saw the Light and angels in it, but they were far away. I asked the father what was holding him back, because Light always comes when spirits are ready to go. Father said that there was a two-year-old Jack inside big Jack who was holding his hands and did not want to let him go. This two-year-old Jack had inside him demon entities that were influencing him. After removing the dark entities from two-year-old Jack, and after some therapy, he was willing to let go of his father, who was released to the Light. Two-year-old Jack was cleansed, healed, and integrated with the grownup Jack.

Soul fragment trapped inside a demon entity: Sometimes patients report their soul parts are totally covered and trapped inside a demon entity; these soul parts, or little ones, feel totally helpless. They are aware only of being in total darkness and completely controlled and restrained by the demon entities. In these cases, fragmented soul parts give the possessing demons more power, and their transformation and releasement become difficult. The angels cannot help as long as the demon entity has any fragmented soul part of the patient or little ones trapped inside it or holding on to it, because they cannot interfere with the patient's free will.

Melissa, under hypnosis, saw a black demon entity in her head. When I called angels to surround that gray blob in the net of Light, Melissa reported that the gray blob was changing colors, into red and black, and that the Light was not surrounding that blob. With years of experience, I learned to recognize that there had to be a part of Melissa trapped inside it or holding on to it. So I called out for any little Melissa who might be there. Melissa described an eight-year-old Melissa trapped inside the gray blob, a demon. She was afraid to come out of the gray demon because she could not trust grownups. The gray demon told her that it was her friend and she should not talk to me or anybody else.

After some therapy, little Melissa came out of the demon. After that, Melissa reported that angels were able to surround the demon in the net of Light. After some therapy, the demon was transformed into the Light and was released to the Light. Little Melissa was integrated with grownup Melissa after the resolution of her trauma.

Past life personality: Sometimes a trauma in the current life can reactivate the memory of the trauma in a past life, causing the soul to fragment; the fragment becomes a past life personality. This soul part holds the memories of a past life trauma. This past life personality may have the same or a different name, different looks, and even different sex, but it is the fragmented part of the patient's soul. This phenomenon is common in cases of multiple personality disorders, but can happen in anybody.

Sara, a patient with an eating disorder, started to diet to lose weight. During this time a part of her soul fragmented, creating a soul part that had memories of a past life when she starved to death. In this life, this past life personality did not want anything to do with dieting. So it separated from the main body of the soul when Sara began to diet and it became a past life personality. After resolving her past life trauma, she was integrated with Sara.

Faith, a patient, had a past life personality named Alexander, a four-year-old boy, who separated from Faith at the age of four, when her father suddenly died. This trauma reactivated the memories of a past life trauma when Alexander's father was killed by enemies when he was four. After the resolution of the past life trauma, Alexander, the past life personality, was integrated with Faith.

Soul Fragments That Leave the Body

Sometimes patients report that the soul fragments leave the body and can go to different places and people, as follows:

- Soul fragments going to another living human being;
- Soul fragments leaving the body during a trauma and returning later;
- Soul parts in possession of a living person on the earth while the main body of the soul has gone to heaven after the death of the body;
- Soul parts going to heaven with a diseased person who had possession of them, although the patient is still living on the earth;
- Soul parts remaining at the location of the trauma that caused the soul to fragment;
- Soul parts in possession of Satan and his demons; and
- Soul parts stored in a warehouse in hell by Satan.

SOUL FRAGMENTATION AND SOUL LOSS

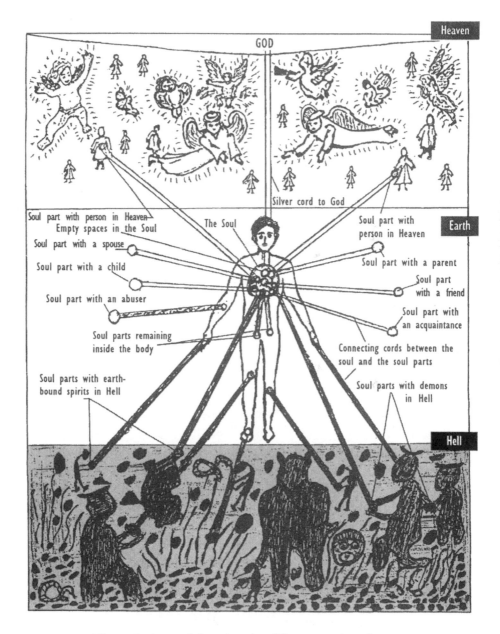

(Compilations of drawings by different patients)

Soul Fragments That Go to Another Living Human Being

A soul fragment can go to another living human being, such as a family member, a friend, an aquaintance, a loved one as a part of mutual soul sharing, an abuser, a victim of physical and sexual abuse, a person wishing to take another person's pain, and a victim of spells and curses.

To a family member: Patients often report finding their soul parts with a family member.

Sondra, under hypnosis, recalled that when her brother became severely ill, many parts fragmented from the main body of her soul and went to her brother so he could recover faster. Although it was a very loving act on her part, it was a mistake because she was not whole in her own body and could not function properly until we brought back her soul parts and integrated them with her.

To an acquaintance: A soul fragment can go to an acquaintance.

Jimmy had a car accident and was taken to a hospital by an emergency squad. Under hypnosis, he saw a cord going to a man from the emergency squad who helped him after the accident. It was brought back, cleansed, healed, and integrated with Jimmy.

To a loved one, as part of mutual soul sharing: Sometimes two people, lovers, spouses, parents and children, or other loved ones, can share parts of their souls and accept a part of the other person's soul in return. Thus, there is a mutual exchange of their soul parts as part of a consenting relationship. It is always a mistake, because they are not whole in their own body.

Sue, under hypnosis, found several cords going to her best friend and had soul parts of that friend with her. This was their way of maintaining their friendship, but the consequence was that they were not whole in their own bodies. Both their parts were returned to their own bodies and integrated with them.

Tina had a hard time getting over her husband after their divorce. No matter how much she tried, she had a hard time going on with her life. Under hypnosis, she found a soul part of her husband inside her. He looked young, the age when they were dating each other. She also saw a cord that was connected with her soul part, going from her to him, which also looked the age when they were dating each other. She got the understanding that they both mutually gave their soul parts to each other when they were dating because they were in love.

After some psychotherapy, his part was returned to his body, cleansed, healed, and integrated with his main body of the soul. Her part was also brought back cleansed, healed, and integrated with her main body of the soul, with the help of the angels. After that session, Tina felt free of him and was able to move on with her life.

To an abuser: A soul fragment can go to the abuser who caused the trauma that led to the soul fragmentation.

Eve, a forty-five-year-old female, was sexually abused by a family friend when she was fourteen years old and had trouble forgetting the experience. She had trouble getting close to anybody and had sexual difficulties in her marriage. Under hypnosis, she saw many of her soul parts with the man who sexually abused her and she also had his soul parts with her. After resolving her traumas, bringing her soul parts back, and returning his soul parts to him, she felt free of that traumatic memory for the first time and was at peace.

To a victim: Sometimes patients report that strong emotions such as anger, hate, jealousy, or the desire to control other people can cause the soul to fragment. The fragment goes out and attaches to the person toward whom these strong emotions are directed—as in cases of verbal, physical, sexual, or ritualistic abuse—which still exert fear and control over the victim.

Alexandria was sexually abused by her uncle. Under hypnosis, she found a soul part of her uncle in her. He claimed that he was there to control her and to make sure that she did not tell anybody.

Sylvester, a forty-five-year-old man, was verbally and physically abused as a child by his father, who had a violent temper.

At times, even now, he expressed a great deal of fear of his father, although they live far apart and did not see each other much. Under hypnosis, he found several fragmented soul parts of his father, who appeared as he was when Sylvester was growing up. Every time he became angry at Sylvester, a part of the father fragmented and went to Sylvester. These fragmented soul parts had demonic influence and were dark. Also, there were many fragmented soul parts of Sylvester inside him who resembled him at a younger age. These fragmented during the physical and verbal abuse. They were cleansed, healed, and integrated with Sylvester after processing their traumas. All the soul parts of his father were cleansed, healed, and integrated with his father. Sylvester experienced a big change, and there was even a change in his father's attitude.

To a person wishing to take another person's pain: How often we hear about people desiring to take the suffering of a loved one on themselves—a mother, for example, praying to receive her child's pain, so the child can be free of it. In this case, a soul part of the suffering person can take all the pain, can fragment, and can go to the person who is willing to have it, and may or may not suffer with it, depending on how the person was wishing.

According to my patients, sometimes our wishes can be granted by God or by Satan, depending on how we are wishing and how we are praying. If we just wish to take the pain without asking God, then God cannot answer it, because He gives us free will. But dark ones are always waiting to bring the full-blown pain and suffering to the person wishing, because through their wish they open their shield. So we should be careful about what we wish and how and who we ask.

Brandy, a thirty-year-old female, under hypnosis, saw a gray blob in her abdominal area. This gray blob had a soul part of her and her father trapped inside it. At this point, she began to experience severe pain all over her body. She realized that it was her father's soul part that was suffering with his pain, which she was experiencing in her body. I asked her father how and why he came into Brandy. He said that as he was suffering with his pain at the hospital, this soul part of him took all the pain and came into Brandy because Brandy was praying to take his pain.

At this point, Brandy was also able to see how it happened. She described that as she was praying to take her father's pain, a part of her soul fragmented and went to her father. Then she felt a Light pushing the pain from her father's feet up through his body and pushing it out of his head, along with his soul part. Also, her soul part that went to her father was also pushed out of his body by the Light. As this happened, Brandy felt the pain leave and a sense of peace came all over her. These feelings were her father's feelings, which were transferred over to her. She waited for the pain to come to her, but it never came, although her father was relieved of the pain. As her father's and her soul parts came out of the father's head, a dark being trapped them and brought them to Brandy's body.

Because Brandy's intent and prayers were out of love for her father, they were answered by God with mercy. It was taken away from her father in a soul part of her father and then was brought into Brandy. But because the soul parts of Brandy and her father were trapped inside the dark being, the grownup Brandy did not have to suffer with it. She realized that God answered her prayers with love and not with suffering.

Brandy's father's soul part was released after some therapy. After the resolution of her trauma, her soul part was cleansed, healed, and integrated with the main body of her soul.

To a victim of spells and curses: Casting spells and curses during black magic or witchcraft can cause the fragmentation of the practitioner's soul. The fragment then attaches to the victim. Usually when this happens, demon entities are attached to those soul parts, giving power to the curse or the spell.

Lena had multiple physical and emotional problems. She believed that a neighbor, Fred, with whom her family had problems, had cursed them or had cast a spell on her and her family. As we were checking Lena for the entities, I called out for Fred. Lena saw him in her head, covered by a dark demon entity. After we removed the demon entity from around him, he still looked very dark and evil. He was very angry and hateful and admitted casting a curse on Lena and her family. I asked him how he did so. He arrogantly said, "It is easy. You just will a piece of your soul to go to the person you are angry at. I focused on the anger and the hate I felt toward Lena until it took a form and then directed it to Lena." As he was describing it, Lena saw how it happened. A soul part of Fred, which was very dark, separated from him and was surrounded completely by a dark demon entity and came into her when her shield was open. Fred said that he asked Satan to help him and, as a result, Satan sent that demon, which gave the power to the anger and curse. After his soul part went to Lena, along with the demon, they could cause different types of physical and emotional problems for her.

Lena saw many soul parts of Fred surrounded by dark entities in her and her family members. I tried to make Fred realize that by casting these spells he was losing his soul parts to others and weakening himself. As a result, he was not only hurting others, but himself too. He refused to listen to me because of the demonic influence in him. So I requested angels to remove all the dark entities and energies from Fred's soul parts that were in Lena, and integrate the soul parts together. After cleansing and healing, his attitude totally changed. He understood how he hurt not only Lena and her family, but also himself because he was not whole in his own body, and all those empty spaces in his soul were filled with the dark entities and energies. He had been totally under the influence of Satan and his demons and all that anger and hate were fed to him by the darkness.

All the fragmented soul parts of Fred were removed from Lena and from her family members. They were cleansed, healed, and integrated with the main body of his soul in his own body with the help of the angels. The angels cleansed and healed his body and shielded him with the Light.

Lena felt a change for the better in her and her family members after that session.

Soul Leaves the Body during a Trauma and Returns Later

Some patients report that during a trauma the main body of the soul leaves the body, leaving a small part of the soul behind to activate the body and to cope with the trauma. The main body of the soul, or personality, returns to the body after the traumatic event. As a result, the main personality—the patient—has amnesia for the event.

Tammy, under hypnosis, recalled that during a sexual abuse, the major part of her soul, or personality, left the body and went far away, leaving a small part of her soul, an alter personality, to activate the body and cope with the sexual abuse. The main body of the soul returned to the body after the traumatic event was over.

As a result, Tammy had amnesia for the traumatic event. Only that alter personality, that small part of the soul, had the memory of the trauma, and it was so damaged that it could not go back and integrate with the main body of the soul. Later, in therapy, after the resolution of the trauma, that soul part was cleansed, healed, filled with the Light, and integrated with Tammy with the help of the angels.

Soul Parts in Possession of a Living Person on the Earth, While the Main Soul Went to Heaven after the Death of the Body

Patients report that sometimes the main body of the soul returns to heaven following the death of the physical body, while missing soul parts are still in possession of living people on earth or in possession of an earthbound entity or a demon entity. This separation serves as a drawback to the person in heaven and causes him or her to operate without full capacity during the stay in the Light.

Martha, under hypnosis, saw in herself a soul part of her father that appeared several years younger than when his body died. As Martha looked up she saw her father in the Light in a white robe.

He apparently went to heaven after the death of his body, while his fragmented soul part was still with her on the earth.

Her father's soul part was cleansed, healed, and integrated with him, in the Light.

Soul Parts Went to Heaven with a Person Who Had Possession of Them, Although the Patient Is Still Living on the Earth

Some patients report their lost soul parts went to heaven after the death of the person who had possession of their soul parts, although the patients are still living on the earth.

Janet, under hypnosis, saw two silver cords coming out of her soul, as we were trying to locate her soul parts. As she traced them, she saw them going to heaven. One cord went to her soul part that was with her deceased child, and the second one went to her soul part that was with a family member who had died several years before. Both parts were brought back, cleansed, healed, and integrated with Janet with the help of the angels.

Soul Parts Remaining at the Location of the Trauma

Some patients tell that sometimes the soul parts remain at the scene of an accident, on a battlefield, or at a location where the trauma occurred. This trauma may be in the current life or in a past life.

Randy, a thirty-one-year-old man, had an obsession to move to different places every few years. He was totally puzzled by his behavior and did not know why he was doing so or how to stop. During a session, under hypnosis, I asked Randy to check his soul and locate any fragmented soul parts. He had many. We brought them back, processed their trauma, cleansed, healed, and integrated them with the main body of his soul.

Just to be sure, I called out for any other part of Randy who may be hiding inside. All of a sudden, in a distant, scared voice, he answered, "Yes, I am here. I cannot find my way home. I'm lost."

At this point tears were pouring from Randy's eyes. He saw a part of him who looked like him as a nine-year-old, on the road in the town where he grew up. This little Randy fragmented when he got lost and could not find his way home. He was still wandering on the road, desperately trying to find his way back.

Big Randy remembered that at the age of nine he did get lost, but later found his way home. In that moment of panic, a part of him fragmented and stayed on the road, still desperately trying to find his way home. We requested the angels to bring that part back to Randy. After we did some therapy with little Randy, he was cleansed, healed, filled with the Light, and integrated with the grown Randy; the reunion was very emotional. He felt whole after the integration.

After the session, Randy shared the insight he received. He felt that this was why he was moving from place to place. He was searching for this lost part, although he was not aware exactly why he was on the road. He always felt something was missing in his life and that he was not whole and he felt kind of empty inside. After that session, Randy's obsession of moving from place to place and his feelings of emptiness inside were relieved.

Paul, under hypnosis, recalled a past life when he was a young and studious resident doctor. He died during his residency because of exhaustion. He left many of his soul parts near his books and in the laboratory because they were an important part of his life.

Rob, under hypnosis, recalled a past life when he was a soldier and both his legs were blown away by a cannon shot. Later, he died of infection. When he saw the Light and angels in it, he refused to go with the angels until he found his legs. He saw angels going to the battlefield and bringing his soul parts, which belonged to his legs. They were still lying there. They integrated those soul parts with his body after cleansing and healing them. The soldier then walked into the Light with the angels.

Nadine had to put her father in a nursing home after he went into a coma. At home, she kept on feeling his presence and sometimes she heard him calling her name. During a session, under hypnosis, as she checked her home, she saw many soul parts of her father roaming in the house. They all looked like her father at his current age. They did not want to be in a sick body, so they fragmented from him and stayed in the house. After some counseling, they all were cleansed, healed, and integrated with his body, with the help of the angels. Nadine did not feel or hear him in the house anymore.

Soul Parts in Possession of Satan and His Demons

Often patients report that Satan and his demons were the possessors of their soul fragments. The soul parts in Satan's possession are not irretrievably lost, despite his apparent power. During the treatment, their parts can be returned from Satan and his demons with the help of the angels.

Gilda, a thirty-year-old female who came to me for a weight problem, saw a soul part from her stomach with Satan. She saw him touching and squeezing that part of her soul; every time he did so, she would feel extreme hunger and would eat compulsively. Her soul part was returned with the help of the angels. They cleansed, healed, and integrated it with the main body of her soul.

Paulina had suicidal preoccupations from time to time. Under hypnosis, she recalled a lifetime when she was kidnapped by some smugglers and was mentally and physically tortured. She would not eat and committed suicide by hanging.

From heaven, as she looked back in that life, she saw that, as she was being tortured, her soul exploded and fragmented into many pieces, which were taken by Satan and his demons. They used them as a memory device, reactivating the memories and feelings of suicide in the current life, from that past life by squeezing them. They also gave her thoughts that she believed were her own thoughts like: "You are no good." "You deserve to die." "Go ahead and kill yourself." "There is no other way." Those soul parts were brought back with the help of the angels, cleansed, healed, and integrated with Paulina after resolving their trauma.

Soul Parts Stored in a Warehouse in Hell by Satan

Under hypnosis, some patients say that Satan has a huge stockpile of soul fragments of different people, not just from this current lifetime but from many past lives. The influence exerted by Satan can extend for more than one lifetime.

Gavin, a thirty-year-old male, had many soul parts missing. While he was under hypnosis, I asked him to locate and trace the cords and see where they went. He saw many black and gray cords coming out of the main body of his soul. He traced those cords from his body into a dark, cold place that he felt was hell, where his soul parts were stored in different bottles or jars symbolic of different time periods and places. He described the whole place as a huge warehouse where soul parts of different people were stored for centuries.

Gavin recalled a past life event when he lost those soul parts centuries ago. He remembered being a young man who wanted to join a group that was doing good social work. He was directed to a club.

When he reached there, he was asked to take an oath that he would serve the club with his mind, body, and soul. As he took that oath, parts of his soul were taken from each of his seven energy centers, which he called *chakras*. He realized he had been tricked into joining a Satanic club. From that life onward, he did not function with his full capacity. We retrieved all of his soul parts with the help of angels, cleansed them, healed them, and integrated them with the main body of his soul.

We also requested the angels to bring all the other soul parts of other people that were stored in that dark place in hell. Gavin watched in amazement as the angels brought all those soul parts back, cleansed, healed, and integrated them with millions and millions of people, to whom they belonged here on the earth and to those who were in heaven. Some people who were working for Satan did not want those parts back, so the angels bound them in space so Satan could not capture them again. According to the angels, those soul parts will be returned to their owners when they are ready to receive them back. Gavin said that angels cannot do anything unless we request them.

Causes of Soul Fragmentation

According to my patients' reports, different types of traumas, usually of a physical, emotional, sexual, or spiritual nature, can cause a soul to fragment. The trauma can be mild or severe. The more intense the trauma, the more dramatic the shattering and splitting of the soul.

Physical Trauma

Physical trauma can be due to physical injury, surgery, or physical abuse.

Lee, under hypnosis, found five fragmented soul parts of himself who were all twenty years old. They fragmented from his back when he had a car accident at the age of twenty. He had constant back pain, which improved immediately after we integrated those soul parts that belonged to his back.

Guy, under hypnosis, found fragmented soul parts of himself who looked like him at age six months and at age two years. Both parts fragmented when his mom was bathing him with very hot water.

Gary was physically abused by his alcoholic mother when he was young. Under hypnosis, he found many fragmented soul parts (the little Garys) inside him. They all claimed to fragment from the main body of Gary's soul during the physical abuse. They were all scared of the mother. Some were hiding and did not want to be found. All were cleansed, healed, and integrated with the main body of Gary's soul after the resolution of their traumas.

Emotional Trauma

Emotional traumas such as mental abuse, rejection, sadness, fear, or grief can cause soul fragmentation. Sometimes it may not be a trauma, but an overabundance of positive emotions, such as joy and happiness. Strange as it may seem, a soul part may leave a soul that contains an overabundance of positive emotions.

Tina, under hypnosis, found a soul part of her mother that fragmented when Tina fell and broke a leg bone at the age of six. Her mother felt guilty that perhaps she was not careful and attentive toward her. A part of her mother's soul fragmented, out of guilt, and went to Tina to help her.

Tracy, under hypnosis, found a soul part inside her that fragmented at the age of fifteen, when she was still grieving over her father's death. She did not get a chance to say goodbye to him. Even twenty years after her father's death, she could not talk about him without becoming emotional and crying. We cleansed, healed, and integrated that part of her soul, after the resolution of the trauma. After that, Tracy felt in peace.

JoAnn found a fragmented part of her soul inside who looked like her at the age of eight. Her family was going to move to another city and she did not want to move and consequently was anxious and sad about it. This anxiety caused the fragmentation of her soul part.

Reva had a six-year-old fragmented soul part in her who separated from her during a severe thunderstorm. The grown Reva was also extremely afraid of thunderstorms. The fragmented soul part of Reva was cleansed, healed, and integrated with her after the resolution of the six-year-old Reva's trauma. After the integration of the soul part, grown Reva's fear of thunderstorms was resolved.

Bertha had several fragmented child soul parts. All of them appeared very happy and giggled a lot during the session. They had no idea why they fragmented. After those parts were integrated with Bertha's main body of the soul, Bertha described feeling happy and childlike at times, having a desire to giggle and laugh for no reason.

Sexual Traumas

The trauma of sexual abuse is complicated, because the abuse is a combination of emotional and physical trauma. Under hypnosis, people often describe being outside their bodies and watching the abuse. Sometimes the main body of the soul leaves the body and goes far away from the scene and a small part of the soul is left behind to activate the body and to deal with the trauma. The main body of the soul returns later, when the abuse is over. This also explains why sometimes the victims have amnesia for the abuse.

Leslie was raped at the age of fourteen. After that she had a hard time trusting men. During a session, under hypnosis, she located several parts of her soul, which fragmented during the rape. Some were inside her and some with her abuser. After the resolution of her trauma, they were brought back, cleansed, healed, and integrated with her own soul. She felt free of the traumatic memories and was at peace afterward.

Spiritual Abuse

Spiritual abuse takes place when a child is purposely exposed to Satanic and other negative influences. The most extreme example is a dedication of the child to Satan. In other cases, the child is taught evil ways and evil approaches to life, such as cruelty and lack of respect for humanity and other living beings. Anything that is negative in dealing with people is sufficient to cause soul fragmentation.

The Basic Operating Mechanism and Purpose of Soul Fragmentation

The basic operating mechanism and purpose of soul fragmentation is the same whether the trauma is physical, emotional, sexual, or spiritual. It is to deal with the trauma without damaging the whole body of the soul.

Sometimes the patients report that they watched the trauma take place while they were outside the body. At other times, the main body of the soul goes far away from the body during the trauma, leaving a small soul fragment to activate the body and to cope with it. As a result, patients have total or partial amnesia for the trauma. When it is safe, the main body of the soul returns to the body and resumes its duties. It is able to function normally with minimum negative effects.

The small portion of the soul that fragmented to cope with the trauma is usually so damaged that it cannot be returned to the main body of the soul. It contains all the memories and feelings of the traumatic event. This small portion of the soul is sacrificed and isolated to protect the main body of the soul. Therefore, the main portion of the soul or main personality has very little knowledge of the trauma, resulting in total or partial amnesia for that event.

Curing that amnesia means rejoining the soul fragment with the main body of the soul. The trauma must be processed and resolved before rejoining the soul fragment with the main body of the soul.

Effects of Soul Fragmentation and Soul Loss

My patients describe many effects of soul fragmentation and soul loss:

- Patients suffering from soul fragmentation and soul loss feel an emotional loss even without looking at and examining their souls under hypnosis. The patients' intuition allows them to recognize the unnatural condition of their souls. They feel spacey, in a fog, and disconnected from life. Patients describe the condition of soul fragmentation and soul loss in their own words:

"I feel like I am not whole."
"I feel empty inside."
"I feel a void inside."
"When he broke up with me, I felt like my heart shattered into a thousand pieces."
"I feel like he stole my soul."
"I feel like I left a part of me with him."
"He has no soul."

393

"I feel like a part of me died with him."
"I feel spaced out."
"I feel disconnected from life."
"I feel like something is missing," etc.

- Patients report that each part that leaves the body weakens them and makes them more subject to psychological and physical illnesses. They can have symptoms from head to toe due to soul loss.
- Patients no longer operate at their full physical, emotional, mental, and spiritual capacity. Soul fragmentation and soul loss diminish their spiritual power.
- Amnesia for certain events or for certain time periods in life is another common complaint associated with soul fragmentation and soul loss.
- Patients describe deterioration of their decision-making ability. They tend to make wrong decisions.
- Patients do things that will hamper their growth, both humanly and spiritually. They are confused about their purpose here on the earth.
- Patients are more subject to outside influences and are more open to possession by earthbound and demon entities.
- Those soul parts that have demonic influence prove to have the most negative effect on the patient.
- The most damaging effects suffered by patients are due to those soul parts that are outside the body. The empty holes and spaces cause weakness in the patients' souls and their bodies, which are filled by the earthbound and demon entities.
- According to my patients, when the soul fragments are with Satan and his demons, it is like trying to drive a car while someone else is controlling the steering wheel. The soul is very controllable, and a large part of our thoughts and actions can be dictated by Satan and his demons. They can affect every part of the patients' existence. Patients have free will, but it is influenced. They believe they are operating on their own, in their own best interest, but it is not true. Others are in control and they do not

even know it. Demons create faulty logic and flawed thinking. They influence the patients' attitudes, behavior, emotions, actions, and every part and organ of their bodies. Patients report that whatever demons do to their soul parts that are in their possession in hell affects them in their bodies here, creating different physical, mental, and emotional problems for them.

- When soul parts are with Satan and his demons, they diminish the patients' planning ability here on earth and even in heaven. Patients do not function with their full capacity.

Maggie had severe pain and cramps in her back and legs. When I asked her to go to the source of the problem under hypnosis, she recalled a past life when she was brutally beaten and tortured. As a result, her back was broken. After her death, when she went to heaven, she saw herself losing many soul parts from all over her body, especially from her back and legs. She saw that those parts were in the possession of the demons in hell. They were wringing those parts like wet rags, thus causing pain, cramps, and stiffness in her back and legs. Those parts were brought back and integrated with Maggie, after cleansing and healing. Afterward she was completely free of her symptoms.

Stuart had stabbing and shooting pain in his shoulders and upper back. Under hypnosis, he saw many black cords coming out of his shoulders and upper back. As he traced those cords, he saw them connected to his soul parts that were with the demons in the darkness. He also recalled a past life when he fell and hurt his back and shoulders. He saw demons stabbing those soul parts with needles, causing the stabbing and shooting pain, which Stuart was experiencing in his shoulders and back. With the help of the angels, those parts were brought back, cleansed, healed, and integrated with him. He was relieved of his symptoms after that session.

Beth felt depressed, trapped, withdrawn, and lonely most of her life. Under hypnosis, she saw several gray cords coming out of her heart and going to the darkness, to her missing soul parts. She saw that demons had those soul parts, which they enclosed in a black box, making her feel trapped, withdrawn, and lonely. She also recalled losing those soul parts in a past life during which she felt depressed, withdrawn, and lonely. After the resolution of the trauma from that past life, those soul parts were brought back, cleansed, healed, and integrated with her with the help of the angels. After that she was relieved of her symptoms.

Tim had problems with snoring for several years. Under hypnosis, he saw many gray and black cords coming out of his throat and nasal passages and going to his soul parts in a dark cold place; they were in possession of the demons. He recalled traumas in several lifetimes, when he lost those soul parts after being hanged, being decapitated, and being shot with a gun in his mouth, blowing out his throat, mouth, sinuses, and nasal passages. These soul parts were in the possession of the demons in hell. He saw demons using those soul parts. They were holding his throat and nasal parts over a fire. Heat caused expansion of those soul parts, shutting down the throat and nasal passages here in Tim's body, causing difficulty in the air flow. Other times, demons were plucking on the connecting cords, causing uneven vibrations and difficulty in smooth air flow through Tim's nasal passages. Those soul parts were brought back, cleansed, healed, and integrated with Tim. After that, according to Tim, his snoring was reduced a great deal.

Amanda had skin rashes and extremely dry skin. Under hypnosis, she recalled a life when she was burned as a witch. In another life she had a severe skin infection. She lost soul parts from her skin from all over her body during these lives; these soul parts were later taken by demons and were in their possession in the darkness. The demons were infusing black, murky liquid through those soul parts and the connecting cords to Amanda's skin, leading to skin lesions, rashes, itching, and dryness. Her condition was relieved after resolving the traumas of those past lives and bringing those parts back and integrating them with her after cleansing and healing.

Ethel had severe arthritis, causing her to have swollen, hot, and inflamed joints. Under hypnosis, she recalled a past life where she was brutally tortured by her enemies and most of her joints were damaged and bones were broken. During that time many soul parts from her joints fragmented and later were taken by Satan and his demons. She saw that Satan and his demons were putting those captive soul parts above the fire and infusing black liquid in her joints through the connecting cords, making her joints inflamed, hot, and swollen. We retrieved and integrated those parts with Ethel after cleansing and healing them, with the help of the angels. Afterward there was a great deal of improvement in her chronic arthritis.

Cindy complained about thinning of her hair and sometimes burning and itching of her scalp. Under hypnosis, she saw several gray and black cords coming out of her scalp and traced them going to a dark, cold place to her soul parts, which were possessed by the demons. She also saw a lifetime when she was being scalped, and another life when she was being burned in a fire. She saw demons infusing some type of black fluid through those soul parts and their connecting cords to Cindy's scalp, leading to burning, itching, and hair loss. Those soul parts were brought back, cleansed, healed, and integrated with Cindy's scalp, relieving her symptoms.

Mike, during a session, scanned his whole body to check for any new entities before we proceeded with a past life regression. He saw himself as totally clear and brightly lighted. After that, we proceeded to find the source of his headaches. He was able to recall and visualize a past life that was responsible for his headaches. But after a few minutes he got confused and blocked, and he was not able to visualize and recall. So I asked him to check his eyes and brain. He saw in his eyes a black blob, who claimed that it was pushed into Mike's eyes just now through his soul part and its connecting cord, blocking Mike's thinking and vision. We transformed that dark demon into the Light and sent it to heaven. Mike's soul fragment was brought back, cleansed, healed, and integrated with him. Mike was then able to recall and relive that life vividly without any problems.

During another session, Mike all of a sudden started to complain of severe pain in his head. As he looked in his head he saw a clamp-type of device with sharp teeth, which was shoved in his head through a missing soul part and its connecting cord. We requested angels to remove and destroy that device and bring and integrate his soul parts with him. After cleansing and healing, Mike's pain was immediately relieved.

Gordon, a thirty-year-old college-educated man, had had problems with talking too much since he was a little boy, causing disruption or saying things to hurt people. He felt that words would come out of his mouth even when he did not want to say them. During the sessions, he sometimes expressed things in such a way that even after a long time I was at a loss as to what he was trying to say. Under hypnosis, he recalled a past life when his tongue was cut off as a way of torture. During that time he lost several soul parts from his tongue, which were in the possession of demons.

Gordon saw Satan and his demons pulling and vibrating the cords that connected those soul parts with his tongue. As a result, his words were shaken loose and he could not say what he wanted to express. Also, they were transmitting negative thoughts and words through the connecting cords, making him say the wrong things or talk too much.

Ashley had problems with her memory. She would read a book and later have a hard time recalling what she had read. She would make a list so she could remember to do things, but would forget to look at the list. Even while speaking, her thoughts would block.

Under hypnosis, she saw that she had many missing soul parts from her brain, which were in hell with demons. They used those soul parts to affect her memory, First they shredded each brain soul part in many pieces and cords like spaghetti, and then they wove the cords and scrambled all the parts, causing confusion and forgetfulness. Other times, the demons clamped the cords of those brain parts, causing the memory blocks.

All those parts were brought back and integrated with Ashley's brain, after cleansing and healing. Afterward there was a great deal of improvement in her memory and comprehension.

Lucy, who had a hearing problem, saw angels bringing several parts of her soul from the dark entities at our request, during one session. She saw these parts being integrated with her ears. She saw demons sending different thoughts and ideas through the connecting cords between her ears and the fragmented soul parts that were with the demons. It was as if they were constantly whispering in her ears thoughts that Lucy thought were her own thoughts. The demons were also clamping the connecting cords off and on, thus blocking her hearing from time to time.

Shirley had pain, burning, itching, blurred vision, and sensitivity to sun and bright lights from time to time. She had many soul parts missing from her eyes, which were in the possession of Satan and his demons. She saw different ways Satan and demons used those soul parts to affect her. They clamped the connecting cords off and on, causing her blurred vision. They also gave her ugly and scary visions through the captive soul parts and their connecting cords. Finally, they caused pain; irritation and sensitivity to sun and bright lights; burning; and other vision problems by infusing black, murky liquid in her eyes through the connecting cords.

After we retrieved, cleansed, healed, and integrated those parts with her, her symptoms were relieved.

Lily had episodes at home where different entities would come out and speak through her from time to time, according to her family. Lily had no memory of what happened during those times. During a session, I asked one of the earthbound spirits inside Lily about how they could take over her body for those short periods of time. The entity said, "Satan and his demons have many soul parts of Lily in their possession. They were infusing some kind of narcotic type of substance through those soul parts and connecting cords to the main body of Lily's soul. As a result, Lily was feeling weak and sleepy and it was easy for us to take over partial control of her body and speak and act through her." After retrieving, cleansing, healing, and integrating those lost soul parts, Lily felt better and more in control.

Gene was a fifty-five-year-old single man who lived an isolated life with no special goals. Under hypnosis, he recalled that in his planning stage in heaven for his present life he did not plan anything at all. If any higher beings suggested that he should make plans for his coming life, he completely ignored them, saying that he did not need to make any plans at that time. He would plan when he was in the body in this life on the earth.

From heaven, when I asked him to see why he had that attitude, he described seeing Satan and his demons possessing many of his soul parts. They were using those soul parts to control his thoughts and attitudes, even in heaven, making him ignore the guidance of the higher Light beings.

Diagnosis of Soul Fragmentation and Soul Loss

There are several ways to recognize if the patient has soul fragmentation and soul loss.

Patients' emotional and intuitive feelings: Many patients feel soul fragmentation and soul loss emotionally. They feel the loss without even seeing their souls under hypnosis. They often express themselves as feeling empty, not being whole, not being at home completely, feeling they have a strong positive or negative connection with someone, or that they are being controlled by somebody. Patients feel that when a loved one died, a part of them died, too. Some feel that after surgery or an accident they have lost something and they are not the same.

In cases of divorce or the breakup of a love affair, people complain that they are still obsessed or controlled by the thoughts of the other person. Sometimes they feel as if the other person stole their soul.

Visual inspection of the soul: The patients are asked to visually examine their souls under hypnosis. Patients often report that parts of their souls are missing. Sometimes patients report that chunks are missing from the edges of the soul. When the soul appears in a geometric shape, they find it easier to detect the missing parts than if the soul is an amorphous blob. Sometimes the soul is seen as having holes, as in Swiss cheese, as if a core had been removed, or as if a tunnel were cut through it.

Frequently, patients state that the parts of the soul are scraped off the edges and the shape appears as being scalloped. The corners or edges may be broken. The soul may appear to have holes, blotches, or empty spaces on the surface.

The patient may miss seeing the holes or empty spaces on visual inspection, especially when they are filled in with outside entities or negative energies or demonic devices. As a result, when the patient looks at the soul, it appears to be fully integrated. In this case, the color of the soul reveals the true situation. It may appear to be grayish, black, or blotchy.

Visual inspection inside the body will also locate the fragmented parts of the soul, as well as earthbound and demon entities who have possession of these fragmented parts of the patient's soul.

Tracing the cords: The patient, under hypnosis, is asked to visually inspect the soul to see if any cords or threads are coming out of it. The patient is asked to trace the cords, which will often lead to the missing soul fragments either inside or outside the body. The fragmented soul parts are still connected with the main body of the soul by these threads or cords.

Angelic help: A fourth method is to ask the angels to inspect the soul and trace the cords for missing parts of the patient's soul and locate them.

Treatment of Soul Fragmentation

It is very important that every soul part be returned to the main body of the soul for the emotional, mental, and physical health of the patient. This integration is also very important for the patient's spiritual development. They must be returned and the past trauma that caused the soul to split in the first place must be resolved, whether the event occurred in the current life or in a past life.

Locating and Retrieving the Soul Fragments

Recovering soul fragments is done with the help of the patient and the angels. The hypnotized patient is asked to visually inspect his or her soul to see if there are any cords or threads coming out of the soul. They may appear as silver, gold, gray, black, copper, brown, or red to the patient. If cords or threads exist, the patient is asked to trace those cords one by one.

Each cord will lead to a lost soul part, either inside or outside the body. It may be in the possession of a relative, friend, abuser, or stranger. It may be in the possession of an earthbound entity, a demon entity, or Satan.

The patient will also recall and visualize the scene of the traumatic event that led to the fragmentation, either in this life or in one of the past lives. The trauma is processed by recalling, reliving, releasing, and understanding the trauma and resolving the conflict. Finally, the fragmented soul part is cleansed, healed, filled with the Light, and then integrated with the main body of the soul with the help of the angels.

Soul parts inside the body: If the missing soul part is found within the body, it may be by itself or may be in the possession of an attached earthbound entity, the soul part of a living person, or a demon entity. The soul part must be freed from the attaching entity. Then the trauma is processed and resolved. At that point, angels are requested to cleanse and heal that part of the soul and integrate it with the main body of the patient's soul. Any earthbound or demon spirits are then released to the Light, after being counseled and transformed. The soul parts of the living people possessing the patient are counseled and returned to their own body with the help of the angels.

The fragmented soul part of the patient in the body may be surrounded and consumed inside a demon. In this case the soul parts feel trapped and helpless. We need to communicate with those trapped soul parts, encouraging them to walk out of that demon entity, which cannot stop them from leaving. We also request the angels to help those little ones (soul parts) to come out of the demon. After they come out of the demon, the demon is transformed into the Light and released to the Light. The little ones (the soul fragments) are cleansed, healed, and integrated with the main body of the patient's soul after the resolution of their traumas.

Past life personality: Sometimes a current life trauma can reactivate the memory of a past life trauma, causing the soul to fragment in this life. This becomes a past life personality. In this instance, the patient needs to recall, relieve, and resolve that past life trauma and then that part needs to be cleansed, healed, and integrated with the main body of the patient's soul.

Fragmentation in a past life: If the fragmentation was caused in one or more past lives, the past life issues and conflicts need to be resolved. Then the soul parts should be located, cleansed, healed, and integrated with the main body of the patient's soul.

The fragmentation cannot be healed without resolution. Even if the soul parts are integrated into the main body of the soul, they might fall out again unless resolution is reached and the soul fragment is cleansed and healed of the trauma that caused the fragmentation.

Soul parts outside the body: In the event that the cords or threads lead outside the body, it is best to ask the angels to retrieve the soul parts. The patient is asked to send his or her mind's eye with the angels when they go to retrieve the part, rather than be passive in the process. It is as if the angels take them along for the ride. This is important for the patients so that they know where the soul fragments have been, who had them, and how the patient was influenced by those lost soul parts.

Soul parts with Satan or his demons: If the soul part turns out to be in the possession of Satan or his demons, it can be retrieved with the help of the angels. Patients are asked to watch the whole process. This helps the patients to see the illusion of the power of Satan and his demons. It also helps the patients to realize this is not a violent process. When a just demand for the soul part is made by the angels on behalf of the patient in the name of God, Satan and his demons must hand over the soul fragment. It helps patients to understand that Satan and his demons have only as much power as the patients permit them to exert, and that people have the power to ask Satan and his demons to return what is theirs.

Patients, under hypnosis, can go directly to Satan and his demons and ask for their parts to be returned, but doing so is not a good idea. Too many people are too easily influenced. Confronting Satan in person, without angelic intervention, is very dangerous. Satan and his demons already have one or more parts of the patients' souls, and through these soul parts Satan exerts great influence on the patients. If the patients attempt to confront Satan and his demons directly, without the help of the angels, they may be tricked into full demonic possession.

Process of Soul Integration

Any soul parts that are with Satan or his demons or with evil people will appear gray, black, brown, or tinged with red or green. The color is caused by negative entities, energies, devices, desires, thoughts, or ideas. These negative or evil elements should be removed before soul integration is attempted.

After the location and retrieval of the fragmented soul parts, the traumas that caused the fragmentation are processed and resolved. Then a complete cleansing is accomplished by asking the angels to remove from the soul fragments anything evil, dark, or negative—a negative entity, energy, a thought, a memory, an attitude, any active or passive devices, or anything neutral that will make the patient less than he or she should be and interfere with his or her purpose. The patient is asked to watch the process. When the angels finish the cleansing, the patient sees the soul part and the connecting cord as the same color as the main body of the soul, e.g., silver, silver tinged with gold, or gold. A soul fragment that is returned to the body without cleansing has a very negative physical, emotional, and spiritual effect on the patient.

Following the cleansing, the angels are requested to integrate those soul parts into the main body of the soul where they belong. When the soul part is in place, the edges must be firmed together and the substance of the two parts joined. One patient described the process as follows: "I saw my soul as broken pieces. I saw fairies/angels pouring clear, golden, liquid Light, which looked like honey, over the cracks, filling the separations between the soul parts. Then they sprinkled angel dust glitter over my entire soul and I glowed."

Foreign Soul Fragments

Hypnotized patients sometimes report finding soul fragments of living people within their bodies. These foreign soul parts from other people appear to the patients as they appeared at the time of the fragmentation. The foreign soul fragments may belong to a relative, a friend, an abuser, or a stranger. It is possible to talk to these foreign soul parts through the hypnotized patients.

The foreign soul fragments usually claim to be in the wrong body because of strong emotions, usually love, anger, hate, jealousy, or revenge. Their purpose is to help, hurt, or control the patient. Often there is a demonic influence that compels or forces them. Mutual soul sharing with a loved one seems like a very romantic idea, but it weakens both parties in the relationship and is very detrimental. Sometimes patients desire to keep the shared soul parts and insist on leaving their soul parts with the loved one in spite of the danger involved. All foreign soul fragments should be returned to their proper owners.

Effects of Possession or Attachment by Foreign Soul Fragments of Living People

The effects of attachment by a soul fragment of a living person on the patient are similar to the effects of an attached earthbound entity. Any emotional, mental, and physical problems the person has in his own body can be inflicted upon the patient when a fragmented soul part of that living person comes in and attaches to the patient.

Robert, a seventeen-year-old teenager, was having a great deal of confusion about his sexuality. Sometimes he had homosexual thoughts and desires with which he did not feel comfortable. Under hypnosis, he saw a soul part of a man who was a homosexual who admitted giving Robert homosexual desires and thoughts. After returning the soul part of that homosexual man to his body, Robert was free of homosexual desires and did not have any sexual confusion.

Dillon, a thirty-five-year-old man, had racing thoughts and depression. He was obsessively worried about his father, who was diagnosed as having manic-depressive illness. Under hypnosis, he found a soul part of his father in him. After releasing the soul part of his father back to his body, Dillon was free of the racing thoughts and depression, which were due to his father. He was also free of his obsessive worry about his father.

Jill, a twenty-eight-year-old female, had paranoid delusions. She had a strong belief that other people were talking about her. She was especially paranoid about her coworkers. I asked her if she had heard the coworkers speaking about her, and she said no. I asked her if she knew anyone else who had heard them talking about her and told her about it. She said no. I asked her how she knew they were talking about her. She said she just knew and was convinced they were, but she did not know why and couldn't prove it. She could not, however, get the thought out of her mind that they were talking about her.

She was becoming very suspicious of everyone. She felt depressed and anxious and was having difficulty sleeping. She was given antipsychotic medication by her previous psychiatrist, but it did not help much.

During a session, under hypnosis, as she looked inside her body she did not find any earthbound or demon entities. However, she saw soul fragments of her coworkers. They were able to converse through Jill. All of them admitted talking to others about Jill because they were angry with her.

They all claimed they were in tune with what they were doing and saying in their own bodies. They still had cordlike connections with their own bodies and souls. They admitted it was their thoughts Jill was picking up and that in their bodies they had been talking about her to others.

We returned these soul parts of Jill's coworkers to their own bodies with the help of angels. They cleansed, healed, and then integrated them with their owners. During this process, the patient was able to visualize exactly where these people were and what they were doing at the moment of integration.

Afterward Jill felt freedom from those obsessive, paranoid thoughts. She stopped taking the medication and was able to sleep well. These improvements took place after just one hypno-therapy session.

Brad, a thirty-year-old white male, had a long history of depression, suicidal preoccupation, panic attacks, inability to function, and difficulty sleeping. He had many complaints about everybody in his family. He felt that they were treating him like a kid and didn't think he could make any decisions on his own. He claimed to have had these problems since he was a little boy. Over the years, he had seen many psychiatrists and had taken different medications without much change.

During a session, under hypnosis, he did not find any earth-bound or demon entities. He reported having fragmented soul parts of different people who were living. When I conversed with the foreign soul parts of these living people through Brad, they all said they loved Brad and were with him to help him. They did not realize they were harming him. Parts of some of his family members came in him when he was a little boy.

I made them understand that, although their intentions to help him out of love were good, their being in Brad was very confusing and damaging to him. Everybody was telling him what to do and it was very frustrating for him. After understanding how they had affected Brad negatively, they were more than willing to leave. Their soul parts were cleansed, healed, and integrated with their respective bodies with the help of the angels. Brad did not have any other entities in him.

During the next session, Brad appeared very happy. He reported he was not depressed or suicidal. He felt free and clear and knew he could be himself now. He was not sure if what he had seen and heard was real or not, but he had no doubts that he was definitely free of his longstanding, crippling symptoms. That is all he cared about.

Jerome, a forty-five-year-old man, had a history of TMJ, or temporomandibular joint syndrome, for several years. He had inflammation of his temporomandibular joints and aching gums. He was treated with prednisone, pain medication, and a mouthpiece. In spite of these treatments, he continued to have pain in his gums and jaw.

Under hypnosis, as we began to release the spirits from him, he began to feel pain and spasms in his jaw and gums. He saw parts of two of his coworkers with whom he was having conflict. They all claimed to have come into Jerome to aggravate and hurt him, because they were angry with him. After some psychotherapy with these soul parts of his coworkers, they were cleansed, healed, and returned to their own bodies with the help of the angels. Jerome's pain and spasms in his jaw and pain in his gums were relieved right after the session.

Treatment of the Possessing Foreign Soul Parts

The first step in returning the foreign soul fragments is counseling with them through the patient. They are helped in understanding that by being with the patient they are hurting the patient and themselves. They are not whole in their own bodies and, as a result, they are not functioning with their full capacity in their own bodies. When the soul parts are ready to leave, the angels are requested to cleanse and heal them. Then the angels are asked to return and integrate the soul parts with the main body of the soul of the proper owners. The patient is asked to watch the whole process.

The patients usually can visualize these people wherever they are at the time of the integration. They often tell where they are, what they are wearing, and what they are doing. Surprisingly, patients after the session have often confirmed these findings with those other people and found that the visualized information was correct.

Results of Soul Integration

While there is no objective measure of the strengthening of the personality as the soul is integrated, patients' subjective comments give an idea of how they have changed. Patients say they feel stronger physically and emotionally, with a definite improvement in the emotional and physical problems they brought to treatment. They are better integrated, saying they feel whole or more "together" after the soul fragments are returned.

They report being better able to cope with everyday problems and decisions. They are more clear-sighted in their daily activities. Subsequently, patients deal more effectively with psychological traumas, having a better perspective and not taking things to heart so intensely as to allow themselves to be psychologically damaged. Patients also report they do not get easily influenced by earthbound and demon entities.

Summary

Over the years, my patients have consistently reported seeing their souls under hypnosis. They describe it as a spark or a ball of silver white Light, in their chest, solar plexus, head, or neck. They describe it as the divine part of their being, the part of the Almighty God that is within all of us. They say there is an emanation from this condensed part of the soul that spreads all over the body, in the shape of the body, like a halo.

According to the patient reports, this soul can have different shapes: round, egg-shaped, shaped like a candle flame or praying hands, or as a free-floating form, like an amoeba. It varies in size, ranging from a small spark of Light to a ball of Light. The size of the soul has nothing to do with the size of the body. It depends on the spiritual evolvement of the person. The greater the spiritual development, the larger the soul.

The soul can be silver-white, white mixed with gold, or pure gold, depending on the person's spiritual development. It can be infested by earthbound, demon, and other entities and may appear gray, black, red, or other colors.

Patients say that their soul is still connected to God with a silver cord and that communication flows back and forth from God to us and vice versa. Through this cosmic umbilical cord our thoughts and prayers are heard.

Often my patients report that their souls are fragmented and not all together and whole. They describe seeing holes or empty spaces in their souls. They recall that with physical, emotional, sexual, and spiritual traumas, which can be mild or severe, the soul fragments. The more intense the trauma, the more dramatic the shattering and splitting of the soul. The soul can even fragment with the overabundance of joy and happiness.

Patients, under hypnosis, see these fragmented soul parts in spiritual or physical form. In spiritual form, the soul parts appear as sparks of Light or pieces of Light that can be small, medium or large. The soul parts can number anywhere from one to many thousands, depending on the severity of the trauma.

The color of these soul fragments appears similar to the soul: silver-white, white mixed with gold, or gold. In cases of infestation with outside entities, they may appear as gray, black, red, brown, or tinged with green, yellow, or orange.

These soul parts, although separated from the main body of the soul, are still connected to it with the silver, silver mixed with gold, or pure gold threads or cords that, like the soul, are seen in the form of spiritual energy. Like the soul, these connecting cords can also be infested with outside entities and energies, and in that case, may appear as gray, black, red, brown, or tinged with green, yellow, and orange.

Hypnotized patients also describe seeing these soul parts as having the physical appearance that patients had at the time of the trauma and fragmentation. These soul parts look and feel exactly the way they looked and felt at the time of the trauma that caused their souls to fragment. These fragmented soul parts—the "little ones"— have all the feelings, emotions, and memories of the traumas that caused them to fragment, even if they happened many years before, as if they are frozen in time or locked into a given age. These soul parts are the same as what we call in traditional psychiatry a subpersonality, an alternate personality, or an inner child. My patients describe seeing them as distinct and separate from them and not just their imagination.

The soul can fragment in the womb, during birth, and later, anytime during childhood, teenage years, and adulthood, until death. Fragmentation can also occur in one or more past lives. These fragmented soul parts sometimes stay in the body, while at other times they can leave the body. It is better for the person when the soul parts stay in the body.

When the soul fragments leave the body, they can go to another living person, such as a family member, a friend, an acquaintance, an abuser, or a victim. The main body of the soul can also leave the body during a physical or sexual abuse, leaving a small soul part in the body to cope with the abuse, and return when the abuse is over. This leaving creates amnesia for the traumatic event for the main body of the soul or the main personality. The memories of the traumatic events remain isolated with the small fragmented soul part, which stays separated from the main body of the soul. Occasionally the soul parts leave the body during a trauma and never return. Sometimes they remain at the location of the trauma that caused the soul to fragment, still feeling confused and distraught.

A soul part that is in the possession of another person can go to heaven after the death of the possessor, while the owner of that soul part is still living on the earth. Conversely, a person can go to heaven after the death of the body while his or her soul parts may still be on earth in the possession of another living person or an earthbound or demon entity.

My hypnotized patients often report that Satan and his demons are also the possessors of lost soul fragments either from the current life or from one or more past lives. Patients sometimes report seeing huge warehouses, somewhere in hell, where people's soul parts have been stored through the centuries in jars or containers symbolic of the time periods.

Satan and his demons use these soul parts of different people to insert negative thoughts, attitudes, visions, and voices through their connecting cords to the person. They can also insert earthbound and demon entities, devices, and negative energies into the patients, through the soul parts and their connecting cords. They also restimulate the memories of past life traumas by massaging the captive soul parts. These memories are then experienced by the patient in their current bodies. Thus they can cause any and every type of physical, mental, and emotional problems and diseases. They can cause any symptoms, from head to toe.

It is crucial to locate each and every lost soul part and cleanse, heal, and integrate it with the main body of the soul. The trauma that caused the soul fragmentation should be resolved before integration; otherwise, the soul parts will separate again.

All the soul parts that are still inside the body should be located and integrated as soon as possible after the resolution of their traumas. Earthbound and demon entities manipulate and exaggerate these little ones' emotions and keep them upset. They are also manipulated to invite the outside entities inside the patient. They also hold on to the possessing human and demon entities, making their releasement difficult.

Locating, cleansing, healing, and integrating the lost soul parts with their proper owners is done with the help of patients and the angels of the Light, including the soul parts that are in possession of Satan and his demons. Under hypnosis, patients can go directly to Satan and his demons and ask for their soul parts to be returned, but doing so is not a good idea. Confronting Satan and his demons in person without angelic intervention is a very dangerous thing for the patient. Satan and his demons already have one or more soul parts of them and as a result the patient can be tricked into full demonic possession.

In our day-to-day expressions and in our music, we describe the condition of the soul without even seeing it: "I left my heart in San Francisco." "When she left, she took a piece of my heart with her." "When he died, part of me died with him." We wonder how is it that our mothers always seemed to know when something was troubling us or when we were not well, although we were miles apart. How do we seem to "know" to call our children or an old friend right when, it turns out, they most needed to hear from us? These "coincidences" are due to mutually sharing our soul parts with loved ones. These soul parts are still connected with our main body of the soul with a silver cord. Through these connecting cords there is a constant flow of feelings and communication from one person to another although consciously we are not aware of it.

Soul-sharing is as old as time. In our human frailty, mutual soul-sharing with a loved one is a natural mistake to make. It is also the reason people continue to be obsessed with their lovers after a breakup or divorce, and why sometimes grieving over a deceased loved one seems never to end.

Based on the reports of my patients, soul-sharing is a dangerous thing to do. It works as a possessing entity in us, as we inherit a measure of the other person's physical, emotional, and personality characteristics. Only when the soul parts are returned to their rightful owners can we be free from problems and obsessions with other people and feel whole, together, and free to get on with life.

By giving our soul parts away, we weaken our souls and leave those empty places open to spirit possession and emotional and physical diseases. We are not whole in our own bodies and cannot function to our full physical, emotional, and spiritual capacity. We should never give pieces of our souls to others, no matter how much we love them.

As I have said repeatedly throughout the book, the problems and diseases of the physical body are in fact the problems and diseases of the soul due to current and past life traumas and due to soul fragmentation and soul loss and infestation and affliction by earthbound, demon, and other entities that occupy the empty spaces.

To heal the body, we need to heal the soul by releasing the possessing entities and reclaiming, cleansing, healing, and integrating the lost soul parts after the resolution of the traumas from the current and past lives.

Chapter VII

Prayers and Remote Healing

Prayers and Remote Healing

Final Protection Prayer

Over the years, my patients have reported different types of influences and interferences by Satan and his demons. Every time, however, according to patients, Light beings were there to help and provide us with different techniques to counteract these demonic interferences. Regardless of their different cultures, religions, and beliefs, patients reported similar information consistently. So far, different techniques provided by the angels of the Light throughout this book were able to counteract about 99 percent of demonic attacks and influences. According to the angels, in the remaining 1 percent of the cases, two other types of methods are used by Satan and his demons to launch an attack.

One attack is launched through the spiritual dimensions in which demons and angels travel freely. This has the effect of bypassing the shield around the patient. In spite of the shield being intact and in place, demons can enter a person's body through other dimensions. According to the angels, they do so from certain spots between those dimensions; they cannot do so from just anywhere. Demons can also shove devices from those dimensions to this dimension and have them appear in us.

These other dimensions are like other universes that have vibrations similar to our universe, but are just a little bit different. In these cases, we should request the angels to stay on guard around those certain spots between the two dimensions.

Another way the demons can attack from a distance, according to the angels, is by simply focusing their thoughts and intents on our thoughts and intents to interfere with them. According to the angels, our intents and thoughts cannot be shielded. They must be protected through different means. The primary way to block the attacks on our thoughts and intents is by focusing on a single objective, as in meditation. People in the highest stage of meditation are absolutely immune to demonic attacks because they literally become a part of the Light (heaven).

Angels suggested that another way to ward off the attacks on our thoughts and intents is by having an intent not to give in to the attacks, not to be possessed or influenced, and to completely reject the works of Satan, his demons, and all the human beings under Satan's influence and accept the works of the God. We can also dedicate our life to God and God's purpose and to the purposes we set up in heaven before we came on earth. When people dedicate their life to God and God's purposes, there is usually constant communication back and forth from God to the person, therefore, the person is always in the Light.

All these suggestions and techniques given by the Light beings through different patients proved to be extremely effective in protecting against different demonic attacks. According to the angels and different Light beings, almost every human being is open for demonic attacks except maybe a few (.5 percent), who have a special divine purpose and have planned from heaven to have around them a special bubble that totally protects them. They are totally shielded internally and externally.

Based on the different techniques and suggestions provided by the Light beings, through different patients, I have put together a daily protection prayer and protection technique to be used at least twice daily, at bedtime and in the morning after waking up.

Protection Prayer

"I pray to God to please cleanse, heal, shield, and protect me, all my family members, friends, coworkers, and all our surroundings such as our homes, workplaces, cars, and places of recreation and everything in them and miles and miles around them from Satan, all of his demons, all human beings under their influences, and all the foreign entities, dark shields, dark energies, dark connections, and dark devices. Please fill, shield, protect, and illuminate all of us and all our surroundings with your love and Light as long as our souls exist, and bless us, enlighten us, balance us, transform us, and guide us in the right direction. Please keep us loving, giving, caring, forgiving, and humble all the time.

"Please cleanse, heal, balance, and open up all of our energy centers and channels of communication with the Light (heaven) as needed and cover and protect them when not needed.

"I form an intent not to be possessed and influenced by any spirits and reject all the works of Satan, his demons, and humans under their influence. I also form an intent to accept the works of God and achieve God's purposes and to achieve my goals and purposes that I planned in heaven by dedicating my life to God."

Protection Technique

"I request the protector angels of the Light to collect and remove all the foreign entities, dark shields, dark energies, dark devices, and dark connections from my body, aura, soul, energy centers, and cord; from all my family members', friends', and coworkers' bodies, auras, souls, energy centers, and cords and from all our homes, workplaces, cars, and places of recreation and everything in them and miles and miles around them. Collect them in the net of Light, lift them up, help them to the Light, or bind them in space.

"Plug all the holes and tunnels in our bodies, auras, souls, energy centers, cords, and in all our surroundings such as our homes, workplaces, and cars with white, liquid Light. Fill, shield, and illuminate all our bodies, auras, souls, cords, and all our surroundings such as all our homes, workplaces, cars, places of recreation, and everything in them and miles and miles around them, with the brilliant, white, liquid Light. Cover these shields with reflective spiritual mirrors and rays of shimmering white Light.

"Please locate all our missing soul parts from this life and from all our past lives from the beginning of time and bring them back. Cleanse them, heal them, fill them with the Light, and integrate them with our souls. Clamp the cords to the soul parts that cannot be brought back at this time. Please cleanse, heal, and shield our souls with the Light.

"Also, locate and remove all the soul parts of other living people from us; cleanse them, heal them, fill them with the Light, and integrate them with whom they belong.

"Please cleanse, heal, and shield all the foreign entities that cannot be removed and all our fragmented soul parts that cannot be integrated at this time with a triple net of Light and metallic shields. Cut all their dark connections.

"Please cleanse, heal, balance, and open up all of our energy centers and channels of communication with the Light (heaven) as needed and cover and protect them when not needed.

"Please put the triple net of Light and metallic shields around us and our surroundings and cars when needed, and remove them when not needed. Please stay on guard around us in this dimension and in all the other dimensions. You have our permission to take any action on our behalf to protect us as long as our souls shall exist.

"Also, please cover all of Satan's command centers and any other centers he may have throughout creation with the blanket of Light and destroy them. Cut their dark connections with Satan and his demons and with everybody and everything in creation, including the whole earth and all the human beings and other living beings and their surroundings. Please fill, shield, and illuminate the whole creation and everything and everybody in the creation, including the whole earth, and each and every human being, living being, and their surroundings with the brilliant, white, liquid Light, reflective mirrors, and rays of shimmering, white Light. Thank you."

Now visualize or imagine a brilliant, dazzling, shimmering, vibrant, white, liquid Light coming from above your head and going through your head and filling and illuminating your whole body, from the top of your head to the tips of your fingers and to the tips of your toes, cleansing and healing every part, every organ, and every cell of your body. Now imagine this Light spreading an arm's length all around you, below your feet, above your head, in front of you, behind you, and on both sides of you, creating a wonderful bubble or shield of brilliant, white Light around you. Now imagine this bubble of Light covered with reflective, spiritual mirrors and rays of brilliant, vibrant, white Light.

You and only you have a right to live in that body and shield. If anybody or anything tries to enter into your shield, you will be aware of it, even at subconscious levels of your mind, and you will have a right to say no to them. Instead of allowing them in your shield, you will direct them to the Light or where they belong.

Just imagine yourself, your family members, friends, coworkers and all of your homes, workplaces, cars, and places of recreation as a blinding, hot, afternoon sun several times a day.

Use this protection prayer and the visualization at least twice a day, especially at bedtime and in the morning after waking up and between times when needed.

(Note: If you wish, you can record this protection prayer on a cassette tape and listen to it every night at bedtime and in the morning after waking up.)

Intent to Become a Channel for God

As I have worked with hundreds of people with these therapies, for about eleven years, different Light beings have given various kinds of helpful information. One suggestion was that those people who want to do God's work and want to help other people can form an intent to become a channel (conduit) for God's love, Light, power, and healing.

One day **Dorris**, under hypnosis, saw a large angel who claimed to be the archangel Raphial, who was willing to answer our questions. So I decided to inquire about how we can become a channel for God. The conversation went like this:

Dr. Modi: "Raphial, please explain to us about what happens when we form an intent to become a channel for God's love, Light, power, and healing."

Raphial: "People need to know that they can be close to God and they are not separated from him. Everyone is special and can become God's tool for healing. God is waiting for us to ask to become his instrument; when we ask, a connection is made between us and God. Through this connection, God can use us as a vessel to send his love, Light, and healing to other people around us, including those people who are being blocked from God due to the dark influences."

Dr. Modi: "Please explain to me why God cannot help them directly."

Raphial: "God gives everybody a free will and cannot help people directly unless they ask for it. But through another person on earth who wants to help fellow human beings and has given an intent to become a channel, God can heal and illuminate other people around that person. And, like a ripple effect, through the channel, God's love, Light, and healing spreads to everyone with whom the channel comes in contact.

"When you become a channel, God's Light can heal and illuminate others through you, and you become like a magnet to somebody else who may want to be like you. When many on earth give the intent to become God's channel, God, with all your help, can continue to heal and illuminate other people around, and thus gradually your whole planet can be healed and illuminated."

Dr. Modi: "What can we do to become a channel for God?"

Raphial: "First, you have to give an intent to God. Intent has to be pure and inspired by love to help others.

"To become a channel, you have to be a loving person. If you have anger, hate, jealousy, ego, and pride,

421

which are often due to dark influences, then you as a channel become blocked by darkness and God cannot work through you.

"If you feel you have become blocked, then you should meditate and pray to be free of these negative emotions and dark influences, so you can become a loving person and always walk on the right path and eventually become a successful channel for God's work."

Dr. Modi: "What is the process of becoming a channel for God's work?"

Raphial: "You need to form an intent only one time in your whole life. You need a minimum of three or more people to form an intent. If there are fewer than eight people, then you need to hold hands while forming an intent. If there are more than eight people, then there is no need to hold hands.

"Then one person in the group can pray for everyone out loud while others can repeat it within. In the prayer, you give the intent to become a channel for God's love, Light, power, and healing, for the benefit of everybody forming the intent and for mankind. Also, ask him to allow you to serve as instruments to overcome the power of Satan, his dark ones, and humans who serve him, as long as your souls exist.

"Everybody should visualize the entire group enclosed in one bubble of Light and the entire group shall be shielded."

Dr. Modi: "How is it different from dedicating your life to God and God's purposes."

Raphial: "Man is an individual being and also a social being, with social interactions with people around him.

"The dedication individually is acting as one single person, and is beneficial to that person only. Forming the channel for God is a social group act and is beneficial to all who are in that group and spreads out to other human beings around.

"When you dedicate your life as an individual, you are the actor; but God is the main actor and director when you become the channel for God's love, Light, power, and healing."

Dr. Modi: "How does it work?"

Raphial: "Everybody who gives the intent together remains connected with each other, although they may live far away from each other. Through their connecting cords to God, they create a wider channel between them, for more Light to come through.

"For example, if three people from New York, Miami, and San Francisco form an intent together to become a channel for God and then go to their homes, they with their connecting cords to God create a triangle among them. Together they create a wider channel and Light can come down in that triangle. So the Light is coming through them, around them, and between them.

"Most of the Light is where the channels are, but people who are geographically encompassed between the channels get filled with the Light as well. The Light of God emanates through people who gave intent to become channels and changes other people around them. It is like throwing a stone in the water and watching the ripples expand out. If there is a stone thrown here and a stone thrown there, the expanding ripples eventually merge with other ripples.

"When several people form an intent together to become channels for God, they combine their energies and together they create a wider cord or channel between them. As a result, more intense Light can come through faster, to help all those around them and between them. Everything and everybody who is in the geographical space between these channels will also be influenced by the Light and the darkness can also be transformed. The more people who give intent, the bigger the area."

Based on the information given by different Light beings through different patients, I have prepared a prayer for forming an intent to be a channel for God, as follows:

Prayer for Forming an Intent to Become a Channel for God

"Dear God, please permit us to serve as a channel for your love, Light, power, and healing, for the benefit of ourselves and for all mankind. Allow us to serve as your instrument to overcome the power of Satan, his demons, and those humans who serve him. We seek to do so as long as our souls shall exist."

Now visualize that the entire group is enclosed in the Light and is totally and completely shielded, creating a wider cord and channel between the group members.

Remote Healing or Distance Healing

In remote healing, healing is achieved through a hypnotized intermediary person, with or without the patient's presence in the treatment room.

Historical Background

Throughout history, every culture and religion on earth had people such as shamans, medicine men, monks, saints, priests, and other healers who could heal people in person or from a distance. These were highly evolved, gifted, and spiritual people who were connected to and in tune with God. They were often aware of their purpose and knew that healing was their mission.

Those shamans, medicine men, and other healers accomplished their healing by raising their vibrations through prayers, meditation, and different rituals, including chanting, singing, and dancing to drum beats. They tuned into higher vibrations and thus connected with the spiritual realm and God. They then released human and dark spirits from the afflicted persons and located and brought their lost soul parts back and thus healed them. They were aware that healing is achieved with the help of God or through God. Even now, there are shamans, medicine men, saints, monks, priests, and other healers in different parts of the world doing similar healings.

Jesus and masters of other religions, while on earth, healed by casting out demons and other spirits and also performed hands-on healings. They all had God's power to heal the sick and afflicted people.

In the early part of this century, an American psychiatrist, Carl Wickland, M.D., worked for thirty years with severely mentally ill people who he thought were possessed by earthbound spirits. His wife, Anna, was a trance medium. He would call out from patients, spirits who would speak through Mrs. Wickland in trance. If the spirits were resistant, then he would use an electrostatic device, moving it up and down over the patient's spine, to dislodge the spirits from them and then they would speak through Mrs. Wickland. Then Dr. Wickland would converse with these spirits, explaining to them about their condition and would release them. He believed that a group of helpful spirits assisted him with this work. He called them the Mercy Band.

In 1924, he wrote a book titled *Thirty Years among the Dead*. In this book he included the transcripts of the sessions and outlined his theory of mental illness caused by spirit possession.

In Brazil, remote releasement is regularly performed at healing centers through the mediums coming from all walks of life. A family member or a doctor can send the name and address of an afflicted person and their possessing spirits are released through a group of mediums.

Today, the role of those shamans, medicine men, priests, monks, and saints is and extended to modern-day psychiatrists, psychologists, hypnotherapists, physicians, and other healers and lay people. These people are spiritually connected with God and have a great desire to help and heal others.

According to the heavenly beings, we as human beings have done well through our humanitarian works during the last several decades and have raised our planet's vibrations. As a result, it is easier to connect with God and other heavenly beings and tap into the knowledge, a gift that in the past was given to only a few special people. God is allowing us to have more and more knowledge and different gifts to heal and help our fellow human beings and to illuminate our planet.

Anyone with great love, faith in God, and the desire to help others can be a part of this knowledge and healing, but to do so takes work and dedication.

Remote Healing in Therapy

Working with these therapies for over eleven years with hundreds of patients, I have come to understand that any psychological and physical problems can be healed, if the patient is willing to heal. I have seen miraculous healings occurring daily. Most of the time I prefer to work directly with the patients because this way, not only do they heal, but they also gain a lot of firsthand knowledge about what caused their problems and how the healing took place. They learn that we do not die with the death of our physical body, and they learn about the spiritual reality of our existence, about God, masters, angels, and our heavenly guides, also about Satan and his demons and how they are responsible for most of our problems. They learn in therapy about how to free and protect themselves from the outside spirits. It also reawakens their inner soul knowledge and they become more in tune with their soul and with God.

I use remote healing in some people who cannot participate in their own healing because they are too sick, e.g., schizophrenics and other mentally ill patients who cannot concentrate long enough to participate in the sessions. I also use remote healing when a patient is bedridden or too weak to participate in the session, or in cases of young children. It can also be used for patients whose eyes and brains are blocked by the dark spirits so that they cannot do the session. In these cases, they can be cleared up through another person under hypnosis, who can release the dark and human spirits from the patient who may or may not be present during the session. After that, the patient can do his or her own sessions.

People often claim it is easier to do the spirit releasement for somebody else than for themselves. When patients try to release spirits from themselves, their perception can be blocked because of the presence of spirits, especially the dark spirits in the eyes and brain. It is like trying to find things in a dark room. Everything becomes vague and confusing, especially when the entities become silent and resistant.

But releasing the spirits through somebody else, after they themselves are cleared, is much easier, because they can look and locate the spirits in another person more quickly. They can also receive information telepathically from the patient's spirits, even if they are uncooperative and do not want to answer my questions.

Types of healing that can be done remotely: Most of the therapists focus only on releasing the possessing human and demon spirits while doing the remote healing. I have learned that we can also heal patients' current and past life traumas by retrieving the soul parts lost during these traumas. The spirits are in the patients because there are holes in their souls and shields due to their missing soul parts, which they lost in the current life or former lives, allowing new spirits to come in. So to do the complete healing, we also need to locate and integrate all the soul parts from the current life and also from the past life traumas. When all the soul parts are retrieved and integrated with the patient's soul, then there will not be any holes and no new spirits can come in. Thus the physical and emotional problems can be healed completely.

Remote healing can be done from the earth level through the hypnotized mediator, an intermediary person who functions as a medium in healing the patient. But I prefer to work when the hypnotized person is in the Light (heaven) at the Akashic plane, a place of knowledge in heaven, that appears to people as a huge library, where all the knowledge and records are available from the beginning of time. All our individual records are also available in our books there. This way we can tap into the reasons for that patient's problems and do the healing faster.

Doing the session from the earth level is like looking from inside out. We cannot see and understand everything and cannot get all the information. From heaven, the person has a broader and complete overview from above, and understanding of what is happening. Also, dark influences and interferences are much fewer at the Akashic plane in heaven, because demons are afraid of the Light and cannot go close to it. As a result, information is much clearer than when the sessions are done from the earth level.

Essential Requirements for Remote Healing

For remote healing, we require three people: the patient who needs the healing, a therapist, and a mediator, who is an intermediary hypnotized person.

Qualifications of the therapist: To do the remote healing, therapists should have a good knowledge of hypnotherapy, including bridge techniques and psychotherapy. They also should have a thorough knowledge of how to release human, demon, and other spirits, resolve the current and past life traumas, and how to locate and retrieve the soul parts and integrate them with the patient. They also have to have spiritual knowledge and understanding about these healings.

They have to be free of all inside spirits and totally protected from outside influences. They should pray and meditate regularly so they can be in tune with God and can get guidance, knowledge, and protection needed to heal patients. They should be totally free from drugs, alcohol, and negative emotions such as anger, hate, jealousy, pride, and ego, which can open the shields, allowing the outside spirits to come in and interfere and block them from God. They should do the therapy with great love, with the patients' interests at heart. They should be aware that God is using them as a vehicle to heal, but all the healings are done by God.

Qualifications of the intermediary, hypnotized person: These are the people who are willing and interested in healing patients. They can be related to the patient and want to help in healing them out of love and also may be karmically involved with the patient, i.e., a relative. They can be just somebody who has volunteered to be an intermediary, to help in healing for different patients because of their desire to help others, and may not know the patients.

These intermediary people should have already gone through their own healing therapies, and should be totally free of all the inside spirits and influences. They have to have an understanding about how the healing takes place. They should be able to tune in to the patient telepathically, so they can perceive and receive the information required for healing.

They should also stay away from drugs, alcohol, and strong negative emotions such as anger, hate, jealousy, pride, and ego, which can open their shields so that new spirits can come in and block them from God. They should also regularly meditate and pray for guidance and protection, so they can become good vessels for healing persons. They should be willing to help in the healing with love and should be aware that really God is the one who does the healing, and they are only the tools for his healing.

Requirements for the patients: The patients have to be willing to be healed and should give permission for their healing to God and to the therapist. They should receive a thorough explanation about the reasons for their illness and how the healing can be achieved through another person. They should be educated to pray to God for healing and enlightenment. Without their permission and knowledge about how healing occurs, the patients fail to gain the knowledge and learn from it, and even can block themselves from healing. The healing will be in vain.

In cases of cancer and other terminal conditions, patients have to want to live and give permission to heal; otherwise, it will not work.

Patient's higher self: We have a physical body and the spiritual body that is our soul. When we call upon our higher self, we are not calling upon our brain, but we are calling upon our soul, which is the piece of God within us. Our Godhead with whom we are connected is also our higher self in the Light. Our soul and our Godhead have all the knowledge about our problems and plans, even though consciously we are not aware of them.

During remote healing, it is very important to get the permission from the patient's higher self to heal the patient every time, even when the patient is consciously willing. This step is especially important in cases when patients cannot give permission because they cannot understand or are not capable of giving permission due to physical or emotional problems or are unwilling to give permission to heal. Remote healing should be done only when there is a definite permission from the patient's higher self.

Family and friends: It is extremely crucial that family members and friends of the patients be educated about what can be done through remote healing. It is important to get their cooperation and involve them in the healing process, through their positive attitudes and prayers.

Failure of Remote Healing

There are several reasons that sometimes remote healing does not work.

Patient: The patient may have chosen and planned in heaven, before being born in this body, to have specific problems because of their actions (karma) in a previous life. If the problems are things that they have to carry out to balance their previous actions and learn lessons from them, then the therapist needs to educate the patient about it and help them understand that they have chosen it. Once they resolve and balance their previous actions and learn the lessons, they can be healed.

Another possibility is that they have planned to leave the body at a certain age and have not planned to heal in this life and as a result are not motivated to live.

Another reason remote healing may not work is that patients are blocked from God. They do not believe that they can be healed and do not have faith in God. They lack spirituality. Connecting with the patient's soul if it is not spiritual is difficult, even if he or she consciously gives permission to heal. We still have all that material body and its problems to work through before a connection can be made with their soul.

Family and friends: Without the proper knowledge and understanding of the process, family members and friends can hinder and interfere with the healing process. The dark beings through them can block the healing process.

The therapist and the mediator: They can be blocked or influenced by the dark beings. Especially if the mediator is blocked, then he or she cannot make a true connection with the patient's soul and higher self.

The therapist and the mediator should pray faithfully for protection and guidance. Also, before doing the remote healing, the intermediary person, under hypnosis, should check himself or herself, and also the therapist, and remove any negative influences and shield themselves and request the angels to stay on guard and protect them during each session.

Hands-on Healing or Transferable Healing

In hands-on healing, a therapist or any other person who has the gift of healing hands and has given an intent to become a channel for God's love, Light, and healing can heal patients in person or from a distance.

In such cases, the healers act as a vessel, and God's Light enters through their crown chakra (an energy center at the top of the healer's head) and flows down through their arms and hands, to the patient who needs the healing.

In this process, through God's Light the problems can be healed and dark beings inside the patient can be transformed into the Light and released to the Light. Reiki healing is an example of hands-on healing.

Remote healing through hands is done telepathically by tuning in to the patient's soul. The healer imagines, or visualizes, that he or she is with the patient and healing him or her by laying hands on the problem areas.

According to the heavenly beings, we can even try to heal people before their deaths, if they are willing, so that they can be clear to make their transition to the Light (heaven). Also, if we can heal some of their karmic problems in this life, they do not have to deal with them in future lives.

Denise, a thirty-five-year-old female, had her first nervous breakdown when she was nineteen years old. She had been diagnosed as having schizophrenia, paranoid type. She had multiple hospitalizations, was treated by many psychiatrists, and was treated with high doses of different types of medications for the past seventeen years.

When she came to me she was taking 900 mg. of Clozaril a day. In spite of the high doses of the medication, she appeared to be very restless, anxious, and preoccupied with her problems. She had auditory and visual hallucinations and multiple paranoid and somatic delusions.

Her older brother knew about these therapies and wanted to know if I could treat Denise with them. After the first interview with Denise, I told her brother that because of her symptoms, I could not do hypnotherapy with her, but if he or another family member were willing to help her, then we could try to heal Denise through them. Her brother was willing to help his sister.

I explained to him about the nature of therapy in detail and advised him that before we attempt to heal Denise, we have to cleanse and heal him, with spirit releasement therapy, past life regression therapy, and soul integration. He turned out to be an excellent subject. After his cleansing and healing, he was able to tune in to Denise and locate and release her possessing human, demon, and other spirits and located and integrated her soul parts after the resolution of their traumas. Then we proceeded to look into her past lives, which were responsible for her problems and feelings and thus resolved her traumas and brought back and integrated her missing soul parts.

After a couple of sessions, working with her brother alone for her, without her presence, I had her sit in the session, also. During the session, what amazed me was that even she was able to locate the spirits in her and recall her past lives without any hypnosis and without closing her eyes.

Session after session, we removed foreign entities, dark devices, dark energies, dark shields, and dark connections from her. Then we brought back her missing soul parts that belonged to those holes and integrated them with her. Her current and past life traumas were also resolved.

Her condition is improving consistently. She is taking only one third of the medication she had been taking; she is less confused, paranoid, and afraid; and she is feeling more integrated and relaxed. She is able to catch her symptoms and request the angels to remove whatever is causing her those symptoms and bring her missing soul parts that are responsible for her symptoms, cleanse them, heal them, and integrate them with her. Thus, she is taking an active part in her healing.

The gift of her brother's love and help made it possible for her to heal. (Read "Schizophrenia" in chapter 10.)

Dick recalled a past life when he was a shaman in North America. He recalled that he healed people by releasing their possessing spirits and retrieving their soul parts and integrating them with the afflicted person.

Before the healing, the shaman meditated and prayed a lot. He and others danced to the drumbeat; thus he raised his vibrations, entered a trancelike state, then proceeded to heal afflicted persons.

He also recalled that sometimes in the night, while meditating, he would tune into the afflicted person's higher self and get the understanding of that person's problem. Then, while still in meditation, the shaman's spirit would go out of his body to the afflicted person, who was sleeping far away. He would perform the healing for the afflicted person while he was sleeping and then come back in his body. The next day, the afflicted person often found himself or herself miraculously cured of the problems.

Many of my patients have reported seeing me while awake or in a dream, helping and healing them. I am often surprised to hear those reports, because I have no conscious awareness of the interactions. Working with this therapy, I have learned that many of us travel out of the body, during sleep, to people and places on earth and to heaven. So I feel anything is possible.

Remote Healing through a Large Demon, After Its Transformation into the Light

Sometimes, during therapy, patients find in them a large demon entity who is a big commander in Satan's hierarchy. They claim to train and command millions and millions of demons on earth. After their transformation, they are more than happy to call out from people on earth all those they trained and commanded, and thus heal millions and millions of people from their physical and emotional problems.

Ben, several years ago, under hypnosis, found many large demon spirits in him who claimed to be big commanders in Satan's hierarchy. After their transformation, they were more than willing to call out all the demons they trained and commanded on the earth.

During each session, Ben described that heaven would open up and he would see the whole hierarchy of heaven: God on the top as a mountain of Light: under God the Godheads or masters of different religions; also different angels miles and miles around; and, at the gate of heaven, the angels Michael, Gabriel, and Christopher, who were helping us.

434

He saw millions and millions of large, medium, and small demons coming from different people and places on the earth as the commander called them out. When they came close to their commander, I would tell them to look at their commander who is all Light and that they can all find their Light, change into the Light, so they can all go home to the Light (heaven).

As they came close, the demons appeared as ugly and scary-looking giants or in other forms and sizes. Then, when they heard me and looked at their transformed commander, they would instantly change into the Light and were helped into heaven by the angels.

The transformed commander would also show Ben people from the different parts of the earth from whom the demons were called out. He was shown how people were healed miraculously from their crippling emotional and physical problems, as these demons came out of them. As far as those people were concerned, their healing was a miracle. Then we were told by the angels to request them to fill and shield all the people who were healed and the whole earth with the Light.

We did similar remote healing once a week, for four to five hours each session, for four months. Every time, heaven opened up and Ben would see the whole hierarchy of heaven. Most of the time we were able to work with one big demon commander in a session, and he would call out millions of those he commanded.

The transformed commander demons also gave us the understanding about how they and others they commanded created certain types of problems, and how they affected the people they were in.

The whole experience during those four months was extremely joyous and humbling. We both had an inner knowing that we planned in heaven to do this work, before we were born into this life.

Chapter VIII

Long Cases

Long Cases

In the following long cases, sources of the symptoms were interwoven in current life traumas, including prenatal and birth traumas; possession by earthbound and demon entities; past life traumas; and soul fragmentation and soul loss. The therapy then became a matter of methodically releasing all the foreign entities, regressing the patient through the current life and the past life traumas that caused the symptoms, and locating, retrieving, and integrating all the missing soul parts. This process required several three-to four-hour sessions, but the results were simply astounding.

Ann

Ann, a fifty-year-old married white female, came to me for past life regression therapy because of multiple psychological and physical problems. Her presenting symptoms and secondary symptoms were as follows.

Presenting or Primary Symptoms

Depression: Ann described having had all her life, chronic depression ranging from mild to suicidal, with the worst symptoms in the fall and winter. She was often quiet, impulsive, and withdrawn, and sometimes became moody.

Chronic fatigue: Ann had felt tired and drained most of her life. She felt like she was always dragging herself around and barely making it through the day.

Poor concentration and memory: She was afflicted with poor concentration and memory for most of her life.

Sleeping problems: For most of her life Ann had sleeping problems, which were more pronounced over the past three to four years. For one year, she slept only three to four hours a night and had early morning awakenings.

Dreams and nightmares: Ann had nightmares most of her life. For one year before she came to me they were so bad that she was afraid to go to sleep. She had many repetitive dreams:

- She dreamed about snakes hanging all over her.
- She dreamed of falling but waking up before hitting the ground. This dream recurred five to six times a year for most of her life.
- She dreamed of being chased by somebody who was trying to kill her.
- She dreamed of feeling that she had to get something done but could not seem to do it.

Anxiousness and restlessness: Ann was anxious and restless most of her life. She was constantly biting her nails and as a result had very little of her nails left.

Panic attacks: Ann had panic attacks with palpitations and difficulty in breathing three or four times a month.

Conversations in her head: Ann had constant conversation in her head. Many nights she could not go to sleep and had trouble concentrating during daytime due to this ongoing "chatter in her head." She felt as though her mind were always racing.

Compulsive eating: Ann had been a compulsive eater most of her life. She weighed about 205 pounds and had a difficult time losing weight.

Secondary Symptoms

On further questioning during the interview, Ann reported having the following emotional and physical symptoms. She had experienced these for a long time, but was able to deal with them to some extent.

Fears: Ann had multiple fears most of her life:

- Fear of being smothered;
- Fear of heights;
- Fear of rainstorms;
- Fear of driving over bridges (particularly if traffic stopped on them);
- Fear and visions of a car accident; and
- Fear of snakes, spiders, and bugs.

Inability to wear anything close to her neck.

Perfectionism: Ann was a perfectionist. Everything had to be perfect and she had to make it so, including the lives of everybody she knew.

Feelings of pressure in her head: She often felt that her head was going to explode.

Headaches: She suffered from headaches most of her adolescent and adult life. These were either tension or sinus headaches.

Aches and pains all over her body: These aches and pains included cramps in her legs for as long as she could remember.

Low back pain and spasms: She had these most of her life. These had been worse since an injury sustained during her freshman year in college.

Pain and lack of strength and mobility in her right hand: At times she experienced numbness and had no grip in her right hand.

Poor circulation in her hands and feet: She suffered with these for most of her life.

Intolerance of heat and hot weather: Sometimes she would faint in hot and muggy weather.

Irritable bowel syndrome: She could not tolerate and digest many foods, especially foods with heavy cream or fat, most of her life. She had instant cramping and diarrhea.

Hyperacidity: At times, because of hyperacidity, she was not able to lie down and sleep. This difficulty became more pronounced about a year before therapy.

Sinus problems: Ann had sinus drainage and headaches most of her life.

Allergies: She was allergic to citrus fruits, dust, grass, and weeds.

Essential hypertension: Hypertension had been a problem since the age of twenty-one. It was 245/165 when discovered. She had headaches, dizziness, upset stomach, and fatigue due to it. She had been on medications since then. Her blood pressure had spiked many times over the years, and as a result she had been hospitalized several times. She was taking Prinivil and Lasix for it.

Tendencies for infections and inflammation: Ann had been prone to infections and inflammation most of her life. During the winter months the problem seemed worse, and she always carried a high sedimentation rate.

Nail infection: Ann had an infection in her fingernails, which were red. This was more pronounced in both thumbs from the age of nineteen and her thumbnails were irregular and rippled. She also had ingrown toenails.

Poor depth of vision: Ann had poor depth of vision most of her life and could not tolerate glasses because they made her dizzy and nauseous.

Hearing: Although Ann did not have any measured hearing loss, she always had difficulty in focusing on listening. Too much peripheral noise made it impossible to filter out and focus on what she was trying to hear. During the interview, Ann had a tendency to turn her head to the right to hear and often asked, "What did you say?"

Music: Ann had always been drawn to music, but never had much confidence in her musical ability. Often she woke up hearing the beautiful music in her soul, but could not remember it long enough to write it down.

Medication: Ann was taking Furosemide, 20 mg.; Prinivil, 10 mg.; Daypro, 600 mg.; Premarin, 0.625 mg.; Elavil (amitriptyline), 10 mg. tab.

During the next session, I made a relaxation tape for Ann with protection techniques and positive suggestions.

First Hypnotherapy Session

I explained to Ann, in detail, about hypnosis and hypnotherapy and what she might discover while she was under hypnosis. I told her about the human spirits, demon spirits, fragmented soul parts, and past lives traumas that may surface during a session under hypnosis. She already had an understanding and knowledge about these concepts before she came to my office and was willing to try hypnotherapy. When she heard about the possession of a person by the human spirits, she felt that she might have many of them on board with her and must be like a motel for these spirits.

We proceeded to look for any attached human and demon entities and fragmented parts of her soul. While under hypnosis, Ann found the following entities inside her:

Father: Ann's father died in 1977 of heart problems. Ann's guilt and sadness opened her up for him to come in.
Effect: Her father was depressed and suicidal. These feelings were transferred to Ann. He also had stomach ulcers, which Ann experienced as stomach acidity.

Brother: Ann's brother died of melanoma six months before she came for therapy. It started in the left arm and later spread over his body, including his brain. He claimed to come in to help Ann.
Effect: Her brother claimed to cause her the tired and drained feelings. He weakened her immune system and increased her depression and feelings of desolation. He had all these symptoms before he died, which were transferred over to Ann.

Cousin Jack: Jack died of Hodgkin's disease at the age of twenty-seven. He joined Ann when she was thirty-seven. She wrote a nice poem about him after his death. Her compassion opened her up for him to come in.
Effect: Jack claimed to cause her depression and weakened her immune system, making her more prone to infections. He had these symptoms before his death and they were transferred over to Ann.

Susan: This ten-year-old girl died in a car accident. She was riding in a car on a stormy night on a bridge when the bridge collapsed. She claimed to have joined Ann when Ann was three years old and was in the hospital having a tonsillectomy.

Effects: Susan claimed to cause Ann to have the fear of driving over bridges, fear of being smothered, fear of car accidents, and the fear of driving during rainstorms. Susan also caused back pain and aches and pains all over Ann's body because different parts of Susan's body were broken. These were Susan's feelings and symptoms, which were transferred over to Ann.

Ray: A sixty-two-year-old man, who was her neighbor. He died in 1971 of a gunshot wound in the head. Ann remembered Ray as creepy and not very nice. Ray claimed that after his death dark demons grabbed him and took him to hell. They burned him in the hellfire and then told him to go to Ann and cause her problems and bring her soul to Satan. He claimed to have joined Ann when she was thirty-one, at a time when she was very unhappy and sad.

Effects: Ray claimed to have headaches, high blood pressure, and felt hot all the time as he felt when he was burned in hellfire. (Ann was feeling extremely hot when Ray was speaking through her.) All these symptoms were transferred over to Ann.

Grandfather: Her grandfather died of old age. He joined Ann when she was twenty-three. According to her grandfather, she invited him in.

Effect: He claimed to cause her chronic fatigue and poor concentration and memory.

Second Hypnotherapy Session

Ann reported feeling more energetic following her first hypnotherapy session and that her depression, concentration, and memory were improving. She was sleeping well all night and for the first time in many years didn't have nightmares. She also lost about seven pounds.

She felt she may have in her the spirit of a teenager, Darla, who died in a car accident. She had helped Darla in a time of trouble. Under hypnosis, Ann found the following entities:

Darla: Under hypnosis, she saw Darla, who claimed to have joined Ann in the funeral home because she liked Ann. Darla claimed to cause Ann the following problems that she had.

Effect: Darla claimed to cause Ann visions, dreams, and fear of a car accident. It was Darla who was recalling her car accident over and over. This became Ann's symptom after Darla joined her. She also caused her headaches and aches and pain all over her body. These were Darla's feelings due to head and other injuries to the rest of her body, that later were transferred to Ann.

Little Ann (fragmented soul part): She appeared to Ann as herself at the age of four. She fragmented and separated because she was sad and unhappy. They had to move to another city and she did not want to move. She was integrated with the grownup Ann after resolution of her trauma.

Soul: Ann saw her soul as a round white Light located inside her chest, around her heart. She saw several threads, or cords, coming out from her soul. She saw them going to and connected with her soul parts in the following people:

Ann's mother: She had Ann's soul part with her. Ann's mother had Alzheimer's disease and cold hands and feet, which became Ann's symptoms too.

Her father: We sent him to the Light during the last session. He had a part of her soul.

Phyllis: A little girl who was in heaven, having died of cancer. Ann did not know her in this life, but had a feeling that she gave this part to Phyllis in a past life.

She saw angels bringing all these soul parts back to her at our request. They cleansed and healed the parts, and filled them with the Light and then integrated them with her soul.

I told Ann to check for any other missing parts from her soul. She saw another cord coming out of her soul. As she traced that cord, she saw it going into the Light (heaven) and to one of the masters, whom she recognized as Jesus. From Jesus she saw that cord going to God. At this point she heard the following message: "Love is the only thing which matters. Believe that God is a loving and forgiving God. He loves everybody unconditionally no matter what you do. You can be strong because strength comes from God through this connecting cord and that we are all connected with God and with each other." She stayed quiet for a minute or so and appeared to be blissful.

After the session, Ann said, "I was totally unprepared for what happened. I was instantly infused by what I would call a cosmic power surge. That is a grossly inadequate phrase. The incredible Light, rush of energy, warmth and love that came in, is beyond description. It was an incredible presence and felt wonderful. I felt like I was supremely blessed, personally, firsthand. There have been two or three times before, once in college and twice during communion, when I felt a fraction of this feeling, but this experience was beyond measure. I wish everyone could experience this."

Third Hypnotherapy Session

Ann reported her depression, chronic fatigue, headaches, aches and pains, leg cramps, fear of driving over bridges, fear of rainstorms, dreams, and fear and visions of car accidents were totally alleviated after the last session.

Her hyperacidity, back pain, and right hand pain were 90 percent improved. Mobility in the right hand was 80 percent improved, while the strength in the right hand was 50 percent improved. Almost all her primary symptoms and many of the secondary symptoms were relieved.

As we proceeded, under hypnosis, to check again for any other possessing entities, she saw several dark-looking demon entities in her back.

A gray demon blob in her back: It claimed to have joined Ann at the age of three, when she was having her tonsillectomy. This gray blob said that during the surgery Ann was out of her body. After the surgery, when she was coming back in the body, the gray blob came in with her.

Effect: The gray blob claimed to cause Ann back pain and stiffness.

A black (demon) cloud: It was also found in her back. It claimed to have joined Ann when she had a back injury at the age of eighteen. She could not walk for a while.

Effect: This also claimed to cause her back pain and stiffness.

A black snake (demon entity) in the back: It claimed to have joined Ann when she fell off of a car hood at five years of age.

Effect: It claimed to cause her back pain, headaches, and breathing difficulties.

A black demon blob in her head and eyes: It claimed to join her at the age of three, when she had an eye infection. Initially it was hard to communicate with it because it had a two-year-old Ann trapped inside it. After some therapy, two-year-old Ann was freed. Afterward the black blob was cooperative.

Effect: The demon claimed to cause her vision problems and headaches and said it tried to block her from the Light.

Two-year-old Ann (fragmented soul part): She was totally trapped and surrounded by that black blob in the eyes. This two-year-old Ann fragmented and separated at the age of two, when her mom was sick in the hospital. She was afraid for her mother.

All the dark demon entities were transformed into the Light and released back to heaven. Little Ann (two-year-old) was integrated with the grownup Ann after the resolution of her trauma.

As Ann was scanning her body, she saw her right kidney slightly enlarged and saw a kink in one of her blood vessels. She saw angels removing the kink and healing the kidney. They also cleansed and healed her back and eyes where the entities were. Then the angels filled and shielded the rest of her body with the Light.

Fourth Hypnotherapy Session

Ann reported that she was doing very well. None of the symptoms had returned. She had lost fifteen pounds and had no back pain and stiffness since her last session. She said that for the last two to three days she had been feeling dizzy and was also feeling dizzy during the session. Under hypnosis, Ann found the following entities:

Dark cloud demon in the head and eyes: It claimed to have joined Ann at the age of ten, when she had problems with her eyes. The entity said that during the last session Ann could not find it because it was hiding under another layer. It claimed it did not let Ann focus with her eyes, did not let her use glasses, weakened her eyes, caused her headaches, and caused her dizziness by pressing on the nerves.

Dark blob demon in the right ear: It claimed to have joined Ann when she had mumps, fever, and earache at the age of seven. It claimed to cause earaches and dizziness by causing pressure in the ears and did not let her hear.

Both dark demon entities were transformed into the Light, after some psychotherapy, and were released back to the Light.

Soul part of her mother: It came along with Ann when she went to visit her in the nursing home two days before. Her mother did not want to stay in her body because it was old and sick. This soul part was partially responsible for Ann's dizziness and memory problem. It was cleansed, healed, and integrated with her mother with the help of the angels. Her mother had six of Ann's soul parts, which were brought back and integrated with Ann after cleansing.

Effect: Memory problems, nervousness, sleepiness, and dizziness were caused by the mother's soul part.

Regression to the Source of Her Weight Problem

I decided to use the bridge technique for regression to the source of her weight problem. I did not use any progressive relaxation. I just asked her to close her eyes and focus on her thoughts and feelings when she thinks of her weight problem. She stated the following thoughts and feelings:

"I feel lumpy and unattractive."
"I feel sad, scared, and want to cry."

"I feel pressure from my neck up."

"I feel like my head is going to explode."

I asked her to repeat those phrases and let these thoughts and feelings take her to another time when she felt the same way. After repeating them three or four times, she slipped into a past life in which she was a man. His name was John. There was a famine and everybody was starving. He had a wife and three small children. He stole food so his children could eat. He was caught and hanged. His last thoughts were, "Who will feed my children?" and "I will never be hungry again."

After the death of his body, he saw the white Light and angels, who took him to the Light. From heaven, while reviewing John's life, Ann saw his whole life flashing in front of her like a movie on fast forward. She saw that he ran away as a teenager because he didn't get along with his parents. He was hungry most of his life. He got married and was good to his wife and children. Lifelong starvation was the main theme of his life.

Soul parts: From heaven, Ann saw many soul parts that fragmented from John's eyes, ears, throat, and brain during hanging; the soul parts were in the possession of Satan and his demons. They were causing her hearing, vision, and memory problems by squeezing the soul parts or clamping the connecting cords. There were also soul parts from his stomach with Satan, who was restimulating her appetite and hungry feelings by squeezing those parts. They were all brought back, cleansed, healed, and integrated with Ann.

Problems coming from John's life: From heaven, Ann recognized the following problems that came from John's life.

- Hanging caused her headaches, fear of suffocation, feelings that her head was going to explode, inability to wear anything close to her neck, dizziness, and pain and poor circulation in her hands.
- Constant overeating, even without feeling hungry.
- Memory, vision, and hearing problems due to lost soul parts from her ears, brain, and eyes due to hanging.

After forgiving others who hurt him and forgiving himself for hurting others and stealing food, Ann felt free of all the physical and emotional problems which came from that life.

Regression to the Source of Hypertension

While Ann was in heaven, I asked her to look back in her past lives and locate the lifetime responsible for her high blood pressure. From heaven, she saw a life of a fisherman on a boat in Tunisia in 1400 B.C.

I asked her to go down in that life. He was a twenty-six-year-old fisherman on a boat. His name was Rahim. During a storm his boat turned over and he drowned.

He described it more like a stroke than like drowning. The pressure of the sea was so intense that all his blood vessels in his head and eyes ruptured. He said that right before he died everything turned red (his eyes exploded), and then everything went black.

Soul parts: From heaven, Ann saw that Rahim lost big soul parts that belonged to his eyes, ears, and brain. They were in the possession of Satan. He squeezed the parts and clamped the cords off and on, causing vision, hearing, and memory problems for Ann. The parts were brought back, cleansed, healed, filled with the Light, and integrated with Ann.

Problems coming from Rahim's life: From heaven, Ann saw the problems coming from Rahim's life:

- High blood pressure, headaches, pressure in the head, and feelings that her head was going to explode (feelings of Rahim when he died)
- Vision problems and poor depth of vision
- Hearing problems
- Fear of choking and of being smothered

Fifth Hypnotherapy Session

During this session, Ann wore a blouse that she was able to button up close to her neck, and it did not bother her. Her blood pressure had remained within normal limits and she was able to cut her medication in half. Her depth of vision had improved since the last session. Her pain, strength, and mobility in the right hand had improved to almost 95 percent. None of the other symptoms came back.

Under hypnosis, while scanning her body for any entities, Ann saw dark demon entities who were hiding at a deeper level.

Dark demon blob in the ears: It claimed it had never been human. It joined Ann when she was twenty-three years old and was sad.

Effect: It claimed to create noise in her ears, which vibrated and created confusion. It also claimed to scramble sound by twisting the nerves until everything got garbled and then she could not focus on what she was hearing.

Gray demon shadow: It was on the right side of the brain. It claimed to have joined Ann when she was two, when she broke her nose.

Effect: It claimed to cause Ann headaches, vision problems, and memory problems.

Regression to the Source of Ann's Hearing Problems

I asked Ann to focus on her thoughts, and emotional and physical feelings about her hearing problems. They were

"Noise bothers me; I cannot hear clearly."
"I feel nervous, shaky, and frightened."

After three or four repetitions, she found herself in another life on a battlefield, where guns and cannons were firing constantly.

She was an eighteen-year-old young man in the Civil War. His name was Jamie. He was shot in the back, was left on the field for a long time, and, as a result, infection set in. He died later in the hospital from the infection, fever, fatigue, and weak-

450

ness. He did not want to shoot guns and did not like the roar of guns or sound of a cannon firing. His last thoughts were, "I will never fight again. I do not like those sounds."

Soul parts: Ann saw many soul parts that had fragmented from Jamie. She saw four parts from his ears, two from his eyes, and one from the brain that were with Satan and his demons. They caused problems by squeezing the soul parts and clamping cords off and on, causing her to have hearing, memory, and vision problems. Her back pain was caused by several soul parts that had fragmented from Jamie's back when he was shot.

There were two soul parts still lying on the battlefield. They fragmented out of fear and caused the problem with hearing, noise, and confusion. All the parts were brought back and integrated with Ann after being cleansed and healed.

Problems coming from Jamie's life: From the Light, Ann recognized the following problems coming from Jamie's life.

- Fear of loud noises. They make her nervous. She becomes confused and anxious and cannot concentrate. She cannot listen because she does not want to hear it again.
- Back pain, as Jamie was shot in the back.
- Chronic repetitive infections.
- Chronic fatigue.
- Bad circulation in her arms and legs.

Sixth Hypnotherapy Session

After the last session there had been a remarkable change in Ann's hearing. She was able to hear and comprehend without any problem. For the first time she did not have to turn her head to one side to try to hear what was being said and didn't have to ask to repeat. She did not have a confused look on her face as she tried to hear and comprehend. Loud noises did not bother her. Her back pain was improved. On an average she continued to lose four to five pounds a week and continued to feel good.

Regression to the Source of Her Sinus Problems

After checking for any attached entities, we proceeded to find the source of her sinus problems. As she focused on her sinuses, she had the following thoughts and feelings:

"I feel pressure in my nose and sinuses."
"It is itching."
"I cannot breathe."
"I am scared."

After a few repetitions of these phrases, Ann shifted into a past life when she was a seven-year-old girl named Jeanette in France in 1682. She was playing in the woods with her brother. There was a fire in the woods and she was trapped in the fire and could not get out. She died of smoke inhalation, feeling burning, itching, and pain in her sinuses. Her last thoughts were, "My nose hurts. I cannot breathe. I am going to die."

Soul parts: Three soul parts were retrieved from her brother and her parents and integrated with her after they were cleansed and healed. Some parts from her sinuses were with demons in the darkness, who restimulated the memory of sinus irritation, pressure, itching, and difficulty in breathing by massaging those parts.

Problems that came from Jeanette's life: From the Light, Ann saw that her sinus problems and the fear of choking and being smothered came from the smoke inhalation.

Second Regression to the Source of Sinus Problems

As she was in heaven, I asked Ann to check her sinuses and see if any negative sensations or feelings were still there. She still had some itching in her nose and sinuses. I asked her to locate the source of that problem from heaven. She saw a life on an Island in 1430. She was nineteen, and her name was Lani. I asked her to go down in that life and relive it.

She was in a tropical country with lots of fruits. The natives used the fruits for many things including foods, medicine, etc.

She had to walk through the jungle to pick the fruit. Grass and weeds caused her a sinus problem.

Lani got married at the age of twenty-three. She had a child, a boy, and died of excessive bleeding, feeling sad about leaving her baby. Her last thoughts were, "I do not want to leave my baby. Who will take care of him?"

Soul parts: From heaven, she saw that as she was dying, she gave a soul part to her son, thinking. "It hurts too much; take it away, we will find each other again." In this life he is a very good friend.

She gave another part to her husband. Both parts were brought back and integrated after being cleansed and healed.

Problems that came from Lani's life:

- Allergies to grass, weeds, and citrus fruits. The allergies were a reminder of the sadness due to the loss of her baby.
- Sinus problems caused from her allergies to grass and weeds
- Hyperacidity due to citrus fruits
- Dislike for the tropics

Seventh Hypnotherapy Session

Ann reported that her allergy to citrus fruits was completely gone. She was able to eat citrus fruits without any problem. Her vision problems were gone and her hearing problem, according to Ann, was about 95 percent improved. She did not feel that her sinus problem was completely gone, although it improved about 80 percent.

Two days before this session, Ann ate some potato soup with heavy cream. She instantly started to have severe cramping and diarrhea, and her sinuses started to drain. So we decided to explore these symptoms.

Regression to the Source of Diarrhea and Sinus Problems

I asked Ann to close her eyes and focus on those thoughts and feelings about diarrhea and let those feelings take her to the source of those problems.

"I am feeling abdominal pressure and cramps."

"My sinuses are draining."

"I feel very restless and anxious."

"I am itching all over."

As she was focusing on those thoughts and feelings, she instantly moved into a life where she was a twenty-year-old male in Belgium. His name was Andreas. He and many other people were taken to some place as laborers by soldiers to build a shrine. They walked barefoot in the hot weather. They were hungry and thirsty and had sores on their feet. Four men, including Andreas, tried to run away. He remembered running through thick woods, itching all over due to weeds, dust, and other plants and trees. (Ann was scratching vigorously all over her body and was very anxious and restless during the session.)

As Ann was going through the session, to my surprise, my feet and body started to ache severely and I began to itch all over. (I wondered if I might be there, too.) While in the woods, Andreas was bitten by a snake and fainted. Soldiers found him and dragged him through the woods to a cave. He was fed thick cereal, or soup with milk. He hated the taste, had diarrhea, and died. His last thoughts were, "I do not like snakes and spiders" and "I will stay away from the woods."

After his death, his soul was completely surrounded and trapped inside a demon, so he could not see or hear anything. It was all black and cold. Then he felt as if he were falling faster and faster and had no control. He became afraid and started to pray to God for help. He saw the Light coming with little baby angels who carried him to heaven.

From heaven, Ann recognized me as one of the four people trying to escape. I was running through the woods, too, and had sores on my feet and was fed the same stuff in the cave.

Soul parts: From heaven, Ann saw that while walking painfully, she lost many soul parts from her feet, legs, sinuses, stomach, and from the whole body, which were in the possession of the demons in the darkness. They squeezed those parts to restimulate the memory and thus caused pain in her feet, legs, and all over the body, sinus problems, and abdominal cramps.

Andreas lost large parts of his soul when the snake bit him. He was completely possessed by a demon at that time.

All those fragmented soul parts were brought back and integrated with Ann after cleansing and healing them. We also requested angels to bring back all my soul parts that I lost during that life and cleanse, heal, and integrate them with me.

Problems coming from Andreas' life: From the Light, Ann saw the following problems coming from that life:

- Allergies to grass, weeds, dust, etc.
- Sinus problems
- Irritable bowel syndrome with instant cramping and diarrhea when she drinks or eats food with heavy cream
- Aversion to walking in the woods
- Pain and spasms in her legs and feet
- A drop in her blood pressure and passing out when she takes medication derived from snake venom

This session was a unique and interesting experience. After the session, my leg and foot pain and itching stopped, too. I used to get a throbbing pain off and on in my legs and feet and had severe allergies to milk and milk products leading to instant cramping, bloating, and diarrhea. I also do not like to walk in areas with high grass and have absolutely no desire to walk through the woods.

Eighth Hypnotherapy Session

Ann reported she is not having any cramping or diarrhea and can eat different foods, milk, and certain grains. Her sinus problems had improved. Soups with a creamy base were easier to digest.

Regression to the Source of Fear of Heights

Ann had repetitive dreams of falling and would wake up screaming. I asked her to close her eyes and recall that dream, focus on it, and expand her awareness into that dream. Ann instantly recalled:

"I am falling and falling. I am afraid; there is nothing to grab on to. I am falling faster and faster in some kind of pit. It feels like I am falling for a long time. I fall on a rock. It is a dark well. There are snakes, spiders, and poisonous bugs. Something bit me on the neck and I feel sleepy and dizzy. I am hungry and thirsty and I have chills. An angel comes and helps me out." [death]

From heaven, as Ann reviewed that life, she recalled that her name was Anya, a twenty-four-year-old female in Europe in 1302. She was a clairvoyant and an abandoned child. She grew up by herself and lived alone in the woods because people thought she was a witch and stayed away from her. But they all came to her when they needed healing. She could heal different types of problems.

She could see and had knowledge of the future. She told the baron that his wife would have a deformed child. He wanted her to fix it so the child would not be deformed. She, of course, could not. So they threw her in a pit with poisonous snakes, spiders, and insects, where she was bitten by a snake and died. The baron, it turns out, was her father and had abandoned her. Her mother was a servant working for the baron. Her last thought as she was thrown in the pit was, "I will never tell again."

Soul parts: From heaven, Ann saw that many soul parts that Anya lost all through her sad and lonely life were brought back from Satan and his dark ones and from the darkness. Many soul parts were also lost from her ears and brain and from all over her body as she was falling and was in the pit. She also gave a part to the baron. All the parts were brought back and integrated with her after cleansing and healing.

Problems that came from Anya's life: From the Light, Ann saw the following problems coming from Anya's life:

- A fear of snakes, spiders, and bugs and allergies to their bites. She had severe reactions to bug bites, which resulted in hospitalization.
- Dreams and nightmares about snakes and dreams of falling

- Fear of heights
- Back pain
- Pressure in the ears and dizziness
- Headaches and feelings that her head was going to explode
- Inability to take blood pressure medications that are derivatives of snake venom came from this life.

She still has ability to "see" and "know," but is very careful about letting this be known.

Ninth Hypnotherapy Session

Ann reported her fear of height had been completely alleviated. She went to a conference and noted that although her room was on the sixteenth floor, she was able to walk up to the window without panic. She was also comfortable riding in elevators and escalators.

Ann said that although she is not nervous or anxious, she still constantly bites her nails. So we decided to explore that problem during this session. She also had a fungal infection in her thumbs and ingrown toenails.

Regression to the Source of Nail Biting and Infected Thumbnails

As she began to focus on her nails, she began to feel nervous, shaky, and hot. Her mouth was dry. She slipped back into a life as a thirty-two-year-old man in Europe. His name was Jacques. He was the choirmaster at a French cathedral. He was a quiet man who led people by his example.

He harbored fugitives in the cathedral following an uprising and smuggled them out at night through a secret passageway under the organ. An informant in the church set him up, and he was captured. He was tortured by being burned with a hot iron on the back and was hit on the head, but he refused to talk. So they chopped his fingers off, one by one. Then his thumbnails were smashed, split, and pulled out. They did the same with his toes. Still he refused to talk, so they beheaded him in the marketplace.

After his death, he found himself suspended in a dark tunnel in which he could not see or hear anything. He was cold and did not feel right. He felt as though something were pulling him down and he was falling. So he prayed to God for help. Instantly he felt something like a falling star coming. They were angels who pulled him out of the dark tunnel and took him to heaven.

Heaven: He saw heaven as with no walls and no floors, but everything was contained. Angels took him to a cathedral, where he saw Jesus. Jesus apologized for Jacques' suffering, as if he had suffered with him, too. Jesus said that it was a big test of his faith and he passed it.

"He is touching my hands. They are comforting and healing. His hands give me the ability to touch people, to comfort them. He gives me healing."

Soul parts: From heaven, Ann saw that Jacques lost many soul parts:

Soul parts to torturers: Every time they cut a finger or toe, they took from those areas a soul part that later Satan and his demons captured and used to reactivate the memories and feelings of torture and pain in Ann's body by touching and squeezing them.

Soul parts from the throat, ears, eyes, brain, and whole face: He lost these soul parts due to decapitation. It was as though a circuit were cut between hearing, seeing, speaking, and memory. There was a disconnection between those functions.

Soul part from his heart: These parts were left in the cathedral and also went to other brothers.

All the parts were brought back with the help of angels, who cleansed, healed, and integrated them with Ann.

Problems that came from Jacques's life:

- Nail biting and infections: Satan and his demons restimulated feelings and memories of torture by touching and massaging those soul parts. Ann then became aware of her fingers and bit her nails.
- Poor eye, hand, and foot coordination

- Headaches, dizziness, hearing problems, vision problems, and memory problems
- Circulation problems in hands and feet due to decapitation and cutting off the fingers and toes
- Attraction toward church music and mass
- Does not want to play organ ever again
- Still has healing touch in this life, too, and uses it generously

Tenth Hypnotherapy Session

Ann reported that she did not bite her nails anymore and her nails were growing. During this and several other sessions, we found the source of her music block. According to Ann, she often dreamed and woke up in the night hearing the most beautiful music in her soul, but could not hold it long enough to write it down. This experience frustrated her a great deal. Under hypnosis, in each transition to the Light, she would hear the music in heaven and would cry quietly, as from a sense of a loss.

Regression to the Source of Her Music Block

Ann recalled the thoughts and feelings connected with her music block and repeated them.

"I can hear the music, but cannot hold it long enough to
    write it down."
"I feel frustrated."
"I feel sad."

After a few repetitions, she regressed to a life in Paris, France. She was a child prodigy who played piano. Her name was Marie. When Marie was six years old, her mother died. Marie and her baby brother, who were very close, were separated and placed in separate orphanages. Marie was very upset by the loss of her mother and brother.

At the age of fourteen, she left the orphanage when a wealthy family took her on as a governess. The family had a piano, which she played for their small children. The family recognized her talent and paid for piano lessons to prepare her for an audition for the Paris Conservatory. At eighteen, she was accepted. At twenty-one, she found out that her brother had been killed. Devastated by his death, she left Paris and gave up her music. Marie died at the age of sixty-three. Her last thoughts were: "I miss my brother. I could have been a good musician." She felt intense sadness over the loss of her brother and music.

After her death, as she went to heaven, she heard the most incredible music. In her review stage, she understood that it is important not to quit and to use what one is given. She would have to come back again soon and do it all over again. She was to find her brother, and she would find her music again.

Effects of Marie's life: In this life Ann always felt empty and sad when she thought of music. She always felt that she lost something and was unsure about her music ability.

People: She recognized her brother from that life as a good friend and a coworker in her current life.

Soul parts: In that lifetime she gave her brother a big soul part that had to do with her music. That part was retrieved and integrated after cleansing and healing, with the help of angels.

Second Life Connected with Her Music Problem

She saw herself as a twenty-six-year-old female in Vienna, Austria, in 1682. Her name was Hanne. She was a woman musician, a rarity in that time. She and others were preparing for a concert of Hungarian music. There was an uprising and fighting. She and a friend, Stefan, for whom she cared a great deal, and others stayed in an opera house for a couple of nights and then decided to flee. Hanne was against running, but Stefan insisted on it. She was hit in the chest and killed. Her last thoughts were, "Why wouldn't he listen?"

As she went to heaven, she heard the music that they were playing on earth, but it was much more magnificent. She was taken to a great big sun (God), where the same music was playing and it felt as though he poured something into her. [music]

People: She recognized Stefan as a friend in this life. Her mother in the current life was also her mother in that life.

Soul parts: Hanne gave to Stefan two soul parts that belonged to her ears because he would not listen. They were brought back and integrated with her.

Problem coming from Hanne's life: An inability to hold the music long enough to write it down.

Eleventh Hypnotherapy Session

During this session, Ann reported that the music that she heard in heaven was the most incredible music. Since the last session, she was given that song, piece by piece, and she got all the words and music. It was as though it were dropped into her lap. Although she had no easy access to a piano, she did not lose the music. When she finally got to a piano, after only a little practice, she was able to play this music. Now she is refining it.

Regression to the Source of the Music Block

This time she regressed back to another life in Salzburg, Austria, as a fifteen-year-old German girl, whose name was Anneliese. Her parents were persecuted for their religious beliefs. She was taken into an abbey, where she became a nun. There she got into trouble for playing the organlike instrument, which only one person was allowed to play. She overate all her life, as a substitute for the music, to fill up feelings of profound emptiness.

She died of a rupture of blood vessels in her head, feeling like her head was going to explode. Her last thoughts were: "It was a good life. I only regret that I could not play the instrument. I feel I was robbed."

After the death of her body, she heard the music and found herself moving toward it. She was surrounded by angels who were playing the harp.

In the Light, in the review stage, she understood the lessons she needed to learn from this life:

- Accept what you cannot change. She felt she learned this.
- Learn to listen to the sound of her soul.
- Unconditional love in the abbey was as in heaven. We should give that to others.

Soul parts: She left three parts at the abbey near the organlike instrument. Her irresistible desire to play it in that life has given her now the feeling of approach and avoidance, which persists.

Connections between two lives: In this life, Ann has always loved Catholic church services and music, although she is not a Catholic. She can also play the organ in this life, but will not play it.

Second Regression to the Source of the Music Block

She regressed to another life, where she was a fifteen-year-old boy in Yorkshire, England, in 1627. His name was William, a shepherd boy who played a wooden flute while tending sheep. He was very talented. He got in trouble with the sheep master for playing the flute and he broke and burned it. It was very painful for him and he never played the flute again.

Connections: Ann is still afraid to play music, but not as much. It's as if she does not want to be "found out."

Twelfth Hypnotherapy Session

During this session, Ann regressed to a past life in a monastery as a thirty-three-year-old monk, whose name was Stephan. He was basically a composer of liturgical music, especially chants. He was a quiet, good soul who lived in his music. He was responsible for writing a great deal of early church music.

At the age of forty-one, he had brain fever. He lost his vision and hearing, but still could write the music because it came from God to his soul through inspiration. He could hold it long enough to write it down. Gradually he lost his mind and memory and became confused. During the last years, he remained isolated. Other brothers took care of him. He died at the age of forty-seven of high fever.

After his death he could hear the music. Baby angels came and took him to the Light. He could see and hear now. Four angels came and got him. In a procession, they all went to the golden throne. There was a huge Light (God). He could not look at it. Everybody was bowing down. He felt a hand on the top of his head, but could not look up. He heard a voice from behind him. He knew it was the voice of Jesus.

Voice: "You have come to receive the Light, which is infused with love and you will take it with you when you leave. Through your music you brought love to the world. You are not through yet; you will do so again.

"A vibration emanates from God. It is energy. The closer you are to God, the more energy you have. Sometimes your energy is so strong that people can see it. God's energy is healing energy. Love and Light are gifts from God and what you give, you get back.

"Music and arts are direct communication from God. He gives us those things because people need to see, hear, and touch. When we incarnate, we lose our ability to see, hear, and touch beyond our normal senses. So God gives us concrete things such as music and art. They are physical manifestations of God's love. That is why music is so important in all religions. It transports us back to the source, back to God. It is a way to know that he is not far away. Music and art are like communication from God.

"Baby angels came to get you because you lost your mind and you were childlike. People with mental illness have pure spirits. Because their spirits separate from reality, that makes them distinct. Blessed are the pure in heart, for they shall see God."

Then angels lifted him. As he turned to go, Jesus embraced him.

Review stage: He understood the following lessons from heaven:

Although he lost his mind and hearing, he still could hear the music because divine inspiration transcends handicaps. Where God is, anything is possible. We have to do the best with what we are given, and faith will carry us. The purer in spirit we are, the more we receive from God. Purity of spirit comes from God. Perfection really does not come from us; it comes from God.

Although he lost his mind and hearing, he still could hear the music inside through the divine inspiration.

Connections between Stephen's life and the current life: Stephan also used to wake up in the night hearing music, but feared he could not hold it long enough to write it down. The message was that Ann has to hold it on faith.

Soul parts: Many soul parts were brought back from the monastery and from hell. They were responsible for his hearing, vision, and memory problems.

Thirteenth Hypnotherapy Session

Ann continued to improve. Most of her primary and secondary symptoms were improving after each session. During this session, we decided to explore reasons for her perfectionism.

Regression to the Source of Perfectionism

I asked Ann to focus on the thoughts and feelings about being a perfectionist.

"I have to be perfect."
"Disorder bothers me."
"I get very frustrated and angry with myself when I cannot fix things."
"I expect myself to be perfect. I cannot make a mistake."

Ann started to feel shaky and nervous inside and regressed to another life in Europe in A.D. 154, when she was a twenty-year-old female. Her name was Annette Dupree, a headstrong, overbearing woman, married to an equally strong-headed man. They fought and bickered, though they loved each other.

On a stormy day, she pleaded in an unpleasant manner for him to stay away from the sea. The argument escalated and he stormed off to the sea with his crew of nine men. None of them returned. She was pregnant, but did not get a chance to tell her husband.

The town people ostracized her. They thought she was a witch and that her arguing killed those men. Her son resented her because he lost his father. She died at the age of forty-two by starving herself to death. Her last thoughts were: "I really messed up. I am really angry with myself. It is all my fault. Next time I will have to do it right. I will not make the same mistake again."

After death: She couldn't see or hear anything. She felt stuck and could not move. It was all dark. Something was surrounding her. She felt cold and lost. She was moving down. She felt like she was going to hell because she was a bad person. She felt hot and thought, "God where are you? I need help." She did not think help would come because she was a bad person. But a sunbeam came and there were angels in it. They reached for her and took her up to the Light and the darkness fell away from her.

Lesson: In the review stage from heaven, she understood the lessons that she cannot fix everything. She is not God. Only God is perfect. Just do your best.

People: Ann recognized Annette's husband in that life as her friend in this life.

Soul parts: Annette gave soul parts to all the people who went on the boat, to draw them back. Several parts were with Satan and his demons in the darkness. Through those soul parts, they reinforced her self-doubt and guilt in her body in this current life. They were all brought back, cleansed, healed, and integrated with her.

Problems coming from Annette's life: In this life Ann was a perfectionist. She believed she had to fix everything for everybody. She was also afraid of arguments and confrontations and was afraid of being yelled at.

Fourteenth Hypnotherapy Session

Ann reported that she had lost about forty pounds in about two and a half months. None of the symptoms had returned and she continued to feel better physically, emotionally, mentally, and spiritually. Although her nail biting and nail infection had decreased a great deal and her nails were growing for the first time, she still had some infection in her nail beds and she still at times was biting her nails. She also had a tendency to hide her fingers by making a fist or by hiding her hands under or behind her or by putting her hands in her armpits.

As we were discussing her nail problems, she got a vision of her fingers being dipped in acid and became very anxious and restless, so I asked her to close her eyes and focus on that vision and feelings. She instantly regressed to a life in a concentration camp in Germany in 1940, where she was a five-year-old girl. Her name was Maria. The following is a transcript of what she said:

Maria: "They took me and my three-year-old brother to a fence and they stuffed us in with a bunch of little kids. We were hungry. When it is time to go to get the food, everybody steps all over us and we cannot go to the food. We are hungry, so my brother and I sneak out in the dark to where the food is, but they catch us. They grab me and pick me up by my hair and take me to a place. They squeeze my fingers and dip them in the hot stuff. [crying] It eats my fingers. They do the same to my brother.

"They tie us to a pole and make other kids look at our hands. There are cats that lick and eat our fingers. They leave us there for days. Then they throw us in a cart like potatoes and they push us in a big building. There is fire, I cannot get away. [crying] They pick me up and throw me in the fire. [screams]—[calm]

"Now I am floating above. I see my brother is here, too. We wait for others to come. A big Light like a sun comes around us and picks us up and then the building goes farther away. We are moving up. There are little baby angels who are flying. They come to get us. They are smaller than I am. We want to fly, too. That looks like fun.

"Suddenly it gets real open. There is a garden. We play there. There are flowers and birds, but no cats. I am glad. They ate my fingers. There are funny-looking things here. They look like white feathers. A man

comes. He is nice. He tells us it is O.K., daddy loves us.
Then he goes away."

Dr. Modi: "What happens then?"

Maria/Ann: "The babies come and take us to a room
where there are people with silver spaghetti hair. They
glow. Everything here glows. They tell us that when we
are ready we can go back down again. But I like it here.
I do not feel hungry. They tell us that we were special
gifts like rosebuds, that children die to teach others of
love and compassion. I do not know what that means.
Then one day we go to the other side of this white
ocean. I am not little anymore. We go to the library.
There are books."

People: From heaven, Ann recognized the two men who put
her fingers in the acid as two important people in her life.

Soul parts: From heaven, Ann saw many soul parts fragmented from Maria's hands, stomach, skin, and heart. They went
to those men who tortured her and then were taken by Satan
and his demons. Ann saw demons using those soul parts in the
following manner:

Soul parts from stomach: Ann saw demons clamping the
cords to her stomach soul parts during the daytime and removing
the clamps in the evening and night and squeezing them. This
made her overeat in the evening and in the night.

Soul parts from fingers: She saw demons squeezing the soul
parts of fingers, making her more aware of them and causing her
to bite her nails. They also froze those parts, making her fingers
feel numb, as if they are not there. Then when they are in water
they get sore. Also, sometimes they infused the black liquid stuff
in the fingers through the cords connected with the soul parts
leading to infection.

Soul parts from skin that were lost during burning: Ann
saw demons keeping these soul parts near fire, making her feel
hot and making her skin dry.

Problems coming from Maria's life: From heaven, Ann saw
the following connections and problems coming from Maria's life:

- Nail infections and nail biting
- Numbness of her fingers off and on
- Eating compulsively in the evening
- Aversion for Jewish people, not like a prejudice, but the feeling that "being Jewish got me killed."
- Could not go to Dachau when visiting Europe
- Could not stand heat (being burned)
- Could not watch concentration camp movies
- Fear of adults and violence
- Fear of losing people and fear of abandonment

After forgiving her tormentors, Satan, and his demons, Ann felt free of her physical, emotional, and mental problems.

Conclusion

Looking at Ann's treatment, we can clearly see that most of her presenting symptoms and some of the secondary symptoms were caused by possessing human and demon entities. Most of the secondary symptoms came from the current life traumas, including prenatal and birth traumas, and including the traumas due to the first birth, when her soul was created by God (read "Prenatal and Birth Traumas," chapter 2), and from past life traumas.

To heal her from her symptoms, we needed to free her from all her possessing earthbound and demon entities and then heal her from current life traumas, including the prenatal and birth traumas, past life traumas, and traumas incurred during the creation of her soul by God.

There was no medication prescribed by me, and no traditional insight psychotherapy was done, and yet, session after session, all her lifelong symptoms, from head to toe, were relieved in about two and a half months.

The process is like an onion: we need to peel the roots of the problems, layer by layer, to heal the soul and the patient completely. A thorough healing is possible, but requires a lot of work, perseverance, and commitment on the part of the patient and the doctor. Ann's case is a good example of success in healing her from her crippling symptoms.

Much of the credit for this great success of Ann's cure goes to hypnotherapy, which included releasing the human and demon spirits, soul integration, and resolving the current and past life traumas. But the biggest credit goes to Ann herself. She was determined to free herself from all her physical and emotional problems and was willing to do whatever it took. She had an intense desire to know and understand the truth.

She followed the treatment plan faithfully—sometimes twice a week, three-to-four-hour sessions each—regularly listening to the relaxation tape with protection, and keeping herself protected and positive. She kept a journal about what happened during the sessions and how they changed her. She took full responsibility for her treatment and healing. She kept an open mind and did not try to intellectualize or rationalize the information that emerged from her subconscious mind.

Ann described the experience of her therapy as follows:

"This therapy has been the most exciting experience of my life. The results have been simply miraculous. All my medical and psychological problems are completely cured. I lost about forty-five pounds. I am no longer depressed. I have peace of mind and a strength of resolve about my life that I have never had before. My fears have subsided and I have a sense of direction.

"In fifty years of my life I have always 'known' about God, Jesus, creation, and eternity as Christians teach it. I have learned this summer to know God, Jesus, heaven, hell, Satan and his demons, earthbound spirits, and angels of the Light firsthand. This therapy has given me a very personal relationship with my Creator. I have met God personally; I have been embraced by Jesus on more than one occasion. I cannot find adequate words within the limits of earthly language to describe to you what it is like to be blessed face to face by God and to be embraced by Jesus. What an incredible peace! I have a wonderful relationship with four of the most loyal guardian angels, the most lovely young ladies that ever were. They stay with me constantly and I know they all are always there for me when I need them.

"I have also learned a great deal about prayer. I always knew prayer is important. I never knew quite how to use it. Dr. Modi taught me how to pray for protection and guidance. Now, sessions later, I have developed an easy communication with God. I know prayers are heard and answered. I know God, and I am so thankful to have that firsthand experience. With God all things are possible.

"This therapy has succeeded in 'fixing' what a lifetime of medical treatments failed to fix. I have learned more about God, Jesus, and spirituality during this therapy than I learned from years of traditional religious education, because this time, it was personal. Thank you, Doctor Modi, for changing my life."

Jerry: A Case of Ulcerative Colitis

Jerry, a forty-year-old man, had a history of severe ulcerative colitis off and on for about four years. He had rectal bleeding, diarrhea, abdominal cramps, and distention. He was in and out of the hospital for this condition. One time he bled so much that he was admitted to an intensive care unit and was given five pints of blood and came close to dying. At this point his doctors suggested a colon resection, which Jerry refused. After that he was off work for a long time. He was anxious and depressed because he could not control his physical condition. He felt very helpless and hopeless. Everything was an effort and he lost all his motivation. Jerry was taking 60 mg. of prednisone daily for his colitis. This made him more depressed, irritable, and temperamental. He came to me to try hypnosis to control his symptoms and also to find the source of his colitis.

Jerry's secondary symptoms, which he had for most of his life, were

Neck and shoulder pain, upper and lower back pain, and pain in his hips and legs: He had had these chronic aches and pains and stiffness since he was a teenager, when he had injured himself while working on a farm. These symptoms became worse with stress and depression.

Arthritis in right hand and fingers: He had pain and stiffness in the fingers of his right hand for several years.

Sinus problems: He had sinus problems from time to time for most of his life.

Headaches: From time to time for several years.

Hearing Problem: Jerry had hearing problems for twenty years. They gradually got worse. Hearing aids were prescribed, but he could not use them. Due to his hearing problems, he had trouble communicating; as a result he avoided people and became a loner.

Crowds: Jerry felt very uneasy in crowds and often avoided being in crowded places.

Conversations in head: Jerry had periodic conversations in his head.

Perfectionism: Jerry was a perfectionist, especially in his work. He felt degraded if he was not better than others.

Second Session

During the second session, I made a relaxation tape with positive suggestions to which Jerry could listen at home. I explained to Jerry about hypnotherapy and what he might find under hypnosis, such as possessing earthbound entities, demon entities, or traumatic memories from one or more past lives as a source of his problems. Jerry was willing to try the method.

Third Session

During this session, we proceeded to locate spirits in Jerry's body. Initially, as Jerry scanned his body, he felt that the whole upper half of his body was covered with a dark entity; as a result he had trouble seeing anything. But in spite of his vision block, he was able to receive impressions, feelings, and information and thus was able to locate and release the following entities:

A dark demon entity: It was covering the upper half of his body. This dark entity had a five-year-old Jerry (a fragmented soul part) and other earthbound entities trapped inside it.

Little Jerry: The five-year-old Jerry was scared. He was encouraged to walk out of that dark being and was freed from the dark entity with the help of the angels. He was cleansed, healed, and integrated with the grownup Jerry after the resolution of his trauma.

Timmy: A one-year-old boy, who died of pneumonia, was also trapped in the dark entity.

Clark: A seventy-year-old man who died of a heart attack, was also trapped inside the dark demon entity.

Timmy and Clark came out of the dark entity after some psychotherapy and were released to the Light.

The dark demon entity was transformed into the Light and was sent to heaven with the angels. The dark being claimed to make Jerry anxious, depressed, tired, and drained. After releasing the demon entity, Jerry was able to visualize clearly.

He saw a very powerful, loving Light being in front of him. Jerry became very emotional and tearful. He felt the love pouring from that being, but it did not say anything. Jerry felt the Light being was very powerful and could heal him in no time. He was confused because it did not heal him. He got the impression from that powerful, loving Light being that by healing him directly it would deprive him of the spiritual knowledge that he was supposed to gain through these treatment sessions. He should go through the treatment because he needed to understand and learn some lessons, grow spiritually, and be healed with the treatment.

Fourth Session

According to Jerry, he felt less anxious and depressed after the last session. Under hypnosis, he realized his vision was not blocked anymore; as he scanned his body he found the following entities in him:

Louise: A twenty-year-old female who was in his eyes. She claimed to have died in a train accident and joined Jerry when he was thirty years old. Her head was crushed, and so Jerry experienced headaches. She was released into the Light after some therapy.

Gray demon blobs: They were in Jerry's legs and claimed to cause him leg cramps. They were transformed and released into the Light.

Soul fragment of his cousin Ben: He joined Jerry because he was angry with Jerry. Ben's soul part was returned to his body with the help of the angels, cleansed, healed, and integrated with Ben's body.

Four-year-old little Jerry (a fragmented soul part of Jerry): He was scared and, as a result, fragmented at the age of four. He was cleansed, healed, and integrated with grownup Jerry after the resolution of his trauma.

Fifth Session

During this session, Jerry reported feeling less anxious and depressed. He was sleeping better and was totally free of conversations in his head. During the next several three- to four-hour sessions, Jerry found many past lives responsible for his colitis. During these sessions, I used the bridge techniques to regress him.

First Past Life

Under hypnosis, as Jerry looked inside his gastrointestinal tract, he saw about two dozen small, medium, and large polyps and about twelve to fifteen ulcers in his colon. His colon looked irritated and inflamed to him. During the session, Jerry had the following feelings about his colitis.

"I want to tear it out."
"I cannot handle it anymore."
"I am angry that I cannot function."
"I feel like screaming."
"I feel like I am being punished for something I didn't do."

After a few repetitions of these phrases, he regressed to a life in Georgia. His name was Jim. There was a war. He saw one of the soldiers being shot by the enemy on the street. Jim tried to carry that soldier to a safe place, but couldn't. He could see the enemy coming closer, so he had to leave the wounded soldier and run.

The soldiers in his troop called him a coward for not saving the other soldier and killed him by shooting him in the back. He died feeling angry and confused, that he was punished for something over which he had no control.

When he went to heaven after the death of his body and looked back in that life, he saw the bullet going through his back and creating a hole in his stomach. From heaven, he also saw that during that trauma he lost from his stomach and back soul parts that were in the darkness with the demons. He was amazed when he realized that whatever demons did to those soul parts there in hell, he also felt happening in his physical body here. He saw those demons affecting him through those soul parts as follows:

Stomach soul parts: He saw demons pouring some type of black, hot liquid through those soul parts and connecting cords, into his gastrointestinal tract, causing burning and pain.

Back soul parts: Jerry saw demons hitting and walking on the soul parts from his back, leading to pain and stiffness in his back here in the present life body.

All the soul parts were brought back, cleansed, healed, and integrated with Jerry. He was able to forgive others and himself.

Second Past Life

From heaven, Jerry located another past life in France in 1400. His name was George. He was persecuted for his religious beliefs. Because of his religious beliefs, his persecutors accused him of being possessed by demons. They beat him with sticks and threw rocks at him, and somebody put into his back a spear, which went through his stomach. Then they took axes and chopped his body, including his gastrointestinal tract, into pieces. When he went to heaven and looked back into that life, he saw most of the town people filled with darkness.

From heaven, Jerry saw that he lost soul parts from all over his body, including his stomach, intestine, colon, and back, which were in possession of Satan and his demons. Jerry saw them walking over those soul parts in hell, causing him pain and cramping here in the current life body, especially in his G.I. tract and back. He also saw demons punching his colon soul parts with a wooden fork, creating polyps in his colon here in his body.

All those soul parts were brought back from the demons, cleansed, healed, and integrated with Jerry with the help of the angels. Jerry had a difficult time in forgiving the people who accused and then killed him. After understanding that most of these people were possessed by demons, which made them act the way they did, he was able to forgive them. He also felt a need to forgive Satan and his demons for causing him so many problems. As he did so, he saw them pulling away from him as if they were losing a hold on him.

Third Past Life

Jerry regressed to another life in a prehistoric time. He was a ten-year-old boy and the upper part of his body, including his bowels, was torn apart, and eaten by a large lizardlike creature.

When he went to heaven, he saw that he had lost many soul parts from his gastrointestinal tract, back, and upper part of his body, which were in possession of the demons. They put those soul parts near fire, causing a burning feeling, distention, and pain in his gastrointestinal tract here in his body. Those soul parts were retrieved, cleansed, healed, and integrated with Jerry with the help of the angels.

Fourth Past Life

Jerry recalled another life, as a woman in Holland in 1610. Her name was Mary. She danced on the street so she could make money to feed her family. One day, as she was dancing, she saw her house on fire. She ran in panic, trying to save her three-year-old daughter, but it was too late. Mary died of smoke inhalation, feeling the burning in her throat, lungs, and gastrointestinal tract. She died blaming herself for her little girl's death.

From heaven, Jerry was very surprised and impressed with the healing power of forgiveness when that little girl forgave her mother without any question. This was a powerful lesson he felt he learned from Mary's life.

He also saw smoke inhalation and being burned in the fire as one of the contributing reasons for his colitis. Mary lost many soul parts, from her gastrointestinal tract and from all over her body, which were in the darkness in possession of the demons who were pouring acid on those soul parts, causing holes in them. This created acidity, ulceration, and deep burning pain in his gastrointestinal tract in his present body.

Fifth Past Life

Jerry recalled another life as an American Indian. He was a thirty-five-year-old man in the early 1600s. He was very arrogant and self-absorbed and treated his family and everybody around him badly because they were not as good as he was. He constantly humiliated them.

One day while hunting, he was attacked and torn apart (including his back, neck, and bowels) by a mountain lion. He died feeling angry at the animal and ashamed that he let the mountain lion get to him. He was supposed to be a great warrior.

From heaven, he understood that he needed to learn a lesson of humility; it was as if the mountain lion was supposed to teach him humility.

From heaven, he saw his colitis and back and neck problems partly coming from this life. He saw that he lost from his colon, intestine, back, and neck many soul parts that were in possession of Satan and his demons. Jerry saw demons putting his intestine and colon parts on a stick and putting them above the fire, just as you would do with an animal. Blood oozed from those soul parts, causing distention, burning, and bleeding in his G.I. tract here in his current body.

Jerry also saw demons hitting the soul parts from his neck and back with rocks, causing pain and spasms in his back and neck in his present body. The demons always took a great deal of pleasure in tormenting him through those soul parts.

Sixth Past Life

Jerry recalled another life time as a man in prehistoric times, when people had no feelings for each other. They had no language and lived by the rule of "survival of the fittest." There was not much to eat. Somebody brought an animal. Everybody wanted it, but only a few big people were eating. They did not even give any food to the children. Jerry attacked one of the men who was eating. The man in turn cut him with a spearlike stick, cutting his abdomen, bowels, and his spine.

From heaven, he saw himself losing from his bowels, spine, and bones many soul parts that were in the darkness with the demons. He saw them putting bubbling liquid on his stomach and colon soul parts, creating gas and causing swelling and distention of his gastrointestinal tract in his current body. What they did to his soul parts in hell, he felt in his body here as distention, cramping, ulcers, and burning. Jerry also saw demons shaking soul parts of his spine and rattling them, causing pain in his back.

Seventh Past Life

After two weeks of therapy, Jerry reported that his diarrhea, bleeding, and stomach cramping were 70 percent to 80 percent improved. He was feeling less depressed and anxious. Even his headaches and neck and lower back pain were mostly gone, and he had only a slight pain in the middle of his back. He cut down his prednisone from 60 mg. to 20 mg. per day. He said that although his bleeding was almost negligible, every time he saw blood in his stool he got anxious.

So I asked him to close his eyes and focus on these thoughts and feelings. His thoughts were

"I feel anxious."

"Little bit of blood keeps hanging on. It won't give up."

"I want this to be gone forever."

"I feel like I am not in control of my life."

After a few repetitions, he regressed to a life in 1720 in Scotland as an eight-year-old girl. Her name was Alice. She was grabbed by a man, a stranger, and was stabbed in the stomach and was cut open. Her insides fell to the ground before the body reached the ground. She felt anxious seeing the blood leaving her body. (Jerry said that he felt the same anxiety when he saw the blood in the stool.)

After death, from heaven, Jerry saw that Alice lost many soul parts from her brain and from the blood that were in possession of the demons. They took the brain soul parts, put them in a container, and stirred them up, causing confusion, fear, and anxiety in Jerry.

Jerry saw the demons with the containers of the blood pouring the blood on the ground, mixing it with dirt. This reactivated the memories of weak feelings, of not being able to go on anymore because there was not enough blood. All the soul parts were brought back, cleansed, healed, and integrated with him.

Eighth Past Life

Jerry recalled another life that was responsible for his colitis, in Mexico as a cowboy. He was killed by a cow poking him in the back with its horn, then was trampled by hundreds of cows crushing and tearing his body.

From heaven, he saw himself losing from his gastrointestinal tract, and from all over his body, many soul parts that were in possession of the demons. They were pouring hot liquid on the colon and stomach soul parts, causing ulcers, burning, gas, and bloating in his current body.

All his soul parts were brought back, cleansed, healed, and integrated with Jerry.

Ninth Past Life

Jerry recalled another life in Canada in 1812 where, while hunting, he was torn apart by a bear. His whole body, including his bowels, was torn into pieces.

From heaven, he saw that he lost many soul parts that were with the demons in the darkness. They were holding the soul parts over fire, causing gas, distention, and burning in Jerry's gastrointestinal tract.

Tenth Past Life

Jerry recalled another life in Scotland as a farmer. A leg was caught in a farm machine with sharp spikes. In no time he was dragged and torn and crushed. He lost soul parts from all over his body, including his colon, that were with the demons. All his lost soul parts were retrieved from the darkness, cleansed, healed, and integrated with him.

Eleventh Past Life

In another life in the USA., Jerry recalled looking at a buffalo that was coming at him. It poked its horn through his abdomen, throwing him around like a rag doll and tearing his insides and the rest of his body. He died thinking, "I never thought I would be killed by these dumb animals." He saw that his whole body was mutilated and his bowels were hanging all over. His lost soul parts were located, retrieved, cleansed, healed, and integrated with him. From heaven, he understood that he needed to learn the lesson of humility.

Twelfth Past Life

Jerry recalled another life in Australia in 1780, where he was chosen to be sacrificed to Satan by his tribe. He was tied to a pole and burned. He had difficulty breathing and could feel his stomach, intestine, and colon swelling up and bursting with the heat even before the flames reached there.

From heaven, he saw that he lost many soul parts from all over his body, including his gastrointestinal tract, to the demons, who were causing him gas, distention, and pain. These soul parts were brought back, cleansed, healed, and integrated with Jerry.

Thirteenth Past Life

Next, Jerry recalled a life in Idaho, USA. as a thirty-five-year-old lumberjack. He was very good at his work, but was arrogant. One day the other workers were careless while cutting a tree and it fell on him, crushing his body. He felt one big branch enter his back and literally cut his body in two, crushing his bowels. He died feeling confused about how this could happen to him. He felt he was too big, too strong, and too great for something like this to happen.

From heaven, once again he understood that the lesson he needed to learn was to be humble. He also saw that he lost many soul parts from his back, intestinal tract and the rest of his body, causing him problems. These were brought back, cleansed, healed, and integrated with Jerry with the help of the angels.

Fourteenth Past Life

Next, Jerry recalled a life in France, when he was a thirty-year-old farmer with a corn farm. There was a famine; people were starving, and tried to steal his corn. While he was trying to chase them away, he hit one lady and cut her legs with a sickle. The people got angry and began to hit him with clubs. One man pushed a sharp stick through his abdomen. He died thinking he should have shared his corn with them.

From heaven, he saw himself losing several soul parts from his stomach and spine to the demons in a dark place. He saw them twisting his spine soul parts, causing pain and spasms in his back in his present body. The demons put his stomach and colon soul parts above a fire, causing burning, gas, and distention in his present body. They were all brought back, cleansed, healed, and integrated with Jerry.

Fifteenth Past Life

Next Jerry recalled a life as an American Indian in 1600. Food was scarce and everybody was starving. So he and others decided to steal food from another tribe. They were caught and one person shot an arrow through his throat.

From heaven, he saw himself losing many soul parts from his neck, shoulders, brain, and stomach due to starvation. They were in the possession of the demons in the darkness. Through these soul parts, the demons were causing him neck and shoulder pain and restimulating his memories of hunger, causing him to over-eat and then feel guilty. They also put his stomach soul parts over fire, causing burning, acidity, pain, and distention. Those parts were brought back cleansed, healed, and integrated with Jerry.

Sixteenth Past Life

Jerry, before this session, was having severe pain in his left shoulder and both hips and was walking with a limp.

Under hypnosis, he recalled a life as a forty-year-old male who had a small, one-person airplane. While flying, something went wrong; the plane went into a ditch. His arms and legs were broken so he could not get out and the plane caught on fire. He could not breathe because there was no oxygen. He felt his gastrointestinal tract swelling up with heat. Parts of the plane were melting and dropping on him, burning holes through his body, especially in his gastrointestinal tract.

After the death of his body, when he went to the Light, he saw that he lost from his left shoulder, both hips, sinuses, throat, brain, and gastrointestinal tract many soul parts that were in possession of the demons in the darkness. They caused him hip pain, left shoulder pain, sinus problems, throat discomfort, ulcers, and colitis. Those parts were brought back, cleansed, healed, and integrated with Jerry.

His hip and left shoulder pain were relieved immediately after the session and he was able to walk without a limp.

Seventeenth Past Life

During this session, Jerry complained of having mild diarrhea for two days. He was slightly discouraged because he had been improving so much.

Under hypnosis, as he focused on his feelings about having diarrhea, he regressed to prehistoric times, when he was a fifty-year-old man. There was no language, just grunting and pointing. The people looked like today's humans but were not refined. They had rugged faces, big jaws, and sloped shoulders.

Food was hard to come by. They were hungry. He killed an animal and although he realized it was sick, he ate part of it anyway. He became sick and started to have diarrhea, vomiting, and upset stomach and died in just a few days of dehydration.

From heaven, he saw that he lost many parts of his gastrointestinal tract, which were in the possession of the demons in the darkness. He saw them pouring acid on them, irritating and burning his inside lining, causing diarrhea, irritation, and discomfort. They were all brought back cleansed, healed, and integrated with Jerry.

Eighteenth Past Life

Next, Jerry recalled a life in North America. He came from England and was looking for a place to settle. Suddenly a tornado picked him up as if he were a toy and tossed him around violently. The pressure of the air was so strong that it tore and broke his bones and tore and blew out his insides, including his digestive tract and eyes and ears. Then he fell on a tree limb with such force that his body was torn into upper and lower halves.

From heaven, he saw that he lost from all over his body, including his gastrointestinal tract, hips, head, eyes, and ears, many parts that were in possession of demons in the darkness, causing him colitis, arthritis, and aches and pains all over the body, plus hearing problems. They were all healed and integrated with Jerry.

Nineteenth Past Life

Session by session, Jerry's condition improved a great deal. His bleeding, distention, and diarrhea improved by 90 percent. He was able to reduce his prednisone slowly until finally he was not taking any at all. He was feeling much better. Under hypnosis, he saw his polyps and ulcers were disappearing, session by session, and had only two polyps and one ulcer left. We also realized that in most of these lifetimes he was a victim suffering from one or another type of traumas and tortures. In spite of the dramatic change, at times he was frustrated as to why he had to go through all these tortures and why God did not heal him faster.

I asked Jerry to focus on that one ulcer and two polyps and how he felt about them. He said: "I feel aggravated and disgusted. I feel like cutting them off. I feel anxious. It feels like a burden and I am tired of carrying it."

After a few repetitions, Jerry regressed to a life in 1530 as an American Indian chief. People from another tribe were stealing things from his tribe, so he and his tribe decided to raid their village.

He saw himself on a horse, watching as his tribe brutally tortured and killed people and burned their homes. As he watched this massacre being committed by his people on his command, he felt sick and realized how senseless it was and that those people did not do anything to deserve this treatment. He had second thoughts about what his people did to the other tribe.

When they returned to their village, people were happy and were celebrating, but the chief could not participate. He felt guilty and responsible for the brutal deaths of those people. He felt burdened, as if he were not worth being a chief, or even a human being.

He saw himself two days after the attack standing at the top of a cliff ready to commit suicide. His last thoughts were: "I want to end it so I do not make any more bad decisions. I do not want any authority or power so I do not make any mistakes again. I cannot carry this burden. Someday I will have to pay for my evil actions." He jumped from the cliff, hit the rocks below, and died.

From heaven, he saw the force of the impact from the fall burst his insides, including his stomach, intestines, and colon, as when a water balloon is dropped on the rocks. His whole body was broken.

Problems coming from this life: From heaven, he saw many problems coming from this life: colitis, hip pain, arthritis, back and neck pain, headaches, perfectionism, obsessive-compulsive behavior, fear of making a mistake, and feelings of being overburdened and anxious all the time without any good reason. He is a loner in this life so he does not have to take any responsibility for anybody and does not have to feel guilty.

From heaven, he saw that he lost soul parts from all over his body, including his brain, shoulders, arms, hips, back, digestive tract and from all his organs like lungs, heart, and liver. These parts were in the possession of the demons in the darkness. They used these parts to create different types of physical and emotional problems by reactivating the memories of that life's problems and traumas.

Twentieth Past Life

Jerry reported feeling much better, as if a burden had been lifted from his shoulders, and feeling less anxious and more at ease. He still felt that there was something more, but did not know what.

Under hypnosis, he saw that one ulcer that had refused to heal had now begun to heal. It was smaller, but not completely healed. His polyps were smaller and less irritated.

As he focused on that ulcer and his feelings about it, he regressed to another life as a twenty-eight-year-old Japanese commanding officer, trying to invade an island. He and his men were captured and taken to a village on the island. The islanders were peace loving and had not faced any violence so far. They gave him a choice of drinking poison or being killed by a spear.

He chose to drink the poison. His last thoughts were: "I feel disgusted and hate myself for what I did. You cannot accomplish anything by being forceful. This type of power is useless."

After his death, from heaven, he saw that he lost many soul parts from his gastrointestinal tract, due to poisoning, and from his brain and heart, that were in possession of the demons in the darkness. They froze his digestive tract soul parts in ice, causing indigestion and discomfort.

Intensive Care Unit Experience

During the initial interview, Jerry said that when he was in the intensive care unit, he came close to dying. He felt that something had changed in him since then, but he did not know what. He had a feeling that he would be O.K. and that he would not die.

So during this session, I asked him to look back from heaven and see what really happened to him in the intensive care unit. He was surprised to realize that he had had a near-death experience. He saw his spirit wandering in the hospital to find a healthy body to go to, but then he changed his mind and came back into his own body.

He saw the same powerful Light being, which he saw during the session, protecting his body and later healing him just enough so he could continue to live without a colon resection. He was given the understanding that there was something else planned for him, although he did not know it yet.

Twenty-First Past Life

Under hypnosis, as Jerry looked inside his colon, he saw that his one remaining ulcer had reduced greatly, but was not completely healed. His two remaining polyps were less irritated, but not gone. He felt discouraged. As he focused on his thoughts about the ulcer, he regressed to a life that he did not want to see. He had a feeling that he had to look at it.

He recalled this life somewhere in the Middle East. He was a seventy-year-old man, a shepherd. He lived by himself outside a city. One day he had an inner vision and knowledge about a nearby city. He was shocked to see how those people were living.

They had no morals and were stealing, fighting with each other, and living an immoral life.

He was given knowledge that he should go and help and teach these people, otherwise the city would be destroyed. But he did not go inside the city to help, because he was afraid that he would be negatively influenced.

Later, he saw that the whole city was on fire. He was dumbfounded and felt a strong sense of guilt, believing he was responsible for the destruction. He realized that the knowledge had been given to him by God, but he did not have enough faith in God to follow his instructions. He felt like a failure and unworthy of God's love.

Totally distraught, he wandered around in the wilderness with no direction. He wanted God to forgive him, but he did not believe that he would be forgiven. As he kept asking for forgiveness, he saw a bright Light being in front of him who told him that he was forgiven. He felt the forgiveness from this being and he promised that he would never doubt God again. He died at the age of ninety. From heaven, he saw that the whole city and people in it were all filled with and surrounded by darkness and that it was Satan and the dark ones that took over and influenced the people in that city, eventually destroying it. God wanted to intervene and help them through him, but could not.

From heaven, as he was trying to review the shepherd's life, he became confused and saw himself as a black blob who possessed people and caused them to do evil things and turn them against God. As he focused on that black blob, he realized he was totally trapped inside a black demon entity. He was a female and her name was Rose. I asked him to move back in time when Rose was living in her body to see what happened.

He recalled a life near Israel. Her family was very poor and did not have food. Her parents were religious and prayed to God for food and other things, but nothing changed. So she began to believe that there was no God. She ran away from home, became a prostitute, and died at the age of seventy-four. She felt empty and bitter. After the death of her body, she felt as alive as before.

She saw both Light and darkness. Because she did not believe in God, she voluntarily went with the darkness. She was totally trapped and surrounded by a dark demon entity and had no control over what happened to her. Together she and the demon went and possessed different people and caused them to do evil and turned them against God. Rose recalled some of the people to whom she was taken by the demon, whom they possessed and affected as follows:

1. They possessed a man and went to his stomach. They caused him stomachaches and digestive problems by squeezing his stomach. He died of stomach problems.
2. They possessed a ten-year-old girl and went into her ears. They squeezed her eardrums, causing ringing in her ears. It drove her crazy and later caused her to commit suicide.
3. They went into an elderly lady and squeezed her heart, causing chest pain. Later she died because her heart stopped.
4. They went to a middle-aged man and moved around in his joints. They caused him arthritis by causing pressure on his joints, forcing them apart.
5. They went into another man, causing him stomach problems. After he died, they floated in space for a while. Rose did not like what they were doing, but she had no control.
6. Then they went in the shepherd who was receiving the knowledge from God about saving the city, but Rose and the demon fed him thoughts telling him not to go to the city, that he would be taken over by evil. When the shepherd went to see what was happening in the city, the demon left and Rose and the shepherd stayed outside the city.

After the demon who was surrounding Rose left her and the shepherd, they watched the city being destroyed. Rose realized how she and the demon changed and affected the shepherd and made him feel scared of going to help people in that city. She felt very guilty and responsible for the destruction of the city.

Later, when the shepherd saw the Light being who said that he forgave the shepherd for not following his instructions, Rose separated from the shepherd. She realized that there was a God and felt that she was forgiven, too. She was taken to the Light by that Light being.

Soul parts: From heaven, Jerry saw that Rose lost parts of her brain and heart, which were with the demons in hell. They closed her heart part in a black box, keeping her away from God, and used her brain parts to restimulate the memory of Rose's life, causing confusion and lack of faith in God.

Jerry was very surprised that even as the possessing spirit Rose, he was totally aware of the shepherd's feelings and thoughts. So in the beginning he thought that he was the shepherd and that they were one and the same.

After this session, Jerry felt completely free of bleeding, diarrhea, distention, and discomfort. Under hypnosis, he saw all his ulcers healed and all the polyps gone, and there was no sign of inflammation and irritation.

Conclusion

As we review Jerry's treatment, we can see that his ulcerative colitis came from the following emotional and physical traumas from many past lives.

Unresolved physical traumas and tortures to his gastro-intestinal tract caused by people: By being poked, punctured, and stabbed by a knife, a spear, a stick, and a bullet; by being cut open by an ax; and by being burned at the stake.

Traumas caused by animals: Being hurt by a mountain lion, a bear, and a large lizardlike creature; and by being poked, punctured, trampled, and mutilated by cows and buffaloes.

Traumas that were caused by natural disasters and accidents: Being blown apart by a tornado, being hit by a tree falling, being torn apart by a farm machine, starving due to a famine, dying in a plane accident, and being burned in a fire.

Self-inflicted traumas: Due to poison, jumping from a cliff, and bowels being destroyed.

Unresolved emotional traumas: Feeling anger, fear, guilt, humiliation, fear of making mistakes, and feelings of unworthiness, causing him gastrointestinal problems.

Also, in most of the lives he recalled being victimized, life after life, and had a feeling of "why me?" until he recalled the last three or four lives, which were recognized as connecting or karmic lives, where he victimized, traumatized, and killed many people. He felt intense guilt about making wrong decisions that led to brutal killings. He felt overwhelming guilt about possessing and influencing the shepherd by not allowing him to follow his inner knowledge and the visions given to him by God. Thus he felt responsible for the deaths of people and the destruction of the whole city.

After he resolved these physical and emotional traumas and issues, by recalling, reliving, releasing, and resolving them and retrieved the lost soul parts and cleansed, healed, and integrated them with him, his ulcerative colitis was completely healed. Even his polyps completely disappeared.

From heaven, during one session, he was given the knowledge that there were about 210 lives that were responsible for his ulcerative colitis, but we were given the understanding that he did not have to look into each and every life. We were allowed to retrieve, cleanse, heal, and integrate all the lost soul parts from the remaining lives out of those 210, without going through each and every life before the thorough and permanent healing could take place. But permanent healing was allowed only after he clearly understood the different lessons about patience, humility, love, and forgiveness he needed to learn by reliving and resolving these lives.

It is interesting to realize that not only were his ulcerative colitis and polyps completely healed, but most of his secondary symptoms—his chronic back, neck, shoulder, hip, and leg pain and arthritis of his hands—were also healed. His headaches, sinus problems, and hearing problems were relieved, too.

Emotionally, he was free of his depression, anxiety, and obsessive-compulsive and perfectionistic behavior. He was able to relate and communicate with his family and other people better and thus has less desire to be a loner.

He understood the destructive nature of inflated ego, anger, guilt, and fear, understood the healing power of forgiveness, and learned to be less arrogant and more humble.

Jerry described his treatment experience as follows:

> "I have gained so much knowledge in the past one and a half months that I feel my life before the treatment was wasted. However, I know it had to be like this, so I could learn what I have learned through these sessions. I look at life so much differently now. I feel at ease, peaceful, and have much more understanding and knowledge of the real truth. Whenever I am in critical need of help, the Light being always shows up as he did in the intensive care unit, in past lives, and during the sessions. I am free of guilt, anger, and arrogance and feel at peace. Not only am I free of my colitis, but I am also free of my chronic back, neck, shoulder, hip, and hand pain and other aches and pains. My headaches, sinus problems, and hearing problems are also cured. I do my best and do not worry about making mistakes."

As we compare Jerry's case with Ann's case, we can see that in Ann's case only one or two past lives were responsible for each symptom and resolving these past life traumas healed her symptoms, session after session.

In contrast, Jerry had to resolve traumas from twenty-one lives to heal just one symptom, his ulcerative colitis.

Although, throughout the treatment, we were focusing on healing just one symptom, his ulcerative colitis, resolving the traumas of those past lives also healed most of his secondary symptoms.

Chapter IX

Different Sources of
Different Symptoms

Different Sources
of Different Symptoms

So far we understand that any symptom, psychological or physical, can originate from earthbound, demon, or other entities, devices, energy absorbers, current or past life traumas, or soul fragmentation and soul loss.

Typically, I find that most symptoms originate from more than one source, and sometimes all of them play an important role in the origin of a single symptom. The process is like an onion: we need to remove the problems layer by layer to achieve a thorough healing. Following are some examples.

Stammering

Norton, a forty-year-old white male, had difficulty expressing himself. It was difficult for him to "find the words," especially when he became excited. As a result, he developed a habit of stammering and repeating phrases. Sometimes he paused in mid-sentence temporarily, unable to find the words to complete the thought.

This condition contributed to Norton's low self-esteem and made him self-conscious. It caused him to lack confidence, resulting in poor communication skills. The condition helped retard Norton's social growth and job performance. In addition, it caused him some embarrassment and insecurity.

Earthbound Spirits

Under hypnosis, Norton found inside him several earthbound spirits who claimed to contribute to his stammering problem:

- A thirty-seven-year-old man experienced a terrible automobile accident at age fourteen. He had damage to his nervous system and vocal cords, causing severe speech problems. He claimed to cause Norton laryngitis and difficulty in expressing himself.
- An eleven-year-old boy, severely abused by overzealous, religiously fanatical parents, developed a stuttering problem. He claimed to cause Norton the stammering problem.
- A four-year-old child severely ill with meningitis, suffered some brain damage, resulting in mild retardation. She had difficulty "finding the words" to complete thoughts, which was transferred over to Norton.
- A twenty-nine-year-old woman who was born partially deaf and had difficulty with sounds. She claimed to cause Norton difficulty in expressing himself and trying to "overclarify" words and sounds.
- A fifty-nine-year-old woman had her vocal cords ruined as a result of an explosion. She caused Norton difficulty in expressing himself and caused him self-consciousness when speaking.

Demon Entities

Norton saw many dark demon entities, who were arranged in layers on the front part of his tongue, with many dark entities in each layer. The layering looked like little tiny sheets of paper. The demon entities in these layers weighed down Norton's tongue and caused him the erratic speech patterns.

Devices

Norton saw the following types of devices which were used by dark demon spirits to cause him the speech problems. All these devices seemed to be present at all times. They did not cause problems until they were activated by the dark ones.

A muzzle: This was similar to the device used to prevent dogs from biting or eating. These leather straps fit over the mouth, interfering with Norton's expression.

A black curtain wall: This small wall was put directly in front of the mouth. Sometimes it stopped sounds from being discharged. Other times it partially blocked the sounds.

A black handkerchief: It was placed in the mouth and when activated, acted like a "gag," on the principle of a steel bit in a horse's mouth.

A malfunctioning microphone: It was placed in the mouth. This device caused some sounds to come out clearly and other sounds to come out garbled.

Past Lives

Norton recalled the following past lives that were responsible for his speech problems.

- A life in Philadelphia as a forty-two-year-old housewife. Her name was Iris. While controlled and dominated by her physically and verbally abusive husband, she stayed cut off from social advancement and growth, living a lifestyle designed by her husband. She was not allowed to speak up and lacked social growth and personal expression. These problems were carried over to his current life, with his soul.

- He was a nineteen-year-old young man in China, a political prisoner. He advocated freedom from excessive government control and oppression. He was shot to death by government officials. He was killed for exercising freedom of speech. He died promising himself: "I do not want to be in this situation again. I will hold my tongue and keep everything in." These last thoughts and decisions were carried over to the current life with his soul.

- He was a twenty-two-year-old soldier in Wyoming. He was captured and tortured by Indians. They put hot pebbles in his mouth and knives into his flesh, slitting the end of his tongue. He died of starvation, feeling shock, panic, fear, and helplessness.

- Norton recalled a life in Siberia as a child. On a thirty-below-zero day, he stuck his tongue to a metal object, causing severe damage to his tongue. The incident caused permanent damage, resulting in a lifelong speech problem. He was self-conscious, had low self-esteem, and had difficulty speaking and communicating; these problems were carried over to the current life with his soul.

- He was a twenty-three-year-old man in Germany in 1550. He experienced a bad fall while horseback riding. His teeth clipped off the tip of his tongue on impact from the fall, resulting in a severe speech impediment. He withdrew from the mainstream and lived in isolation.

- He recalled another life as a man in England. He had an extremely high fever from a strep infection, causing some brain damage and resulting in a partial loss of hearing and speech problems. These problems were transferred over to his current life with his soul.

- He was a young soldier in France. While in battle, he was shot through the cheek, grazing the tongue and exiting through the other cheek. This incident reduced his speech to grunting sounds. He died of infection after three years.

- He was a politician and his tongue was cut out because of different viewpoints.

- He recalled a life as a clergyman, where he was tortured and his tongue was cut off by an opposing tribe because they disagreed with his beliefs.

- He had a life where he was captured by an enemy. He was bound, gagged, and tied for many days. As a result, circulation around his mouth and tongue was cut off. He couldn't speak again. He could make only grunting sounds.

- In another life he was kicked in the head and face by a horse. His teeth were knocked out and he had deep cuts in his tongue. His speech patterns were affected and he couldn't sound words correctly.

Norton's last thoughts, decisions, speech problems, and physical and emotional symptoms from these past lives were carried over to the current life with his soul and created a speech problem for him.

Soul Parts

During each of the past lives, Norton lost many soul parts that were later captured by the demons. They used these soul parts to affect Norton in a variety of ways:

- By touching and squeezing the captive soul parts, the dark beings restimulated the memories of the speech problems in those lives, causing him to stammer in the current life.
- The demons would wrap or cover the soul parts with tape (as if taping the mouth shut) whenever they wanted to stop the word flow.
- The demons would cover the soul parts with their hands (as if holding the mouth shut) whenever they wanted to stop or inhibit expression.

Norton described the following changes in him:

"I have much more self-confidence in my ability to communicate, especially in challenging situations. Words seem to come in my mind more easily than before and I am not struggling as much to 'find the words.' I have a positive perspective about my ability to express myself and I am less self-conscious than before."

Weight Problem

Dawn had a weight problem that was caused by earthbound entities, demon entities, soul fragmentation, and past life traumas.

Earthbound Entities

Under hypnosis, Dawn found the following earthbound entities responsible for her weight problem.

Matthew died of cancer of the stomach. He could not eat anything because he threw up all the time. He died craving food. His experience became Dawn's problem after he came into her.

Juda was a twenty-year-old female who died in Spain, of starvation. There was a famine and they had to eat straw. She was just skin and bones.

Job was a slave who was hanged for stealing food because he was hungry.

Bertha was a forty-year-old woman who weighed 450 pounds. She was hungry all the time, so she ate constantly.

David was an eight-month-old boy who was left alone and consequently died of starvation.

Jose was a forty-year-old man who died in Mexico of starvation during a famine.

JoAnn was very sick and had severe sores in her mouth; as a result she could not eat anything. She died of starvation, thinking of food.

George died of starvation, feeling hungry and thinking of food.

Joseph worked in a slaughterhouse in 1846, slaughtering pigs. There was no food, so he stole ham from the slaughterhouse. People killed him by thrusting a sword into his stomach. He claimed to cause Dawn's desire to overeat, her craving for pork, and high blood pressure.

Jezebel was a seventeen-year-old female who was a king's concubine. She was put in a dungeon, where she starved to death.

John was an eighty-year-old man who died of starvation because everything was dry and hot and there was no food. He died feeling hungry and thinking, "I wish I could just eat."

Most of these above entities mentioned that they were sent to Dawn by Satan and his dark ones, who told the entities they could eat through her.

Grandmother used to wake up in the night and eat. Dawn started to eat in the night after grandmother's spirit came in Dawn. After releasing the grandmother, Dawn did not wake up in the middle of the night to eat.

Feelings of hunger, desire to overeat, and other physical and emotional problems that these spirits had were transferred to Dawn after they joined her.

Demon Entities

Dawn found many demon entities in her stomach who were responsible for her weight problem.

Many dark demon entities in the stomach: They all claimed to make Dawn hungry by squeezing her stomach and gave her a desire to overeat.

Dark demon blob in the eye: It claimed to make Dawn crave sweets and overeat and block her vision. After its transformation into the Light, this dark demon entity remembered who and where it was before it joined Satan.

"I was in the garden in heaven as an angel. I chose to stay with God. One day Satan called me from the other side of the Light. He told me to try an apple he had. At first I did not want to listen to him, but later I became curious. As soon as he touched me, I became dark. Then he took me to hell and told me I would be hungry all the time. Then I was trained to go inside people and make them hungry."

There were many other dark demon entities who claimed to give her the desire to eat constantly.

Past Lives Responsible for Dawn's Weight Problem

Dawn recalled the following past lives that were responsible for her weight problem.

Jack Johnson was a forty-five-year-old man in Dublin, Ireland. There was war and he was starving because there was no food. Soldiers chased him on horseback because he stole food and hit him on the head and killed him. He died promising himself that he would never be hungry again and he would never be in the same situation again.

Makipa was a nine-year-old black girl living in Uganda who was taken away on a slave ship along with many others. They stayed on the ship for ten months and were given very little to eat. Makipa was extremely scared and could not eat anything.

After they reached America, the slaves were sold, but nobody wanted to buy Makipa because she was too skinny and weak. She kept thinking, "I wish I was fat, so somebody would want me, too." She was bought by a lady whose sons later sexually abused her over and over. She starved most of her life and was killed at the age of fifteen by one of her masters.

Fran was a twenty-eight-year-old black slave on a tobacco farm. The slaves worked hard, but were given very little to eat. Fran was starving all the time. She had an infant whom she hid in an outhouse. She tried to breastfeed the baby, but there was no milk. Her master found the baby and killed the mother and the baby. Fran died feeling sad. She promised herself that she would never be hungry again.

In the current life, during her delivery, part of her soul fragmented due to anxiety. This soul fragment's name was Fran and had memories of Fran's life, which were activated due to the birth of her baby.

Hussen was a ten-year-old boy living in Nairobi working for royalty. He and others worked hard, but were not given much to eat, while all the masters just ate and ate. As a child Hussen promised himself that when he grew up he would do whatever it took to be like royalty.

At the age of thirty, Hussen gathered others and killed the masters and took over. As he watched them being killed, he felt sick to his stomach and realized what was happening was wrong. He felt extremely guilty.

He became the King Hussen. He was surrounded by harem girls who were constantly feeding him, but he could not get rid of his guilt. Hussen hated himself for what he did and could not enjoy himself. He ended up committing suicide by drinking poison.

Connection: In this life, eating makes Dawn feel alternately good and bad, up and down.

Dawn's emotional and physical feelings of hunger and last thoughts and promises of never to be hungry again, from those past lives, were brought back to the current life with her soul. In this lifetime, she often found herself eating even before she felt hungry because she did not like the feelings of hunger.

Soul Fragments Responsible for the Weight Problem

Dawn had many fragmented soul parts that were inside and outside her body, contributing to her weight problem.

Many fragmented parts of Dawn, at the ages of a few days, two months, one year, and two years, were hungry and were partially responsible for Dawn's problems.

Four-year-old Dawn was fragmented and separated when she ate laxatives thinking they were chocolates. Four-year-old Dawn continued to crave chocolate and sweets, and grownup Dawn, in turn, was craving and eating sweets.

Ten-year-old Dawn was fragmented and separated because she believed she was skinny and ugly and kids made fun of her. She wanted to eat and gain weight. She gave grownup Dawn the desire to overeat.

A past life personality named Makipa was a fragmented soul part of Dawn, a past life personality, who remembered being taken on a boat, as a slave at the age of nine. She starved for months on the boat as described above.

Past life personality named Fran was a twenty-eight-year-old soul part of Dawn who held a memory of starvation in a past life as described above.

In her past lives, Dawn lost many soul parts that were in possession of demons in hell. They used those soul parts to affect Dawn as follows:

- They restimulated the memories of starvation and hunger in Dawn from her past life by touching those soul parts
- By squeezing the soul parts from her stomach, they made Dawn feel hunger here in her body.

Headaches

As we look at Ann's case in chapter 8, we see that her headaches, feelings of pressure in her head, and feelings that her head was going to explode came from the following sources.

Earthbound Spirits

Ann found the following earthbound entities in her, which were responsible for her headaches. All these spirits had some type of disease or trauma to their head and their pain was transferred to Ann after they joined her.

Ralph was a neighbor who was shot in his head and died.

A brother died of cancer with metastasis to the brain, causing headaches.

A cousin died of Hodgkin's disease with metastasis to the brain, causing headaches.

Susan died in a car accident in which her body, including her head, was crushed.

Darlo also died in a car accident in which her body, including her head, was crushed.

Demon Spirits

Ann had many demon spirits in her head and eyes who claimed to cause her headaches and vision problems.

Past Lives

Under hypnosis, Ann recalled several past lives when she had headaches and feelings that her head would explode. Those feelings were carried over with her soul to the current life, creating similar problems for her.

Harry was hanged. He had headaches and the feeling that his head was going to explode as he was dying. Those unresolved physical feelings were carried over to Ann's life with her soul.

Rahim drowned in the sea during a storm. The blood vessels in his head and eyes exploded, giving him headaches and feelings that his head is going to explode. These unresolved physical feelings were carried over to Ann's life, giving her headaches.

Anya was thrown into a pit with poisonous snakes, spiders, and insects. As she hit the bottom of the pit, she hit her head. She developed a severe headache and felt as though her head were going to explode as she was dying. These feelings were carried over to Ann's life with her soul.

Jacques was tortured by being hit on the head and by other methods and finally was beheaded. He felt severe pain and pressure in his head and feelings that his head was going to explode, which were carried over to Ann's life.

Anneliese, a nun, died of ruptured blood vessels in her head, feeling as if her head were going to explode. Those feelings were brought to Ann in her current life.

Soul Parts

In all these lifetimes, due to different traumas, Ann lost many soul parts that were in possession of the demons in hell. They were restimulating the memories and feelings of the head traumas by massaging the soul parts, which Ann was experiencing here in her body.

Birth Trauma

During a regression to her birth, Ann recalled having the feeling of pressure in her head and feelings that her head was going to explode, when the doctors applied forceps to bring her head out.

After releasing all the earthbound and demon spirits and resolving the trauma from birth and past lives, and by locating and integrating all her lost soul parts, Ann's headaches and feelings that her head was going to explode were relieved completely.

Temporomandibular Joint Pain (TMJ)

Shirley started to have jaw pain when she was eighteen years old. A few years later, her jaw began to make loud clicking sounds and would pop out of place. Later, the popping became painful. Often her jaw would lock open. She went to a TMJ clinic. Doctors put her on muscle relaxants, painkillers, antiinflammatory medication, and sleeping pills. She also began to drink to kill the pain.

Doctors fitted her with splints that made her lower jaw protrude. The pain became so severe that all the hair around her face turned white in four months. She stopped going to the TMJ clinic, but continued on pain pills.

In 1987 her jaw locked shut. She was in immense pain. She could not eat, drink, talk, or brush her teeth. She went to the hospital for surgery on her jaw. After surgery some of her problems were relieved, but the jaw did not heal properly and she developed scar tissue.

After the surgery, she had problems chewing because her teeth did not meet, and had limited opening of her jaw. She experienced swelling around her jaw line. Doctors suggested another surgery, but she refused.

Under hypnosis, she found the following reasons for her jaw problems.

Earthbound Entities

Shirley had earthbound entities who were responsible for her TMJ pain as follows:

Bill was a drug addict who was beaten and killed by gangsters because he owed them money. His head, jaw, and every other part of his body were broken, causing him headaches, jaw pain, and aches and pains all over his body, which were transferred to Shirley.

Andy, an old friend who was a drug addict, was in her jaw because he did not want her to talk about him.

503

Demon Entities

Shirley had many dark demon entities in her jaw in different layers. They all claimed to cause her jaw pain.

Devices

Shirley had the following devices put in her jaw by the demons to cause her TMJ pain:

- She had a device like a rubber band on both sides of her jaw, restricting her jaw movements.
- Another device was like a staple remover, but with many teethlike projections in her jaw, causing her pain.

The jaw pain was greatly reduced and jaw mobility improved after releasing the earthbound entities, demon entities, and devices.

Past Lives

Under hypnosis, Shirley recalled the following lives that were responsible for her TMJ symptoms.

Rhonda was a female who fell from a horse. Her jaw, face, and whole body were crushed.

Mike was a soldier whose whole body, including his face and jaw, was torn apart and eaten by wolves. The day after that regression, the swelling in her jaw area was completely gone and her teeth could meet.

Soul Parts

In both lives, Shirley lost many soul parts from her jaw, that were in possession of demons. They were restimulating the memories of jaw pain from those lives by squeezing and massaging those parts, causing Shirley to feel pain and spasms.

After recalling, reliving, and releasing the traumas of these past lives, particularly the one in which the soldier was eaten by wolves, the change was immediate and amazing. When Shirley woke up the day after that regression, all swelling along her jaw line was gone. A friend asked her that very day if she had had a face lift! Her back teeth met, something that hadn't occurred since her surgery. Four different doctors had recommended surgery to remove the scar tissue and fix the bite. The problem was corrected without any surgery, after removing the earthbound and demon entities and devices, and by recalling and resolving the two past lives. Shirley described her progress as follows:

"I look ten years younger without the swelling and evidence of pain. I have no problem in chewing because my teeth meet now, and I can eat what I want."

Obsession to Masturbate
with Violent Sexual Fantasies

Alphonso, a thirty-five-year-old single male, had had an obsession to masturbate with violent sexual fantasies since he was twelve years old. In high school and college, girls did not seem to be interested in him and he felt rejected by them. As a result, he would masturbate with fantasies of dominating, controlling, and having forceful sex with the girls who rejected him.

According to Alphonso, he did not have fantasies of a normal sexual relationship with a woman. His fantasies were of having forceful sex by controlling and dominating women, and were always self-limited. He never hurt anybody by acting out those fantasies and desires. Sometimes, at work or at other inconvenient times, he would have an urge to masturbate and the negative fantasies would flash in his mind, but he was able to control his desire.

He had no desire to get married and had a very low opinion of women in general. He always felt that most women have an agenda: all they want is to have a baby, a house, and a husband to work as a mule and earn money for them. He was very critical and judgmental of everybody, always suspicious and distrustful of women and even men. As a result, he was a loner most of his life.

Over several hypnotherapy sessions, Alphonso found several sources of his obsession to masturbate with violent sexual fantasies.

Earthbound Entities

Alphonso had many earthbound entities who gave him an obsessive desire to masturbate with violent fantasies.

Dark Demon Entities

Alphonso found many demon entities in him who claimed to make him angry, critical, judgmental, suspicious, and impatient and gave him an obsessive desire to masturbate with violent fantasies.

Past Lives

Alphonso recalled many past lives that were the sources of his obsession:

1. He was a fourteen-year-old young man in a Viking-type culture. His name was Lorath. A daughter of an important person led him on and they were caught together. He was castrated because it was assumed that he forced himself on her. After his castration, he felt constant embarrassment, humiliation, anger, and frustration toward men and women and lived a wretched life. At the age of eighteen he killed one of the men who castrated him. He in turn was killed by other men who were friends of the victim.

   After the death of his body, part of his spirit went to heaven while another part of his spirit was tricked and taken to hell. As he was in hell, he saw dark energy sticking to him like an armor and he felt powerful and strong. The spirit of Lorath was sent back to his village, where he possessed and tormented another man who castrated him. Lorath made him lose his temper and get into fights. He squeezed his testicles when he was around women and drove him crazy with lust. He gave him the desire to drink and beat his wife. He drove him to kill somebody and, as a result, he was executed. Lorath then possessed another person and then another. He felt he caused a lot of damage to the village people and their society.

This part of Lorath, a past life personality of Alphonso, was still working for the darkness and gave Alphonso the obsessive desire to masturbate with violent fantasies.

2. Alphonso recalled another life as a member of the Spanish royal court in 1200. He was very ugly, but was very influential and rich. He was angry that women did not want to be with him, so he abused and raped women whenever he wished. Finally, he was poisoned by some court nobles who were fed up with his abuse.

3. He recalled another life in Russia in 1500. He specialized in torturing women physically and sexually. It was his job, and he took a great deal of pleasure in doing so.

4. Alphonso recalled being a wealthy merchant. In another life, he lived with a caravan in the desert. He was not good-looking. He had a few slave women and was very rough, abusive, and degrading during sex and even killed women just to be mean. He felt women were a necessary evil. He considered them necessary for men's sexual pleasures, but thought they were dangerous to have around. He did not trust women. He was killed by the sister of a woman he had killed.

5. Alphonso recalled another life in Africa, where he used women as slaves and abused them physically and sexually.

6. In another life, he was a man in Scandinavia. Women were kept on an island and were used for men's pleasure and as breeding stock.

7. He recalled another life in Germany in pre-Christian time. Women were seen as common property and were not treated as people.

8. In another ancient life he was a sixteen-year-old pagan priest-in-training in South America. A young woman was kidnapped and selected for a sacrifice in a religious ritual by a high priest, who had sex with her, tortured her, and then killed her. As he was watching this incident with other priests, he felt turned on and very confused. Other senior priests told him it was O.K. to have an erection and climax. That was part of the ritual. This type of sacrifice was performed several times a year, and he and other priests masturbated while watching a woman being sexually abused, cut, and killed by the high priest.

9. Alphonso recalled another life in London, when he was a pimp and had several prostitutes working for him. He considered them his property and was controlling and physically and sexually abusive toward them.

Soul Parts

From heaven, Alphonso saw that after the death of his body in these past lives, he lost thousands of soul parts that were in possession of demons in hell. He saw demons using these soul parts to cause him problems in his body here, in the following ways.

- They restimulated in Alphonso the memories and feelings of anger, control, domination, and sexual abuse from those past lives by touching those soul parts. These memories and feelings traveled into Alphonso through the connecting cords, during his fantasies.
- They gave him the obsessive urge to masturbate with violent sexual fantasies by massaging those soul parts, especially the soul part that belonged to Lorath's testicles, which he lost due to castration.

- They also interjected in Alphonso negative thoughts, anger, and fantasies through those missing soul parts and their connecting cords.
- All those soul parts were brought back, cleansed, healed, and integrated with Alphonso.

Devices

Alphonso saw a large crabclaw type of device placed around his pelvis and testicles, which was remotely squeezed by the demons when he was at work in the afternoon and at other inconvenient times, giving him negative fantasies and a desire to masturbate.

Conclusion

As we can see, most of these lives had the same common theme. After the life when he was unjustly castrated, he did not trust women and felt anger toward them. Lifetime after lifetime he degraded, dominated, and sexually and physically abused them.

After that first life when he was castrated, demons were able to restimulate his anger toward women and the desire to dominate and hurt them sexually and physically, lifetime after lifetime, by squeezing the missing soul parts. He had no control over those feelings and desires. He was like a puppet in their hands.

After releasing all the earthbound and demon entities, removing the devices from him, and resolving those past life problems and bringing and integrating all the lost soul parts back after cleansing and healing, there was a great deal of improvement in his condition. He had less desire to masturbate and his negative fantasies were replaced with the desire for a normal, healthy sexual relationship.

Alphonso described the changes in him:

"I notice a difference in the way women are now willing to make eye contact, smile, and talk briefly or at length, even though

we have just met. Somehow my behavior, body language, or 'vibes' are different, as the violent and horribly abusive lives are weeded out and neutralized. Also, my dream life is manifesting normal, loving attitudes toward women, loving them in a normal romantic-sexual situation. Dreams about this have been virtually non-existent in my whole life.

"*I always felt these evil and horrible thoughts and desires were part of me. There was nowhere to run, no way to escape, and no way to uproot and destroy them. I was doomed to live with and be tortured by them all my life, and they would forever stand between me and a normal, happy life with normal, happy people. I would only grow more lonely and isolated as my dark thoughts gain more and more control. I now know the dark entities and their dark thoughts are no more difficult to remove than a dandelion from my lawn, using these treatment methods and that they cannot live rent-free in my mind forever.*"

Panic Disorder

Throughout this book, I have described many case histories of patients with panic attacks. Some were caused by earthbound spirits, while others were due to past life traumas. I find earthbound spirits are one of the most common causes of panic disorders. Sometimes, patients find multiple reasons for their panic attacks.

Geneva, a thirty-seven-year-old female, had had panic attacks since early childhood. These attacks would surface when she was in certain situations, e.g., in the doctor's office or in a superior's presence while at work. The panic attacks would also occur without an explainable reason in the morning when she first awakened.

The situational panic attacks would always occur in the doctor's office, no matter how routine the visit. As she waited her turn to see the doctor, she began to grow tense. She developed a tightness in the chest and neck area. Her heart rate would accelerate and her blood pressure would rise above normal limits (100/68). Sometimes the blood pressure would rise up to 170/110. As a result, her doctor put her on blood pressure medicine. She had the feeling of being overwhelmed. She became very frightened as her anxiety intensified and her voice became high pitched. Sometimes her mind ran wild with irrational fears. These symptoms remained with Geneva until she was ready to leave the doctor's office.

In the morning when Geneva first got up, she felt a stirring (uneasy) sensation in the chest area. She became extremely anxious and her blood pressure would rise above normal limits. Uneasy thoughts of having to face "another difficult day" would enter her mind. She felt defeated and depressed. Her outlook was gloomy. As her anxiety intensified, she felt a tightening in the chest and neck area, which resulted in even higher levels of blood pressure. These symptoms remained with Geneva for a few minutes to an hour before they went away. During the treatment, Geneva found several sources for her panic attacks as follows:

Earthbound Entities

Under hypnosis, Geneva found many earthbound spirits in her body, who were responsible for her panic attacks.

- One man threatened a kid with a machine gun, subsequently firing the gun at the kid as he crawled low in the gravel and dirt, feeling panic, anxiety, fear, and rapid heartbeat.
- A young employee of a hardware store was held up at gunpoint by robbers and killed. Fearing for his life, the employee experienced full-blown panic before his death.
- A college student on the way to a job interview was stalked, threatened, and killed by two bullies. He felt fear, panic, and palpitations before his death.
- A man walking along a dark road happened upon a burglary in progress. Fearing for his safety, the man tried to leave the scene. The burglars noticed him and began to stalk him. He felt panic, fear, helplessness, anxiety, accelerated heartbeat, and finally was killed.

- After mending fences, a farmer was sitting in his truck. Down the road the farmer saw a man with a pistol. The pistol was pointed right at the farmer's head. The pistol flashed, the farmer screamed and felt fear, anxiety, panic, shaking, trembling, and elevated heartbeat before he died.
- A policeman on foot patrol was stalked and attacked by two youths. Struggle ensued and the policeman felt anxiety, fear, accelerated heartbeat, and some panic before his death.

All these earthbound spirits experienced fear, anxiety, and panic attacks before the death of their body. Those symptoms were transferred to Geneva after they came on board in her.

Demon Spirits

Geneva had many demon spirits in her who claimed to cause her panic attacks.

Devices

Geneva found many dark devices that were responsible for her panic attacks as follows:

- Dark curtains or dark shields were used to block her from the Light—thus resulting in irrational fear, panic, etc.
- An inflatable device was placed inside her body. Whenever any anxiety occurred, the dark beings inflated the device, causing her to feel pressure in her chest and neck area, feeling squeezed and frozen tight, causing her blood pressure to elevate.
- A sleeve type of device was placed over certain arteries. Dark beings tightened the device on the arteries, elevating her blood pressure.
- A paper "pincher" clip was placed over the artery, causing the blood pressure to rise.
- A movie projected on her mind and certain fictitious stories fed by the dark beings caused unexplained anxiety and fear in Geneva.

- A microphone device was used by the dark beings to communicate feelings of fear, anxiety, and inner stirring in Geneva.

Current Life Trauma

A situation in the current life contributed to Geneva's fear of doctors as follows:

When Geneva was four years old, she developed a bad infection in the left ear. With some urgency, her mother took her to a children's doctor. The doctor advised people around her to "hold her down." People came around her and held her arms and legs down. The doctor was applying a device that cleaned out her ear. The pain was excruciating and she screamed out for help. She struggled for her freedom without success. She felt helpless, frightened, and panicky. She felt violated by the doctor and his nurses. This chilling experience went down to the depths of her soul.

Prenatal Trauma

Geneva's mother had panic attacks when she was pregnant with Geneva. These panic feelings were transferred to Geneva while she was in the womb and she experienced them as her own.

Past Life Traumas

Geneva recalled many past lives that were responsible for her panic attacks as follows:

- She was an eight-year-old boy in Germany. His name was Fritz. He was physically abused by his new stepfather on a regular basis, early in the morning. This abuse caused Fritz to have problems with anxiety, panic, fear, restless sleep, racing heart, shaking and trembling, lump in throat, helplessness, etc., in the morning. He died at age eleven of bacterial infection in the throat.
- She was a Civil War soldier who became anxious the night before a battle that cost him his life. While waiting to fight

early in the morning, he experienced panic, irrational fears, accelerated heartrate, and helplessness. These negative feelings were compounded by his criticism of his superiors' battle plan, resulting in increased anger and bitterness. Wounded in the battle, he died in the late evening from a broken neck and a fractured skull.

- She was a twenty-year-old male in London, England. His name was Jeremy. He experienced a ship fire that became a raging inferno. Facing being burned to death or drowning, Jeremy plunged to his death in the Atlantic Ocean. During the fire his emotions ran wild, feeling full-blown panic, racing heart, feelings of being trapped, feelings of being helpless, feelings of why me (I'm so young), etc.
- She was a forty-year-old male slave for royalty. According to the royalty, slaves reaching forty years were no longer useful. As a result, he was forced out on a tightrope that stretched over a lion's den. Before plunging to his death, he suffered feelings of panic, hopelessness, raging fear, and a racing heart. He felt helpless and betrayed.
- She was a forty-two-year-old coal miner, who chose to be a union sympathizer (instead of a coal company supporter). He was tied to the top of a railroad car and blown up with dynamite. Before being blown up, he experienced full blown panic, fear, and helplessness.
- She was an American Indian fighter who was killed in early morning.
- She had twelve other lives of going into battle in early morning, feeling severe panic attacks.
- She had four lives as a resident in a state institution, where she was abused in early morning.

The unresolved feelings of fear, helplessness, and panic from all these past lives were carried over to Geneva's current life with her soul, creating similar problems for her. Many of these past lives' traumas and deaths occurred during early mornings, leading to panic attacks after waking up in the morning in the current life.

Soul Parts

Due to the traumas in the current life at a younger age, while in the womb, and in all the above past lives, Geneva lost many soul parts. They were all captured by the demons. Geneva, under hypnosis, saw these demons massaging her captive soul parts and thus restimulating the feelings of panic, fear, and helplessness, which traveled through the connecting cords to her current life body, creating similar problems for her.

All those soul parts were brought back, cleansed, healed, filled with the Light, and integrated with the main body of Geneva's soul, with the help of the angels.

Geneva described her progress as follows:

"My early-morning anxiety and inner stirrings have improved a great deal and my blood pressure remains to normal limits when I wake up. I feel more calm and relaxed in stressful situations that would previously upset me and cause me to have panic attacks. My blood pressure stays within normal limits during tense situations and I am not taking blood pressure medication anymore. I am less anxious and my voice remains strong and at the same pitch under pressure. Overall, there has been a great deal of improvement in my condition."

Distorted Perceptions Creating the Blocks

One of the by-products of these therapies, besides the healing of patients' psychological and physical symptoms, is their spiritual awakening. Especially after removing all the earthbound and demon spirits and devices, patients often describe becoming more intuitive and psychic. They feel more aware and connected with their inner self (soul within), higher self, Godhead, and God. They are able to tune in to them more easily during prayers and meditation and receive guidance directly. They are aware of their heavenly guides and guardian angels and able to receive guidance and spiritual help from them. They sometimes become clairvoyant and clairaudient and are able to see and hear beyond their normal sight and hearing.

They have more understanding of the nature of the universe and their place and role in it. Under hypnosis, they are able to go to heaven and see and understand things from the higher perspective.

They become more aware of their spiritual nature and their purpose for this life. They can tap into any knowledge, personal or general, while in heaven at the akashic plane, a place of knowledge, like a library, where all our individual and universal records are available, everything from the beginning of time.

They become aware of their God-given gifts and how to use them. Some people can not only heal their psychological and physical illness, but also learn to heal others by becoming an intermediary person who can remotely locate and remove earth-bound and demon spirits and retrieve and integrate missing soul parts for people who for some reason cannot do their own sessions. By understanding the higher knowledge, they become more spiritual. Unfortunately, some people are unable to do the sessions because their eyes and brains are being blocked by the entities. In some cases, patients are able to locate and release entities and even do the past life regression by receiving the information from their inner self (soul), but are unable to clearly see and recognize Light and the Light beings. Some, after their death in a past life, can receive the knowledge from their inner self and heal, but are unable to go to heaven or see or communicate with a Light being. Some, because of their fear of seeing and communicating with a Light being, including God, experience a lot of interference and deception and are given wrong information by the dark beings during the session.

Over the years, in my work with these therapies, patients have given different reasons for such difficulties, including distorted perceptions about God and the Light, feeling angry and resentful toward God, feeling unworthy of God's love, fear of punishment by God, inability to trust a Light being, and belief that they do not deserve such privilege. These problems often have many sources.

Lee was able to release the spirits and do the past life regression therapy by receiving the information from his subconscious mind (his soul), and heal from most of his psychological and physical problems. But he was unable to see, hear, or communicate with his guides, angels, and other Light beings; go to heaven after the death of his physical body during the past life regression therapy; or tap into heavenly knowledge from the akashic records. These blocks made Lee's therapy painfully slow and difficult and he often felt frustrated and discouraged.

He believed it was impossible to find the Light during hypnotherapy. Each time he tried, a barrier would come up and prevent him from making the connection. These blocks came in as feelings of fear and unworthiness. Each time he attempted to go to the Light, a barrier served to reinforce his belief and increase his frustration.

Sometimes Lee experienced a fear of going to the Light because he felt that he would be punished by God. Consequently, he chose to avoid the Light. Feelings of unworthiness entered Lee whenever he felt he was undeserving of God's love. He felt that he would be cheating if he entered the Light, because he had not earned this privilege. His feelings of fear and unworthiness were accompanied by feelings of guilt and doubt. Each time these feelings surfaced, Lee would take on more doubts. As a result, he had created a self-defeating cycle for himself during the therapy.

During the therapy, Lee found the following reasons for his distorted perceptions and blocks.

Earthbound Entities

Lee had in him many earthbound spirits who were angry with God and had doubts about going to the Light. Some spirits were afraid and felt unworthy about going to the Light. All these thoughts and feelings of the earthbound spirits were transferred to Lee, and he experienced them as his own. Spirits also caused him distraction and an inability to stay focused during the therapy.

Demon Spirits

Lee had many demon entities who created blocks by putting up many dark shields that blocked him from the Light. They transmitted messages to him that prevented him from going to the Light. The messages were (made him believe)

"You cannot find the Light."
"You are unworthy of going to the Light."
"You don't care enough to go to the Light."
"It's not worth the effort—stay away from the Light."
"Something might go wrong for you if you go to the Light."

Devices

Under hypnosis, Lee found the following devices, causing him problems during the sessions:

A black shield: This device was used by the dark beings to block him from the Light. Whenever he attempted to go to the Light, the shield would block him from the Light and interfere with his communication with the spirit world.

A microphone: A device used by the dark beings to feed him negative messages. Whenever he tried to go to the Light, a message from the microphone might say, "You are not worthy" or "You are not quite ready for this yet," etc.

A dark mirror: It was used to distort his perception. Whenever he would look for the Light, the dark beings would hold the mirror in front of him and it would reflect phantom feelings of fear, unworthiness, and doubt, about going to the Light.

A tape recorder: This device was set to come on and send messages of fear, doubt, and unworthiness whenever Lee got close to finding the Light.

A clamp: The demons used a clamp type of device to clamp his connecting cords with his guides, thus blocking the information and communication from his guides.

Past Lives

Under hypnosis, Lee found many past lives that were responsible for his problems:

- He was a vigorous, energetic priest who went quickly downhill after a foot injury that rendered him almost immobile. He did not respond to treatment and died of pneumonia, feeling resentful and angry with God, and had doubts about God's ability to help people.

- He was a priest in Egypt who became disenchanted with the church after discovering corruption. He attempted to "blow the whistle" on higher-ups, which resulted in his banishment to a lonely and remote outpost. His health failed and he died of a heart attack at thirty-nine, feeling angry and disappointed with God. In this life, Lee has problems connecting with organized religion and has crippled communication with God.

- He was a corrupt religious figure in France, who breached trust by selling promises in exchange for personal gain. He became intoxicated and fell from a balcony to his death. He was taken to hell and became a possessing entity for fifty years. He felt too guilty and unworthy to enter the Light, and those feelings were carried over with his soul to the current life.

- He had a life as a Catholic priest in Paris, France. He was a good, hardworking, dedicated priest, who was wrongfully accused of embezzlement. A trial and a guilty verdict resulted in a life sentence on Devil's Island. He died feeling resentful and angry toward God. Lee recognized his difficulty in communicating with God and his indifference to spiritual growth coming from this past life into the current life.

- He had a life as a young woman in China who accidentally killed a plant that the "locals" believed to be sacred. She suffered guilt and died believing she was out of favor with God. She felt guilty about entering the Light, unworthy to be in God's presence, and had a fear of not being forgiven by God. These unresolved feelings were carried over to the current life with his soul.

- He was a soldier captured by the enemy and was tortured, starved, beaten, and mistreated. He prayed to God for intervention, but died feeling rejected and angry with God for not saving him. These unresolved feelings were transferred to his current life.

- He had a life in England as the mother of a sick child. She prayed to God for the child to get better, but the child died. She felt angry, deserted, and resentful toward God. These unresolved feelings were carried over to his current life with his soul.

- He had a life as a psychic, whose duties required long leaves of absence from family. He and his family were very close. While away from family, outlaws killed all the family members. He retaliated by hunting down the outlaws and killing them. He died feeling angry and resentful toward God. He also felt unworthy to enter heaven. He promised never to be a psychic again, and that determination was carried over to the current life.

- He had a life as a child healer, who healed with berries and plants and by laying on hands, and had many successes. Some died anyway, because it was their time. The child misunderstood the reason for their deaths and stopped the healing because he had doubts about his abilities to heal. He blamed God for his misunderstanding of some deaths and felt unworthy because he stopped healing. These unresolved feelings were transferred over to his current life, creating the problems for him.

- He had a life as a tribe's messenger, who traveled to a village with a message that would save the people from an enemy. The message was delivered too late. Many were killed and taken prisoner. He died feeling unworthy of God's love, unworthy to enter heaven, and felt God would not forgive him. These feelings were carried over to his current life.

- He had a life as a psychic channeler who delivered information from the Light. Many who did not follow his advice died. The psychic was blamed and was killed. He died feeling angry and resentful toward God and felt betrayed by him, and those feelings were transferred to his current life; in this life he felt indifferent to psychic activity.

- He had a life in which darkness was intentionally channeled for sexual favors, a grand lifestyle, and financial gain. He died feeling unworthy and guilty about going to the Light. He felt that there would be no forgiveness. These unresolved feelings were transferred over to the current life, creating problems during the treatment.

- He had a life as a twenty-two-year-old female healer (healing hands) in Japan. She had many successes in healing until an invasion by a tribe that relegated women to slavery. The healer was beaten and imprisoned because of her gifts. She died feeling angry and made a decision never to have these gifts; that anger and that decision were carried over to his current life with his soul.

- He was a nine-year-old boy in China who was able to see and communicate with angels and was dependent on them for direction on exploring trips. One time he became lost, was captured, and was made a slave for the remainder of his life. He died feeling deceived by the angels and promised never to work with them again. These feelings and decisions were carried over to his current life with his soul, creating problems for him during the therapy.

- He was a preacher in England, who lived an unbalanced life due to possessing entities. He was booted out of church and later went crazy. He died in a dungeon, feeling guilty and unworthy of entering the Light, afraid that he would be punished by God.

- He had a life in Greece as a philosopher who channeled information from the Light. People disapproved of his actions. He was captured, ridiculed, and put to death by poison. He died promising himself never to work with the spirit world again because he was killed. These feelings were brought to this current life and created a block during the therapy.

- He had a life in China, several thousand years B.C., where he channeled by going into a trance and speaking the words of a heavenly being. People did not believe or trust the channeled messages from heaven. They felt he was "of the devil," and incarcerated, tortured, and killed him. He died promising himself never to channel again.

- He had a life where he had the ability to heal by being able to see and locate spirits and recognize diseases in people's bodies. He had a few incorrect observations and became discouraged. Doubts set in and he stopped using these gifts completely and promised never to have those gifts again.
- He had a life when he was able to see angels and other spirits. Others in power doubted him and stopped him from seeing by putting acid in his eyes, blinding him. Trauma of losing his sight was so great that the visions also stopped. He died angry, promising himself never to see the spirits again.
- He had a life when he was heavily influenced by dark beings who told him that he could find the Light by staring at the sun for hours. He did so and became blinded. He died believing the Light had deceived him and promised never to trust the Light again.
- While in heaven, upon leaving God, after his creation, he tried to look back at him and became blinded by his Light and felt angry with God.
- He had a life as one of the first humans on earth. His soul was infused in a body that was already created by God. He lived for a time in peace and joy. After some members of his community entered a forbidden place (garden), his life changed as he took on some darkness, which surfaced as jealousy, possessiveness, and hostility. He married, had seventeen children, lived several hundred years, and died (willed his spirit back to the Light), feeling unworthy of God's love and fearful of entering the Light. These feelings were brought back to his current life.

The unresolved emotional, mental, and physical problems and his last thoughts, decisions, and conclusions from all these past lives were carried over to Lee's current life with his soul, creating problems for him all through this life and during the therapy.

Soul Parts

During other lives and this life, Lee had lost many soul parts that were in the possession of demon entities. By touching these soul parts, they could restimulate the feelings of fear, anger, guilt, and unworthiness that would travel through the connecting cords to his current life body, here.

Due to his determination, perseverance, hard work, and a strong desire to connect and communicate successfully with God, his higher self, guides, and angels, Lee was able to resolve and remove his misperceptions and blocks. He described his progress as follows:

> *"Overall, there is a great deal of improvement in my ability to stay focused during hypnosis. I am able to see and communicate with my guides and angels and tap into different knowledge from the akashic plane without feeling anxious. I feel better about my relationship with God and other Light beings and feel closer to them."*

Hearing Problem

Ann had difficult focusing on listening. Too much peripheral noise made it impossible for her to filter out and focus on what she was trying to hear. She had a tendency to turn her head to the right to hear, asking, "What did you say?" As we look at Ann's case in Chapter VIII, we can see that her hearing problems came from the following sources.

Demon Entities

Ann found in her the following demon entities that were responsible for her hearing problem.

Demon entity in her right ear joined Ann when she had mumps and claimed to cause her earaches, dizziness, pressure in the ear, and hearing problems.

A dark demon blob in the ear claimed to create noise in her ears, which vibrated and created confusion for Ann. It also scrambled sound by twisting the nerves so everything became garbled. As a result, she could not focus on what she was hearing.

Past Lives and Soul Parts

Ann recalled the following past lives that were responsible for her hearing problems.

John was hanged and lost from his ears soul parts that were in possession of the demons. They created hearing problems for Ann by clamping the connecting cords between her soul parts and her ears.

Jamie was shot in his back in the Civil War and later died of infection. He did not like the noise of guns and cannons firing. He lost from his ears many soul parts that were in the possession of demons, who were clamping the connecting cords between the soul parts and ears, causing Ann's hearing problems.

Jamie also lost from his ears two soul parts that were still lying on the battlefield. They fragmented out of fear and caused the problem with the hearing, noise, and confusion.

Anya was thrown into a pit. While she was falling, she lost parts from her ears that were with demons who were causing Ann hearing problems and pressure in the ears by clamping the connecting cords.

Jacques was tortured and beheaded for harboring fugitives. He lost many soul parts from his ears, throat, eyes, and brain. It was as though a circuit had been cut between hearing, seeing, speaking, and memory. There was a disconnection between those functions.

Hanne, a young female who was a musician in Vienna, was killed in an uprising. She gave two soul parts from her ears to her friend because he would not listen to her.

Stephan, a monk, was a composer of chants. At the age of forty-one he had brain fever. He lost his vision and hearing, but he still could write the music because he heard it within his soul. He lost from his brain, ears, and eyes many soul parts that were responsible for Ann's vision and hearing problems.

Devices

The demons were using clamp types of spiritual devices to clamp the connecting cords between Ann's soul parts and her ears. They were removed and destroyed by the angels on our request.

After removing all the demon spirits and devices, by resolving the past life traumas and integrating all the lost soul parts, Ann experienced a complete cure of her hearing problems.

Tertiary (New) Symptoms

Tertiary symptoms are the new symptoms that manifest during the treatment. They arise from multiple sources, as follows:

1. **Attachment by new earthbound and demon entities**: The possessing earthbound and demon spirits can cause a great deal of damage, which takes some time to heal even after releasing the spirits from the patients and cleansing them. During that period, patients are vulnerable for new spirit entry. New earthbound and demon spirits bring their new symptoms with them. Clearing and cleansing the patient once may not be enough. The patient has to work continuously to prevent reentry. This requires a lot of discipline. Just by being human, we all can open ourselves for spirit attachments because we may get sick, be injured, grieve, have other strong emotions, drink, or use drugs.

2. **Layering of spirits in the body**: Sometimes patients report that the spirits are arranged in multiple layers, one over the other in their bodies. In this case, although the original entities and their associated symptoms were relieved, deeper layers of human and demon entities may surface, bringing new (tertiary) symptoms along.

It may seem like patients are getting worse or the treatment is not helping. But the fact is that the problem is already there, and as we remove one layer of spirits and the problems associated with them, a new set of spirits, which was buried under the first layer, now comes to the surface, bringing the symptoms associated with them, which the patients experience as new symptoms.

We need to continuously check and release the spirits till the patients are totally free.

3. **Soul fragments that remained inside the body**: These look and feel as the patients looked and felt at the time of the traumas and have the memories and feelings of the traumatic events. These soul fragments, or little ones, may begin to experience all the physical and emotional feelings of the trauma during the therapy, and in turn the patients begin to experience all those symptoms that were dormant before and are recognized as the tertiary symptoms.

4. **Soul fragments that left the body**: Those fragments that are in possession of Satan and his demons can be used to insert new earthbound and demon entities, devices, energy absorbers, thoughts, visions, attitudes, behavior, and physical and emotional feelings into the patients, causing them to have new or tertiary symptoms.

Therefore, it is very crucial that every soul part be brought back, cleansed, healed, and integrated, regardless of how small or large and whether inside or outside. Without this, the patient will be constantly influenced and permanent healing will not be possible.

5. **Energy absorbers**: Demons can send energy absorbers through the patients' soul parts and their connecting cords. These in the patients, around the patients, or covering their cords to the Light, can drain their energy and make them feel tired and sleepy and thus create the new or tertiary symptoms.

6. **Devices**: New devices can be inside the body or outside the body, including the remote devices that are sent by Satan and his demons through the patients' captive soul parts and their connecting cords. They can cause multiple symptoms for the patients, which become the new or tertiary symptoms.

7. **New entities, energies, and devices being pushed into the patients from other dimensions**: This is done through certain points between dimensions of similar vibrations in spite of all the shields being in place and intact. They can create new or tertiary symptoms for the patients. Angels should be requested

to stay on guard at those points between another dimension and this dimension.

8. **Past life problems**: Tertiary symptoms may arise from past life problems that surface when the overburden of the spirits is cleared up. Then the patients become aware of symptoms that are coming from past lives. The symptoms were already there, but were buried under the spirit-caused problems that needed to be resolved. To do the complete healing of the patient, these past lives and related problems must also be resolved and healed.

My patients report that current and past life traumas and problems create holes and weaknesses in our souls due to soul fragmentation and soul loss, which create an opening in us for spirits to come in. Unless these past life problems are resolved by past life regression therapy and the holes and weaknesses are healed by retrieving and integrating all the lost soul parts, patients will continue to be influenced by the entities and it will be a never-ending process during the treatment, and complete and thorough healing will not be possible.

It is extremely important to heal those past life problems to keep the spirits away and to have a thorough, complete, and permanent healing. This requires continued treatment. Unfortunately, many patients do not stay long enough in treatment to complete the healing needed because they feel free from their acute presenting and some secondary symptoms in just a few sessions.

Recovered Memories of Abuse

These are the memories of sexual, physical, or psychological abuse that occurred during childhood but were forgotten by the patients; later, several years after, they recall these memories of abuse with or without therapy and with or without hypnosis.

These cases of recovered memories of abuse have created a great deal of controversy. Some claim that all these recovered memories are the total truth, while others think that all memories are false. Both sides of the debate have extreme feelings.

Different Sources of Memories of Abuse

Working with hundreds of patients for about eleven years, with different therapies, I find that there are multiple sources for the memories of abuse:

- Abuse in the current life
- Abuse in one or more past lives
- Memories of abuse of a possessing earthbound spirit
- Memories of abuse of a possessing soul fragment of a living person
- False memories of abuse fed by the demons

Abuse in the current life: Some patients, under hypnosis, recall memories of abuse that occurred in their current life. Under hypnosis, sometimes they describe that during the sexual or physical abuse, the main body of the soul leaves the body and goes far away from the body, leaving a small part of the soul to activate the body and cope with the trauma. As a result, the patient has partial or total amnesia for the abuse.

This small soul fragment, also known in psychiatry as the inner child or subpersonality, contains all the memories and feelings of the traumatic event. It is so damaged that it cannot be returned to the main body of the soul. It is sacrificed to isolate and protect the main body of the soul. This small soul fragment, although separated from the main body of the patient's soul, is still connected to it with a cord.

The main body of the soul, when safe, returns to the body and resumes its duties and has total or partial amnesia of the abuse. It is able to function normally, with minimum negative effects due to the trauma.

Also, during the abuse, patient's protective shield opens up, allowing outside human and dark spirits to come in. The dark spirits trap and surround the fragmented soul parts completely and block the connecting cord with negative energy, leading to total amnesia for the abuse.

Later in life, some event can open up these memories of abuse, e.g., watching a television show or a movie showing abuse, or reading or hearing somebody talking about an abuse.

In therapy, the patient is encouraged to recall, relive, release, and resolve the trauma and forgive the abuser. The fragmented soul part, after cleansing and healing, is integrated with the main body of the soul, with the help of the angels.

Ruth claimed that she does not remember much before the age of twelve and was bothered by this lack of memory. She was afraid of men and could not trust them. She had a nagging suspicion that maybe she was sexually abused, but she was not sure. Under hypnosis, as she was scanning her body she found several fragmented soul parts of her from age six to age eleven. They said they fragmented when they were being sexually abused by a man in the neighborhood. They were still suffering with pain and did not trust grownups. They said that, during the abuse, the rest of Ruth's soul left the body and went far away while they coped with the abuse. As a result, grownup Ruth had amnesia for the abuse. After resolving their traumas, all fragmented soul parts were cleansed, healed, and integrated with the main body of Ruth's soul. After the session, Ruth was not afraid of men and was able to trust them.

Abuse in one or more past lives: Sometimes, memories of abuse can be from one or more past lives and can surface in the current life. Here, patients often think that the abuse happened in the current life. In these cases, the confusion and problems can be solved by doing past life regression therapy and resolving the trauma, and bringing back all the missing soul parts that were lost during those past lives and are in the possession of the demons. By massaging those soul parts, they restimulate the memories of the past life traumas in patients' current life bodies. Those soul parts are cleansed, healed, and integrated with the main bodies of the patients' soul, with the help of the angels.

Maya, a thirty-three-year-old female, always had a nagging feeling that she was sexually abused as a child, but did not have any clear memories of the abuse. She also had a recurrent dream, even as a child, of being a little girl and being sexually abused by a man; she would wake up in a panic. In the dream, she could not see the face of the man.

In therapy, under hypnosis, I asked her to focus on her dream and recall the whole story. She recalled that she was in another life and another body as an eight-year-old girl who was sexually abused and killed by a soldier. After resolving the trauma of that life, she did not have that dream anymore and felt at peace.

She did not recall being abused in the current life.

Memories of abuse of a possessing earthbound spirit: Sometimes memories of abuse turn out to be the memories of a possessing earthbound spirit. Memories of abuse and related symptoms of the spirit can be transferred over to the patient, and the patient recalls them as his or her memories. These memories can also manifest in the patient's dreams and nightmares.

In these cases, the memories of the abuse and associated symptoms can be resolved by releasing the spirit from the patient.

Rosy, a twenty-five-year-old female, had a severe fear of men and difficulty in relating to them. She also had a dream about being sexually abused from time to time. She wondered if she was sexually abused by somebody.

Under hypnosis, when I asked her to go to the source of the dream and feelings, she saw a fifteen-year-old girl in a concentration camp in Germany. She was sexually abused by many soldiers and finally killed. This girl turned out to be a possessing spirit who was still recalling her sexual trauma and fear of men and transferring them to Rosy.

After releasing the spirit, Rosy was not afraid of men and was able to relate to them better.

Memories of the abuse of a possessing soul fragment of a living person: Sometimes memories of abuse of a soul fragment of another living person who is inside the patient can be transferred to the patient, who recalls them as his or her memories.

In this case, after the resolution of the trauma, this soul fragment of another living person is cleansed, healed, and integrated with its owner, with the help of the angels. After releasing that soul part of another person, the patient can be free of the memories and symptoms of the abuse that belonged to the other person.

Tanya, a nineteen-year-old college student, had a feeling that she was being sexually abused by one of her family members. But she did not know for sure and wanted to find out under hypnosis. She also had dreams about a man coming to her room in the night and fondling her.

Under hypnosis, as I asked her to go to the source of her feelings and the dreams, she found a soul part of her best friend Sandy in her. Sandy claimed that she was sexually abused by her grandfather when she was ten years old. These memories and feelings of Sandy were transferred to Tanya and manifested in her dreams. After the resolution of her trauma, Sandy's soul part was cleansed, healed, and integrated with her soul in her body, with the help of the angels. After releasing the soul part of Sandy to her own body, Tanya was free of those dreams and feelings of abuse.

False memories of abuse fed by the demons: Sometimes memories of abuse can be fed by the demons who are inside the patient. In this case, the problems can be resolved by freeing the patient from all the possessing entities.

Other times, the memories of abuse can be fed by the demons from outside. They have the patient's soul parts in their possession. Through these soul parts and their connecting cords between the soul parts and the patient's soul, the demons send the false memories, thoughts, and visions of abuse of their own making to the patient, and the patient recalls them as his or her own.

In these cases, in therapy, we need to bring back all the soul parts of the patient that are in possession of the demons outside and integrate them with the patient after cleansing and healing them. This is done with the help of the angels of the Light. After that, the patient can be free of memories of the abuse.

Marla, a thirty-eight-year-old female, had vague thoughts, visions, and dreams of being sexually abused by different people, although she had no conscious memories of being abused.

In therapy, under hypnosis, as Marla tried to locate the source of the problem, she found in her head a dark demon who claimed to give her the dreams, thoughts, and visions of the abuse. It also said that other demons in hell had her soul parts in their possession and were feeding her false memories, visions, and thoughts of the sexual abuse through her soul parts and their connecting cords to her.

After releasing all the entities from her, retrieving all her lost soul parts, and integrating them with her, after cleansing and healing, she did not have any thoughts, visions, or dreams of sexual abuse.

Sometimes the memories of the abuse can come from more than one source in the same patient.

Treatment: The memories of the abuse and the associated symptoms should be treated as described in each category.

When the abuse occurs in the current life by other people, it should be resolved by recalling, reliving, releasing, and resolving the trauma, and forgiving the abuser. In the treatment, patients should be helped in putting those traumatic events behind them and moving ahead with their life.

Forgiveness is the most important part of the therapy and healing. Sometimes further trauma is caused to both parties by taking legal action and pursuing justice or money for the damages. It keeps the anger, hurt, and desire for revenge fired up, wounds remain open, and the healing cannot take place. The whole point of therapy is healing the patients; without forgiveness, healing cannot occur and the patients cannot be at peace with themselves.

So, in therapy, we will be defeating the whole purpose of healing by encouraging legal action against the abuser. It is a lost cause and does not serve any purpose in therapy. The therapist and the patient should focus on healing rather than blame. Through forgiveness, not only the patient can heal, but also the abuser.

Schizophrenia

Before describing this case, I would like to give definitions of some terms, for understanding.

Schizophrenia: A disturbance that lasts for at least six months and includes at least one month of active-phase symptoms, that is, two or more of the following: delusions, hallucinations, disorganized speech, grossly disorganized or catatonic behavior, and negative symptoms (DSM IV).

The following definitions are taken from Kaplan and Sadock's *Synopsis of Psychiatry*.

Psychosis: Inability to distinguish reality from fantasy; impaired reality testing with the creation of a new reality.

Reality testing: The objective evaluation and judgment of the world outside the self.

Hallucinations: False sensory perception as associated with real external stimuli; there may or may not be a delusional interpretation of the hallucinatory experience.

(a) **Auditory hallucination**: False perception of sound, usually voices, but also other noises, such as music; most common hallucination in psychiatric disorders.

(b) **Visual hallucination**: False perception involving sight, consisting of formed images (for example, people) and unformed images (for example, flashes of light); most common in medically determined disorders.

(c) **Olfactory hallucination**: False perception of smell; most common in medical disorders.

(d) **Gustatory hallucination**: False perception of taste, such as unpleasant taste caused by an uncinate seizure; most common in medical disorders.

(e) **Tactile hallucination**: False perception of touch or surface sensation, as from an amputated limb (phantom limb); crawling sensation on or under the skin (formication).

(f) **Somatic hallucination**: False sensation of things occurring in or to the body, most often visceral in origin.

Illusion: Misperception or misinterpretation of real external sensory stimuli.

Delusion: False belief, based on incorrect inference about external reality, not consistent with patient's intelligence and cultural background, that cannot be corrected by reasoning.

Paranoid delusions: Includes prosecutory delusions and delusions of reference, control, and grandeur (distinguished from paranoid ideation, which is suspiciousness of less than delusional proportions).

(a) Delusion of persecution: False belief that one is being harassed, cheated, or persecuted; often found in litigious patients who have a pathological tendency to take legal action because of imagined mistreatment.

(b) Delusion of grandeur: Exaggerated perception of one's importance, power, or identity.

(c) Delusion of reference: False belief that the behavior of others refers to oneself; that events, objects, or other people have a particular and unusual significance, usually of a negative nature; derived from idea of reference, in which one falsely feels that one is being talked about by others (for example, belief that people on television or radio are talking to or about the patient).

Delusion of Self-accusation: False feeling of remorse and guilt.

Delusion of Control: False feelings that one's will, thoughts, or feelings are being controlled by external forces.

(a) Thought Withdrawal: Delusion that one's thoughts are being removed from one's mind by other people or forces.

(b) Thought Insertion: Delusion that thoughts are being implanted in one's mind by other people or forces.

(c) Thought Broadcasting: Delusion that one's thoughts can be heard by others, as though they were being broadcast into the air.

(d) Thought Control: Delusion that one's thoughts are being controlled by other people or forces.

Over the years, working with these therapies, I have come to recognize that the patients who have auditory, visual, and other hallucinations and different types of delusions are often clairvoyant, clairaudient, clairsensient, and psychic people. They can perceive beyond the five physical senses. The voices they hear and people and things they see, which other people cannot see or hear, may be real human, demon, and other spirits whom they are seeing, hearing, and feeling.

These spirits who talk to the patients may be inside the body or outside. The spirits who are inside the patients can directly talk to them or to other spirits who are inside the patients or outside. These visions, voices, and thoughts are also fed to the patients by the demons in hell who have possession of one or more soul parts of the patients. Through these soul parts and their connecting cords, the demons can transmit visions, thoughts, and feelings into the patient's body, who receives them as their own. Some of these patients are also very sensitive and are aware of the feelings in their bodies, which are called somatic delusions.

Because other people around them, including the psychiatrist, do not see, feel, or hear beyond their five physical senses, they think that the patients are imagining things and have lost reality.

Antipsychotic medications work to some extent in these patients because they also sedate the possessing spirits, but as soon as the medication is stopped or reduced, the symptoms return. Shock treatment may work sometimes because the spirits may be shocked out of the patient's body, but they return and go inside the patient again because their shields are often porous and weak. As long as those spirits are there in them, they will continue to be sick.

I have successfully treated some schizophrenic patients with these therapies. Unfortunately, most of the schizophrenic patients are so fragmented, afflicted, influenced, and controlled by these spirits that they cannot focus long enough to do the work.

These patients sometimes can be healed with the help of a mediator, who can be a family member or a friend who wants to help the patient, or a person who is a good hypnotic subject and wants to help others as described in "Remote Healing." These mediators first have to go through their own cleansing and healing with these therapies and have to have a good understanding of these therapies.

Denise, a thirty-five-year-old female, had her first nervous breakdown when she was nineteen years old. She had been diagnosed as having schizophrenia, paranoid type. She had multiple hospitalizations, was treated by many psychiatrists, and was treated by high doses of different types of antipsychotic medications for seventeen years.

When she came to me she was taking 900 mg. of Clozaril per day. In spite of the high doses of the medication, she still appeared to be very restless, anxious, and preoccupied with her problems. She had auditory and visual hallucinations and multiple paranoid and somatic delusions:

- "I feel that people on T.V. and people in general are stern, strict, mean, and nasty to me, and are talking about me."
- "I feel that signs on billboards look stern and strict, as if they are perfect and they are against me."
- "I feel like people do not like me. I am afraid of people, especially men."
- "I feel like other people's thoughts and actions can penetrate me."
- "I feel like a puppet on strings. Somebody tells me to mimic and I do."
- "I feel like something separated me."
- "I feel like I can get other people's problems."
- "I feel like I am losing my soul."
- "I feel like I have holes in the back of my neck and right shoulder blade."
- "I feel like something entered my body."
- "I feel like somebody took a piece of me."
- "I feel like I have different animals in me."

- "When our car hit a deer, I felt like a part of the deer came into me."
- "I feel like I have prongs on my head."
- "I feel like my breasts are chopped off or deflated."
- "I feel like there is a knife in my vagina, cutting it, or that my vagina is missing."
- "I feel like my right hand is not there."
- "I feel like my nose is missing."
- "I feel like I have a mask on my face."
- "I feel like my tongue is loose."
- "I feel like I have a wooden leg."
- "When I look in the mirror I see somebody else."

Her affect (the feeling tone) was that of being anxious and restless. Sometimes it was flat. At times, when she looked at you, she looked as if she were looking through you. She had poor concentration. Her memory was fair. Her judgment and insight into her problems were poor. She had trouble relating and trusting other people.

Her older brother found out about these therapies and wanted to find out if I could treat Denise with them. After the first interview with Denise, I told her brother that because of the severity of her symptoms, I could not do hypnotherapy with her, but if he or another family member were willing to help her, then we could try to heal Denise through them. Her brother was willing to help his sister.

I explained to him about the nature of the therapy in detail and that before we attempted to heal Denise, we had to cleanse and heal him, with spirit releasement therapy, current and past life regression therapy, and soul integration. He turned out to be an excellent subject. After his cleansing and healing, he was able to tune into Denise and locate and release her possessing human, demon, and other spirits and locate and integrate her soul parts after the resolution of their traumas. Then we proceeded to look into her past lives, which were responsible for her problems and feelings and brought back and integrated her missing soul parts that she lost during those past life traumas.

After a couple of sessions, working with her brother alone for her, without her presence, I had her sit in the session, too. During the session, what amazed me was that even she was able to locate the spirits in her and recall her past lives without any hypnosis and without closing her eyes. I realized that when she had that staring look, as if she were looking through you, she was really in a state of focused concentration as in hypnosis and was tuning in to another dimension and reality. Later, I was able to work with her alone, directly, and then, whenever her brother could come, we did the fast healing through him. I realized that all those feelings and symptoms she was experiencing were really due to spirits, devices, past life traumas, and experiences due to soul loss.

I realized that she was shifting back and forth in this dimension and other dimensions and had a hard time remaining grounded. She was also able to see, hear, and feel the spirits, and was also able to see and feel her soul parts leaving or something or somebody else's parts coming into her. You will see that every symptom and feeling she described was exactly what was happening to her and not just her imagination. Actually, she was very much in touch with reality about what was happening, but could not understand it, and became confused, scared, and upset.

During the sessions, through her brother and also directly with her alone, we found the following sources for her symptoms.

Energy Field (Aura) and the Shield around Her

Her energy field and shield appeared as a cheesecloth with holes all over, making it easy for the spirits to enter her body and affect her. So I requested the angels to put a special triple net and metallic shield all around her. The angels also put a crystal space-type helmet over her head and face down to her neck. These shields protected her from further infestation.

Earthbound and Demon Spirits

Denise had in her many human and demon spirits, whom we released over several sessions. One of the human spirits she recognized was the person she used to see when she looked in the mirror. After releasing that spirit, she did not see that face in the mirror anymore.

There were many areas, in different parts of her body, where there were demon and other spirits who were packed in different layers. So we requested the angels to remove each and every entity, through each and every layer, in different parts of her body and fill those spaces with the Light. Then we requested the angels to locate and bring back all her soul parts that belong to those empty holes where entities were packed in layers. They were cleansed, healed, and integrated with the main body of her soul.

She also had many spirits of different types of animals in her, including a deer. They were all released.

After this, the shield around her appeared stronger and had fewer holes.

Devices

Denise had many dark devices all over her body, giving her paranoid delusions, confusion, and other physical, emotional, and mental symptoms.

Black helmet on her head: This blocked her from the Light. It also short-circuited her brain and energy was not flowing within.

Black screws in her vertebral arteries. These inhibited the blood flow in her brain, causing her confusion.

Black balls on her psychic antennas: These psychic antennas are lodged in the temporal lobes of the brain and are present in everybody. Most people do not pay attention to them, so they do not work in them. Psychic people can raise the antennas telescopically, pay attention to what is going on, and then they shut them down.

In Denise, the demons put two black heavy ball-type devices on those antennas; a demon in hell controlled these devices. The demons had soul parts of Denise from her brain in their possession. They stretched a soul part in the form of a movie screen and projected visions, thoughts, feelings, and stories of their own making, which would travel from her soul part through the connecting cords to her brain here in her body, giving her paranoid and confusing thoughts, visions, and feelings.

Black rods and clamps in her back: They caused her back pain.

Black plugs like hearing aids in her ears: They interfered with her hearing and listening to the relaxation tape. The demons also altered or selectively blocked her communication with others.

Device like a face mask: Denise had many of these face mask type of devices in her face, in layers. They gave her a robot type of facial expression. Through them, they also either restricted her facial expressions or exaggerated them.

Black wire type of devices between her brain and eyes, ears, mouth, and tongue: They caused interference with her vision, hearing, and speaking.

A black rod in her right forearm: This extended from her elbow down to her right hand. There were also black wires going from her hand to her brain, which inhibited appropriate perception from her brain to her hands. They infused black fluid in her right hand, causing numbness in her right hand, making her feel as if it were not there.

Black devices in her stomach: These would squeeze her stomach and make her feel hungry.

Black wire type of connections between her stomach and hypothalamus: They were in her hypothalamus, stomach, and thyroid glands, making her feel hungry and lowering her metabolism.

Devices in vagina, uterus, fallopian tubes, and ovaries: Black wire type of devices in her vagina, uterus, tubes, and ovaries connected to her brain. They created numbness in her vagina, making her feel as if it were not there.

Black iron rod in front of her right leg: It gave her feelings as if she had a wooden leg.

There were many, many similar devices all over her body in layers. They were removed and destroyed with the help of the angels. They also brought back her missing soul parts that belonged to her body where the devices were. They were cleansed, healed, and integrated with her.

Past Life Traumas

There were many past life traumas that were responsible for her symptoms of different types of somatic delusions.

Feelings that her nose and face are missing: She had the following lifetimes with different types of traumas to her face and nose.

- She was a man nosing in other people's business; as a result, her nose was cut off.
- She was shot by an arrow, which went through her face and nose.
- She was a man on a horse trying to get away, but was shot in the face.

Denise had these thoughts and memories in this life and thought that it happened to her in this life, causing her confusion.

- She was a soldier during the Civil War whose face and head were blown off by a cannon.
- She was a chemist working with a mixture of something. She was trying to experiment, but it exploded on her face and disfigured it.
- She was burned as a witch in Salem. She wanted to look down at the fire to show the town people that she was not afraid, as a result, her face was burned first.
- She was a Chinese war prisoner whose face was blown off by a shotgun because he refused to give information.
- She was a queen, very beautiful and seductive, who was having affairs. As a result, her husband cut her face and nose.

Feelings that her breasts were chopped off: She had the following lifetimes that were responsible for her symptoms.

- She was a maiden in a life when a knight raped her and cut her breasts off.
- She was a beautiful princess who was having an affair with a soldier; as a result, her breasts were cut off.

Feelings that her vagina was missing: Denise had the following past life traumas that were responsible for these feelings.

- She was a prostitute when she was shot in the vagina and killed.
- She was raped in another life and her vagina was cut off.
- She was supposed to serve men sexually, but she refused. As a result, they raped her, cut her vagina, and then killed her.

Feelings that her right hand was missing: Denise had traumas in the following lifetimes responsible for her feelings that her right hand was missing.

- She was in a battle in trenches. She raised her right hand to surrender and was shot in her right hand.
- She killed her baby, who was conceived as a result of rape in a past life.
- She put nails in somebody's hands in a past life. She felt guilty about it.

Feelings that she had a wooden leg: The following past life traumas were responsible for those feelings in her right leg.

- A tree fell on her legs in a past life and crushed them.
- An animal tore her leg apart in a past life.
- She was a pirate in a past life whose leg was blown off by a cannon in a ship battle. He used a wooden leg.

All her emotional, mental, and physical feelings due to different traumas and her last thoughts, decisions, and promises during these lives were brought back here with her soul into her current life, creating problems for her.

Soul Parts

Denise lost many, many soul parts due to different traumas in this life and her past lives. These lost soul parts were mostly in the possession of the demons in hell. These soul parts contained the memories of physical, mental, and emotional traumas from those past lives. They used these soul parts of Denise in different ways to cause her different types of emotional, mental, physical, and spiritual problems.

- They squeezed Denise's soul parts that she lost from the above past lives and restimulated emotional, mental, and physical feelings and memories that she felt during those past lives. These feelings traveled through the connecting cords and she felt them here in her current body. They created in her the feelings that her nose, right hand, ears, and vagina were missing, her breasts were chopped off, her tongue was loose, she had a wooden leg, etc.
- Missing soul parts from the back of her neck and other parts of her body created holes in her soul, which she was able to sense. But everybody thought she was just imagining these things. After we brought those soul parts back and integrated them with her, she did not have the feeling that she had a hole in the back of her neck, and other parts of her body.
- The demons in hell used her soul parts as a movie screen, projecting visions, paranoid thoughts, and fears, which traveled through the connecting cord to her brain here in her current body. She received them as her own and acted on them.
- They used her soul parts in hell as a microphone and talked to her constantly, criticizing her, putting her down, giving her negative thoughts about other people she was with, and also giving her commands about what to do. These communications traveled through the connecting cords to her ears, here in her current body, and she heard them as her thoughts.
- The demons used her soul parts, which were in their possession in hell, to send human, demon, and other spirits,

dark devices, and dark energy through these soul parts and their connecting cords into her body. They created more problems for her.

- They used soul parts that she lost from her face in different past lives. They used her different soul parts and their connecting cords to her face, and forced her to make faces and have facial twitches, and made her feel like a puppet. They did so by pulling her strings (cords) and telling her to mimic people.

- The demons used her soul parts that she lost from her breasts, in different past lives, when her breasts were chopped off. They squeezed those soul parts and restimulated her feelings and memories of her breasts being chopped off, in her current body. They also put those soul parts from her breasts on fire, which caused them to swell up like balloons and then poked those soul parts with needles, causing them to deflate. These feelings transferred to her current body, making her feel as if her breasts were deflated.

- They used her soul parts from her right hand, nose, and vagina and inserted black liquid, a negative energy, through the connecting cords to her right hand, nose, and vagina in the current body, which made them feel numb and as if they were not there or were missing.

- They used her soul parts from her ears and clamped the connecting cords off and on, so her hearing would be blocked in the middle of the conversation with other people around. Then they interjected words that they wanted her to hear, thus confusing her about what people were saying.

- The demons in hell used different soul parts that she lost in different lifetimes while feeling inferior, angry, afraid, remorseful, confused, unworthy, etc. By squeezing them they restimulated those feelings in Denise, here in her current body causing her problems.

Session after session, we removed foreign entities, dark devices, dark energies, dark shields, and dark connections from her.

Then we brought back her missing soul parts that belonged to those holes in her soul and integrated them with her. Her current and past life traumas were also resolved.

In this case, we can clearly see that all her visual, auditory, and other hallucinations and paranoid, somatic, and other delusions were not just her imagination. They were real, due to possessing spirits, dark devices, dark energies, missing soul parts, and current and past life traumas. She was the one who was truly in touch with reality, but did not understand that reality and did not know what to do about it. Light beings, through my patients, have often mentioned that mentally ill people are closer to God because they are more in touch with reality.

Her condition is improving consistently. She is taking only one third of the medication she had been taking and is feeling more integrated and relaxed and less confused, paranoid, and afraid. She is able to catch her symptoms and request the angels to remove whatever is causing her those symptoms and bring her missing soul parts that are responsible for her symptoms, cleanse them, heal them, and integrate them with her. Thus, she herself is taking an active part in her healing.

Working with Denise, and her brother for her, shed a new light on the understanding of schizophrenia and gave me hope, not only for Denise, but for all those schizophrenic patients who are often declared by psychiatrists and society to be hopeless and incurable. The gift of her brother's love and his help made it possible for her to heal. Denise described her progress as follows:

> "When I was sick, even before I had my first breakdown (when I was nineteen years old), I felt that everyone believed that there was something wrong with me and I also thought the same. When near other people, especially men, I would freeze and be a nervous wreck. These feelings generalized until I was afraid of everyone and everything. I thought that no one liked me. I was scared, insecure, nervous, paranoid, and schizophrenic. I could not handle even my schoolwork. I became very confused and thought that everyone was talking about me. I could not look at anyone. I thought I was responsible for other people's problems e.g., even if someone just

sneezed. I had five psychotic breakdowns and was hospitalized each time. I was in a personal care home for about eight and one-half years. Dr. Modi has helped me more than all the other psychiatrists I saw in seventeen years. She provided a relaxation tape, which has helped me tremendously. When I hear Dr. Modi's voice on the tape, I am no longer scared and I can relax.

"Working with Dr. Modi, I have learned to face my problems. Her hypnotherapy has given a great deal of help and hope to me. I am a happy person now. I can walk into a restaurant without being paranoid. I am less afraid, nervous, insecure, and paranoid. My self-esteem has improved a lot. If there is a problem with someone, I do not blame myself. I keep telling myself that I am not perfect and do not need to be perfect.

"I am not afraid of people anymore, especially men. After eight and one-half years, I have moved back home with my family and I am getting along much better, which is very important to me. My face, nose, tongue, breasts, vagina, and legs feel much better now.

"Dr. Modi taught me how to pray for healing. Anytime, if any of these feelings return, instead of feeling helpless, I right away pray to God and Christ and request the angels to remove whatever is responsible for those feelings (e.g., spirits, devices, negative energies, or other people's soul parts), and bring back my missing soul parts that are responsible for these problems. I ask the angels to repair my shield and put a crystal shield around me and within minutes, I am free of my problems. Thank you, Dr. Modi, for helping me, and giving me my life back."

Dissociative Identity Disorder (DID) or Multiple Personality Disorder (MPD)

According to *Diagnostic and Statistic Manual of Mental Disorders*, fourth edition (*DSM IV*), diagnostic criteria for dissociative identity disorders (multiple personality disorder [MPD]) are

A. The presence of two or more distinct identities or personality states (each with its own relatively enduring pattern of perceiving, relating to, and thinking about the environment and self).

B. At least two of these identities or personality states recurrently take control of the person's behavior.

C. Inability to recall important personal information that is too extensive to be explained by ordinary forgetfulness.

D. The disturbance is not due to the direct physiological effects of a substance (e.g., blackouts or chaotic behavior during alcohol intoxication) or a general medical condition (e.g., complex partial seizures).

Note: In children, the symptoms are not attributable to imaginary playmates or other fantasy play.

Psychopathology of Multiple Personality Disorder

In patients with dissociative identity disorder (multiple personality disorder), I find the following psychopathology.

Trauma: These patients often give a history of physical, emotional, and sexual trauma which is often severe, repetitive, and sometimes sadistic.

Weakening of energy field: Each physical, emotional, and sexual trauma weakens the energy fields around the patients, allowing outside spirits to come inside their bodies; these spirits remain inside the patients as possessing entities. They can be earthbound spirits, demons or other entities, and fragmented soul parts of living people, that is, of family members, friends, and abusers.

Soul fragmentation: With each trauma, personality or soul consciousness may fragment into many parts, which become the subpersonality, alter personality, or inner child. Fragmentation can happen at different ages with different sets of traumas. These fragmented soul parts or personalities can either stay inside the body or leave the body.

Soul parts that stay inside the body: Soul parts that remain in the body look and feel exactly the way they looked and felt at the time of the trauma and fragmentation, as if they were frozen in time or locked into a given age. They hold the memories and affect of the traumatic events.

Patients say that sometimes, during a trauma, the main personality goes back somewhere inside the body and hides while one of the alter personalities or soul fragments copes with the trauma.

Sometimes patients say that during a trauma the main body of the soul or the main personality goes out of the body and only a soul fragment or alter personality deals with the trauma. The main body of the soul or personality comes back after the trauma is over. In this event, the patient may or may not have the memory of the trauma.

Fragmented soul parts that go out of the body: Fragmented soul parts can leave the body and go to different people or places:

- Fragmented soul parts can go to a family member, an abuser, a friend, an acquaintance, a stranger, or to other victims in a group abuse or ritualistic abuse.
- Fragmented soul parts can remain lost at the place where the trauma took place because they do not know how to go back to the body or do not want to go back to the body.
- Some fragmented soul parts are grabbed by Satan and his demons, who use those soul parts to create various problems for the patients.

Different Types of Alter Personalities

In cases of dissociative identity disorder (multiple personality disorder), I find the following types of alter personalities:

Pure soul parts of the patient: Some alter personalities are different fragmented soul parts of the patient who look exactly as the patient looked at the time of fragmentation during the trauma. They know they were created or born during the trauma, that they are part of the patient, and that the body is theirs.

Pure earthbound spirits: Some alter personalities are spirits of diseased people who did not make their transition to the Light (heaven) and somehow came in the patients when their shields were open due to physical or emotional traumas. They have different names, sometimes different sex, and have different physical and psychophysiological characteristics. They know that they are outside spirits and that the body is not theirs. Sometimes they lie and claim the body is theirs and they are part of the patient.

Pure demon spirits: Some alter personalities claim to be Satan's disciples, and that they are sent there by Satan. Sometimes they also lie and claim they are part of the patient and create problems during the therapy. They are often responsible for self-mutilation and suicidal and homicidal attitudes and behavior.

Pure soul fragment of another living person: Some alter personalities claim to be a part of another living person, who can be a family member, a friend, an abuser, or a stranger. They know they are not a part of the patient and the body is not theirs, but can lie and pretend that they are part of the patient in spite of different identities.

An earthbound spirit with dissociative identity disorder (multiple personality disorder): Sometimes alter personalities in patients turn out to be earthbound spirits who had dissociative identity disorder (multiple personality disorder) while living in their physical bodies. When they joined the patients, not only did they bring their own problems to the patients, but also the problems of all those alter personalities in them. In this case, it becomes a difficult and long process of treatment.

Ivana, a patient with multiple personality disorder had an alter personality, a possessing earthbound spirit whose name was Star. Star claimed to have a multiple personality disorder when living in her physical body. Ivana was in the hospital for treatment, when Star, in the same hospital, committed suicide. After the death of her body, Star's spirit joined Ivana because she liked her.

Treatment was extremely difficult in this case, because we had to work with Star's alter personalities first, before we could release Star from Ivana.

Soul fragment of the patient attached to an earthbound spirit: Some alter personalities are formed by earthbound spirits who are covered by the fragmented soul parts of the patient. For some reason, the earthbound entities forget everything about themselves after they come in and attach to the fragmented soul parts of the patient.

Also, because a part of the patient is attached to them, they have all the memories of the patient's trauma. They think they are part of the patient and the body is theirs in spite of the different name, age, sex, and physical and psychophysiological characteristics.

This explains how one person can have five, ten, twenty, or more personalities, with different names, ages, sex, physical characteristics, and psychophysiological responses, who claim to be part of the patient.

Amanda, a patient with dissociative identity disorder (multiple personality disorder), had an alter personality who was a man called "Mr. Furious." He often came out when anybody bothered Amanda and acted as her protector. In spite of his different sex, he insisted that Amanda's body was his and was a male body. I showed him a mirror and asked him what he saw. He saw his face with a mustache, obviously not Amanda's face. He said he was created when Amanda was five years old and his job was to go after people who hurt Amanda. I asked him to move back to time before he was created and to recall if he had any prior history. With great shock and surprise he recalled the following:

"I heard a little girl crying as I was passing through a house, so I decided to check what was going on. It was Amanda at the age of five. She was lying on the bed and a man was forcing her to play sexual games. She was scared and crying. I could not tolerate it. I tried to pick her up, but could not. I tried to punch the man, but couldn't. I touched her to comfort her and somehow ended up inside her; then I could kick that man through her. A part of Amanda covered me for some reason and I forgot all about myself. How could I fit in this little girl's body? I am a big man."

I asked him to move further back in time and remember what else happened. He recalled that his name was Joe. He was in a fight and was shot. They put his body in an ambulance while his spirit wandered around feeling confused about what happened. As he was walking, he heard Amanda crying, so he went there and ended up inside Amanda.

Amanda's soul part was separated from Joe. Joe was sent to the Light, after some therapy, and Amanda's soul part was cleansed, healed, and integrated with Amanda after the resolution of the trauma. According to Amanda and her other alter personalities, "Mr. Furious" was not there anymore.

A soul fragment of the patient attached to a soul fragment of another living person: Some alter personalities are fragmented soul parts of another living person, which are attached to the fragmented soul part of the patient.

Lina had an alter personality in which a soul part of her was attached to a soul part of a neighbor who was still living and abused her when she was ten years old. He was there to control and scare her and make sure she did not tell anybody. The part of the neighbor was separated and integrated with his own body, and part of Lina was integrated with her after the resolution of her trauma. That alter personality did not exist anymore.

A soul fragment of patient attached to a demon spirit: Some alter personalities are formed when a patient's soul part is attached to a demon entity. These alters are often known as "the angry one," "the evil one," "the monster," "the devil," "the beast," etc. They are often responsible for patients' suicidal, homicidal, self-mutilating, and self-destructive behavior.

Claudia had an alter personality who was called "the beast." All the other alters were afraid of him, because he was mean and evil looking. He was responsible for a lot of cutting and burning and, at times, for homicidal rages.

When I tried to communicate with him, he became very angry and used obscene language. He turned out to be a dark demon entity who had a part of Claudia attached to it. It claimed to make Claudia drink and take drugs and cause her suicidal, homicidal, and self-mutilating behavior.

The demon entity was separated from the fragmented soul part of Claudia and was transformed into the Light and sent to heaven. The fragmented soul part of Claudia was cleansed, healed, and integrated with Claudia after the resolution of her trauma.

After that session, Claudia's behavior improved a great deal and there were no further episodes of suicidal, homicidal, and self-mutilating behavior.

Past life personality: Sometimes the trauma in the current life can reactivate the memories of a past life trauma. This part of the soul consciousness can fragment and become a past life personality that becomes and functions as an alter personality. Sometimes these alter personalities are aware that they are part of the patients' consciousness from a past life. Other times they do not remember. They can have the same appearance as the patient or can look different, as in the past life.

Malinda had an alter personality who claimed to be created when Malinda suffered sexual abuse. The experience reactivated the memory of sexual abuse in a past life that caused that part of the soul to fragment from the main body of the soul. This alter personality held the memory of sexual abuse from that past life. She often came out to cope with sexual abuse in the current life, while the rest of the soul or main personality left the body to return only when the abuse was over. This alter personality had the same appearance as Malinda, at a younger age, but had a different name. She had a connecting cord with the main body of Malinda's soul. After she resolved her trauma from this life and from the past life, that alter personality was cleansed, healed, and then integrated with the main body of Malinda's soul, or the main personality.

Treatment of Multiple Personality Disorder (MPD)

Treatment of multiple personality disorder requires a lot of time, patience, hard work, and determination on the part of the patient and the therapist. Complete healing and integration are possible in a much shorter timespan than in the traditional treatment of multiple personality disorder, by using the following treatment method.

Psychiatric history: Several sessions are spent taking a thorough psychiatric history, making diagnosis, and developing an understanding about the patient and different alter personalities.

Pure earthbound spirits: Locate and identify all the earthbound spirits who do not have an attached soul part of the patient, and release them to heaven. They are not a part of the patient and cannot be integrated with the patient. This process will also free the patient from all the physical, mental, and emotional symptoms that were due to these earthbound spirits.

Pure demon spirits: Locate and identify the demon spirits who do not have any soul part of the patient attached to them. They need to be released to heaven after their transformation into the Light. If there is no time for their transformation and they do not cooperate, they should be lifted out of the patient's body and should be bound into space with the help of the angels of the Light, so they cannot influence the patient or attach to anybody else.

Pure soul parts of another living person: All the foreign soul parts of other living people, who do not have any fragmented soul part of the patient attached, should be located, identified, and returned to their respective owners' bodies with the help of the angels. These soul parts will need some psychotherapy before returning them to their own bodies.

Pure soul parts of the patient: These pure soul parts are alter personalities that resemble the patient at a younger age when the trauma occurred and caused the fragmentation of the patient's soul. We need to process and resolve their traumas and, when appropriate, they should be integrated with the main body of the soul or main personality after cleansing and healing. It is important to integrate them with the main body of the soul or main

553

personality as soon as possible; otherwise the earthbound and demon spirits will manipulate them and take advantage of their vulnerabilities, creating more problems and allowing new spirits to come in.

An earthbound spirit with dissociative identity disorder (multiple personality disorder): This alter personality is an earthbound spirit who also had multiple personality disorder while living in the physical body. In this case, treatment becomes difficult and a long process. Here we have to work with all the alter personalities of the possessing earthbound spirit first, in order to successfully release it from the patient.

Alter personality, where soul part of the patient is attached to an earthbound spirit: This alter personality often insists that it is a part of the patient in spite of a different name, age, sex, color, physical characteristics, and psychophysiological responses. We need to separate the earthbound spirit from the patient's soul part with the help of the angels and release it into heaven after some therapy. We need to work with the soul part or personality of the patient by helping it to recall and resolve the trauma and then integrate it with the main body of the patient's soul or personality after cleansing and healing, when appropriate.

Alter personality, where a patient's soul part is attached to a demon spirit: In this case, the patient's soul part needs to be separated from the demon entity. The demon spirit should be transformed into the Light and then released to heaven.

Then we need to work with the patient's soul part or personality. The soul part is helped by recalling and resolving its trauma. In an appropriate time, it should be integrated with the main body of the patient's soul or personality.

Alter personality, where a patient's soul part is attached to a soul part of another living person: The patient's soul part must be separated from another living person's soul part. We need to send the soul part of the other person back to his or her own body after some psychotherapy and cleansing and healing, with the help of the angels.

Then we need to work with the patient's soul part and resolve its trauma. Then the part needs to be cleansed, healed, and integrated with the patient's main body of the soul or personality when appropriate.

Past life personality: This alter personality is formed when a current life trauma reactivates the memory of a past life trauma, leading to the fragmentation of the part of the soul that holds the memory of that past life trauma. This alter personality may or may not have the name, age, sex, color, and physical characteristic of that past life personality.

The past life and present life traumas need to be recalled, processed, and resolved. Then that past life personality or the soul part needs to be integrated with the main body of the patient's soul after cleansing and healing, in appropriate time.

Retrieve all the lost soul parts: Patient's soul parts that left the body after fragmentation should be retrieved and integrated after resolution of the traumas and cleansing and healing. This is usually achieved with the help of the angels.

Remove and destroy all devices and energy absorbers: This is also achieved with the help of the angels.

Past life regression therapy: Past life regression therapy should be done to locate the source of the current life problems that lead to dissociative identity disorder (multiple personality disorder). Traumas and conflicts from different past lives should be recalled, relived, and resolved. All the fragmented soul parts that were lost during those past lives should be brought back, cleansed, healed, and integrated with the patient. This is done with the help of the angels.

It is extremely important to reintegrate every fragmented soul part, or alter personality, of the patient with the main body of the soul or main personality. Together the patient is stronger than when fragmented. These fragmented soul parts are vulnerable to more manipulation by foreign entities, whether they are demon, earthbound, or fragments of living people, creating more problems for the patient. Fragmentation also creates openings in the energy field, weakening it and allowing more outside spirits to come in, thus making the treatment a never-ending process.

In therapy with dissociative identity disorder (multiple personality disorder) patients, after the initial few sessions, I first locate and release all the outside earthbound and demon spirits and fragmented soul parts of the other living people who are pure. They are not part of the patient and cannot be integrated with the patient. But they do create tremendous problems for the patient, physically, emotionally, mentally, and spiritually, and create a lot of problems during the therapy and unnecessarily prolong the healing.

Then I work with the alter personalities, which are the pure soul parts of the patient. I work with alters where a part of the patient is attached to an outside entity, separate them, release the outside entities, and integrate the patient's part, after cleansing, healing, and resolving its trauma as soon as possible. This is usually done in the same session; otherwise, outside entities will manipulate them and create more problems for them and for the patient. I usually work with two or three alter personalities in one three- to four-hour session, and integrate them beginning with the ones who are creating the most physical, emotional, mental, spiritual, and social problems for the patient.

I strongly feel that multiple personality disorder is a spiritual crisis. A thorough healing is possible, but requires hard work, patience, and a great deal of determination on the part of the patient and the therapist.

Dreams

Throughout the history of mankind, dreams have been considered important, although the understanding and interpretations of dreams differs from culture to culture. In psychiatry, Sigmund Freud put a heavy emphasis on the value of dream interpretation in understanding the patient's emotional state. According to Freud, our repressed emotions manifest in dreams. He stressed that analysis and interpretation of dreams can be key to the understanding of the patient's subconscious mind and patient's problem. In current psychiatry, dream analysis is used by many psychiatrists in treating the psychiatric problems, but dreams are mostly considered symbolic.

Contrary to the popular belief that most dreams are just symbolic, I find that most dreams are very straightforward. Dreams are free of much symbolism, with only a small part to be considered symbolic. I find that there are different sources of dreams:

- Dreams about present life
- Dreams about past lives
- Dreams caused by possessing earthbound entity
- Dreams caused by possessing demon entity
- Dreams caused by demon entity from outside the person
- Telepathic or communication dreams by a living person, by an earthbound entity, by a being of the Light, or by an alien entity
- Dreams about out-of-body experiences
- Prophetic, precognitive, or future dreams
- Symbolic dreams
- Inspirational dreams
- Dreams of a soul fragment

Present Life Dreams

Some of the dreams reported by my patients are connected with the issues and problems of the present life and also may be symbolic.

Nora had many earthbound and dark spirits in her, especially in her eyes, which blocked her vision. She was still able to release the entities by receiving the thoughts of the entities. But the process was slow. After a few sessions she reported having a dream as follows:

"The dream was a mixture of work and people I know and don't know. In the dream my boss told me to find some paper for her.

"As I went to look for it, I saw papers everywhere. There were people around with their shoes and boots scattered all around. I told them they had to pick up all their own stuff and clean it up so I could find what I was hunting for."

In the therapy, we realized that her dream had to do with her current situation. Her boss symbolically was her higher self who wanted her to find the paper, meaning the knowledge. She had trouble in finding the paper (the knowledge) because of all the other papers (problems) and all the people around (the spirits) and their shoes and boots and other stuff (problems of the spirits). In the dream she took charge and told everybody (the spirits) to leave with their stuff (problems) so she can find the paper (the knowledge).

Soon after that dream, she was able to release her possessing spirits faster and was able to see clearly during the sessions. During one session, as she was in the Light (heaven) and looked back into that dream, she realized that in her dream she was actually communicating with the spirits inside her and asking them to leave so she could be clear and find the knowledge she was looking for.

Dreams about Past Lives

A fairly large number of the dreams that my patients report turn out to be past life dreams. They are usually about some type of unresolved traumas and issues from the past lives. The patient's subconscious mind is attempting to resolve them while sleeping. These dreams are often recurrent, sometimes from early childhood. Throughout this book, different examples of past life dreams have been mentioned. Others include the following:

Mili had longstanding headaches, shoulder and neck pain and stiffness, and throat infections and drainage for most of her life. She also told of having recurrent dreams as a child about Indians covered with paint all over their bodies, breaking into her home and kidnapping her. She often woke up feeling scared.

During a session, I asked her to focus on that dream and expand her awareness of it. As she focused on the dream, she recalled the rest of the story.

Mili remembered herself as an eleven-year-old girl in 1732 in North America. Her name was Nora Miller. She lived in a cabin with her parents and a brother. One day Indians with paint all over their bodies came and started to shoot fire arrows. The cabin caught on fire and they killed her brother, father, and mother. They grabbed her, put her on a horse, and took off. On the way they stopped, stripped off her clothes, and raped her one by one and made fun of her. As one Indian was forcing her to have oral sex, she became sick and threw up on him. He was outraged and cut off her tongue. She bled a lot and blood drained down her throat. They took her to their village. She could not eat. She was kicked and beaten by the chief's wife, causing injury to her head and neck. She became sick from the infection of her tongue wound, and as a result died in a few days.

Mili died experiencing pain and drainage in her throat, and feeling anger and hurt, but was unable to express them. The unresolved, unexpressed physical and emotional feelings were carried over to this life. The recurrent dreams were an effort of the subconscious mind to resolve the unresolved traumas and issues during sleep.

After that regression, her headache, neck and shoulder pain, and throat irritation, drainage, and infections were all relieved.

Dreams Due to the Possessing Earthbound Entities

Another large number of the dreams reported by my patients turned out to be the memories of their possessing earthbound entities. It is the possessing spirits who are reliving their traumatic experiences and death while the patient is sleeping and experiencing them in their dreams.

Andy was a forty-year-old man who was normally very polite, conscientious, and honest. He complained of feeling detached, distant, callous, and uncaring for over a period of about two months. It bothered him a great deal. He felt like he was restricted and surrounded by a dark curtain or barrier. He also described having a dream in which he was a mobster, killing people as follows:

"I am standing over five beds (I believe there are five people sleeping in beds) machine-gunning the people. I see the gun recoiling in my hands and I see the people bouncing slightly from the impact of the bullets."

Andy was upset over this dream. He felt that although he never did anything to hurt anybody, he felt at times that he could be a mobster and hurt people.

Under hypnosis, I asked him to focus on the dream and expand his awareness. It turned out that he had a spirit of a mobster who appeared very dark and was surrounded and trapped by a dark demon. This mobster admitted he killed five men with a machine gun while they were sleeping. Later he was killed by another mobster. Andy said that the spirits of the five people who were killed were in the mobster, possessing him because they were angry with him for killing them. They all admitted giving Andy feelings of being cold-hearted, callous, detached, and uncaring. All of them were released to the Light. Afterward, Andy felt free of those feelings and that dream.

Dreams Caused by Possessing Demon Entities

Some of the dreams are caused by the possessing demon entities. Later, during a session releasing entities from inside these patients, these demons often confirm and brag about giving the patients dreams and nightmares. Interestingly, after releasing those entities, the patients do not have those dreams and nightmares.

Shane had recurring dreams and nightmares about evil-looking creatures chasing and tormenting him most of his life. Later during treatment, under hypnosis, Shane saw inside him many evil-looking, dark beings who looked just like the ones in his dreams; they bragged about giving Shane nightmares and took a great deal of pleasure in doing it. After releasing those demon entities, Shane did not have these dreams and nightmares anymore.

Dreams Caused by Outside Demon Entities

Many people, especially children, report seeing and dreaming about evil, black, or scary-looking figures. Their reports are often dismissed as simple imagination because these dreams are hard to prove.

Brandy had a dream about a big black, evil-looking being. She woke up scared and saw that being standing at the door. The next morning her children talked about having a dream about the same evil-looking dark entity and when they woke up they saw it standing in their room.

Later, under hypnosis, Brandy saw inside her the same being, who admitted going from room to room in the house, giving everybody nightmares. It then came inside Brandy when her shield was open.

Stella had a dream about a large black being sitting on her chest. She felt as though she were frozen and had a difficult time breathing. She wanted to scream but couldn't. She had an inner feeling that it was Satan. She found herself screaming in her mind, "Michael! Gabriel! Please help me!" She felt a Light being come and push that dark being away from her. This dream was very real and vivid for Stella; she had no doubt that she was really attacked by Satan and was helped by the Light beings as a result of her request.

Dreams about Out-of-Body Experiences

Many of my patients described having dreams about being out of their bodies and traveling to different places all over the world, to other planets, and even to heaven. In these cases the inner self or soul travels out of the body, but remains connected to the body with a silver cord. According to my patient reports, we all travel out of the body during sleep, but most of the time we do not remember doing so. Patients also report that many of us even go to heaven while sleeping, where we meet with others who are on the earth and in heaven, to plan for future events in this life and also plan for future lives.

Jeff had had a recurrent dream since he was a kid. He described the dream and that place:

"There is grass and low, tended shrubs in front of the temple steps, forming a wide, bordered path of grass up to the dozen or so wide, white steps leading up to the pillared, outward-curving entrance to the temple. As I go to the top of the steps, there is a porch in front of the pillars. Through the pillars, there is a doorway, high with a curved top, opening on a long, high-ceilinged room; immediately in front of the entrance is a wide staircase going down to another room. My impression is that this lower chamber is holy for spiritual purposes. It has a secluded, protected feeling, and I go there once in a while.

"There is a bright hall with a high, vaulted ceiling, which has the feeling of knowledge and wisdom. The height of the ceiling is great, much greater than it appears from the outside, and the hall is much wider and longer than it seems. The walls of the hall are embedded with drawers and lined with shelves with all the knowledge of the universe within. You can float up, down, and sideways to find what you need. Sometimes I know where to look; sometimes there are guides to help. It is very bright in this hall. The Light comes from above the walls. If you go up far enough, you are on a limitless plane of Light, where there is even more knowledge."

During one session, after the death of his body in a past life regression, he went to a place of knowledge in heaven called the akashic plane. He described seeing a white, marble, dome-shaped temple type of building. From heaven, he realized that during those recurrent dreams, he was having out-of-body experiences (OBE) during his sleep, as he was traveling to this white, marble, dome-shaped temple at the akashic plane in heaven.

Telepathic or Communication Dreams

In telepathic dreams, either a living person, an earthbound entity, a being from another planet, or a being of the Light is trying to communicate, to give a message or information to the dreamer.

Telepathic or Communication Dream by a Living Person

Angelo said that at the age of sixteen he was sleeping at his brother's home, about sixty miles from his parents' home. They were sleeping in separate rooms at opposite ends of the house. In sleep they both dreamed about their father calling them. They both woke up and went to the door, thinking that maybe their father had decided to come to visit the brother, but there was no one at the door.

That night Angelo's sister also dreamed about their father being in a coffin.

A person who worked for them also dreamed that night about Angelo's father, who was trying to nail the boards on the windows and the doors, as if to make a coffin. Even their priest dreamed about Angelo's father, who in the dream was asking for some kind of help.

The next day, Angelo's father choked on food and died. It seemed as though his father had a premonition of his death and was desperately trying to communicate with different people in dreams and ask for help.

Telepathic or Communication Dream by an Earthbound Entity

Nina had a friend whose husband, Tim, died suddenly. A few days later she had a dream about him that she described:

"A few days later, Tim visited me in my dreams. It was a very, very real experience. He asked me to give his wife a message. He said he had been trying to reach her through her mother, but he could not get through to her. He asked me to tell her that he was with her the other night. When we were done visiting, he walked out my kitchen door and I said goodbye and closed the door. I immediately woke up. I knew this was not a dream, it was a real experience. I agonized over whether I should tell my friend or not. I was afraid I would upset my friend. But the feeling would not leave me and I knew I had to tell her. I phoned and told her. Tim's wife told me that the other day she had been driving her car and crying and asking over and over, why? Why did it have to happen? She even had to pull off the road. As she was sitting there, the door flew open, by itself, and, as she shut it, a great peace came over her. This confirmed that she knew he was with her."

Telepathic or Communication Dream by a Being from Another Planet

Daisy had dreams about contacts with beings of another planet who were very friendly, loving, and comforting to her. She believed she had known them before and was not afraid of them. During these dreams, these beings gave her a lot of spiritual knowledge.

She also remembered having UFO contacts two or three times, when she was taken to a spacecraft for advanced spiritual preaching by shadowy figures. She again had a strange feeling that she had known them before.

During a session, I asked her to move back in time, when she knew those beings. She regressed to a life thousands of years ago on another planet, where she looked like those beings and she and those beings planned to do some work together at this time on the earth to help humanity. She was supposed to be their contact on the earth.

Telepathic or Communication Dreams by a Light Being

Grace was going to have surgery for cancer of the uterus. That night she had a dream in which she saw Jesus, who told her that she would be all right and that he had special plans for her in the future.

Prophetic, Warning, or Future Dreams

Prophetic dreams are dreams in which the future events are foretold or foreseen. They can also be warnings about future events.

Frank had recurrent dreams about war and missiles being fired everywhere. He had a strong feeling that it was going to happen within months. He started to dream about it several months before the invasion of Kuwait by Iraq.

Gene had a recurrent dream about having a collision with a Chevrolet. At times he even had visions of the accident while he was wide awake.

One day, as he was driving home from the airport, cars ahead of him suddenly stopped, crashing into each other. He applied the brake as hard as he could and was able to avoid hitting the car ahead of him. But then all of a sudden he felt another car hit his car from behind. As he looked in his rearview mirror, it was exactly the same Chevrolet he had seen in his dreams and visions.

Inspirational Dreams

Ann, from time to time, heard beautiful music in her soul in her dreams, but was frustrated after waking up, because she could not hold the music long enough to write it down. During the treatment, she recalled that her block came from several past lives. After resolving those problems, she was able to write the music down after waking up. She also realized that she got the inspiration to write the music from the Light (heaven), through her soul during her dreams. Sometimes when she played the music on the piano in public, people would come to her and say, "It seems as if you play the music from your soul."

Symbolic Dreams

There are some dreams that are symbolic and require an interpretation. Interestingly, working with patients, I am finding that these dreams were sometimes given from heaven and their meanings were confirmed with a Light being later on, during a session.

Cindy had a dream about being in a classroom to take a test. There were thousands of other people there to take the test. After she received the test booklet, she glanced through it and got up and left the classroom without even attempting to take the test. She saw that almost everybody in the room also left after her, with the exception of one or two.

Later, during a session, one of her guides from heaven said it was a warning for Cindy that she is here to take a test in the classroom of earth. There are many on earth here who are taking the test, too. But their test completely depends on Cindy. If Cindy does not take her test, she will deprive many on earth from taking the test because their work depends on Cindy's work.

Joe was a hypnotherapist who was doing spirit releasement work, including releasing demon entities. Although he had total faith in God (heaven) and Light beings for their help during the work and was not afraid of doing this work, he would occasionally wonder about it. One night he had a dream that he described as follows:

"I was in an arena with a bull. There were thousands of people around who seemed to be enjoying themselves. The bull was charging at me and attacking me. I felt sure that I was going to die and I covered my face with my hands. To my surprise, nothing happened, I was alive and O.K. The bull kept charging and attacking me, again and again but it couldn't even touch me."

Later, during a session, one of his guides from heaven said the dream was given to him to relieve him from concerns of any harm coming to him through this work. The bull in the dream represented Satan, while people in the arena represented the evil people working for Satan. The guide said that although Satan, his demons, and evil people under their influence will try to attack him and harm him, as long as he stays in the Light and follows the heavenly guidance, no harm will come to him.

Dreams of a Soul Fragment or Inner Child

Carla, a thirty-five-year-old female, had a recurrent dream about being sexually abused by somebody. In the dream she could not see the face of that person. Carla would often wake up crying, almost like a little girl. She did not have any memories of any type of sexual abuse.

During a session, as she scanned her body, she found a fragmented soul part of her, who resembled her when she was six years old. This little Carla was scared and did not trust grownups because a grownup person, a next-door neighbor, hurt her. She admitted that it was little Carla who was remembering her abuse and pain and crying when grownup Carla was sleeping.

That six-year-old Carla, the soul fragment, was cleansed, healed, and integrated with grownup Carla after the resolution of her trauma. Afterward Carla did not have that dream.

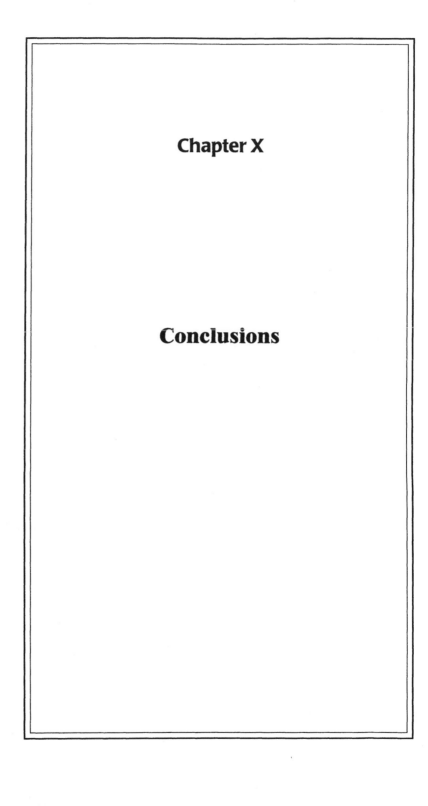

Chapter X

Conclusions

Conclusions

My Research and Conclusions

After treating hundreds of patients with spirit releasement, soul integration, and past life regression therapies over a period of several years, I became aware of certain patterns. I realized that regardless of my patients' backgrounds and their presenting symptoms, the reasons for their problems were essentially the same; the approach to treatment was also identical. Consequently, I decided to examine my cases systematically.

Method: I took the charts of one hundred patients whom I treated with spirit releasement, soul integration, and/or past life regression therapy. In each case I separated the presenting or primary symptoms from the secondary symptoms, and noted the tertiary symptoms during the treatment.

Presenting or primary symptoms: These are the symptoms that brought the patients to my office for the treatment. Patients report these symptoms during the first session; they are usually acute symptoms.

Secondary symptoms: These are the symptoms that patients have had for a long time, but were not the reasons for seeking treatment. They are usually chronic symptoms.

Tertiary symptoms: These are new symptoms that come up during the treatment.

Example

Fay, during the first session, while I was taking a psychiatric history, said that she had been experiencing severe depression for six months. She reported having insomnia, poor appetite, chronic fatigue, lack of motivation, and poor concentration and

570

memory. She had been having periodic suicidal thoughts and panic attacks for several months. She had not been able to function properly day to day at home or at work. These were her presenting, acute symptoms for which she was seeking treatment.

She said that she had been a perfectionist all her life, but now could not do anything right. She also had a fear of water and of high places for a long time, but she could live with those fears by avoiding high places and water. She also reported chronic arthritis and allergies to dust and pollen since childhood. These were her secondary, chronic symptoms, and she had been able to deal with them.

During the treatment, Fay developed headachese due to an earthbound entity who surfaced after we released the first layer of entities. This was identified as a tertiary symptom.

When patients come to me for treatment, I inform them about the various treatment methods. If they are willing, I use the above treatments. Over the years I came to realize how common spirit attachment and soul fragmentation is, and how they can create emotional, mental, physical, and relationship problems. I also realized that the problems caused by outside spirits are really not the patients' problems. As a result, I first do the spirit releasement session with my patients. Then, after releasing all the outside entities and their associated symptoms, the symptoms left are the patients' own symptoms. It is like doing differential diagnostic tests to find out where the symptoms are coming from and doing the treatment at the same time.

Preparation of Different Tables

I separated the psychological and physical symptoms in both the primary and secondary symptom categories for all one hundred patients and prepared the following tables:

- Presenting or primary psychological symptoms
- Secondary psychological symptoms
- Presenting or primary physical symptoms
- Secondary physical symptoms

- Earthbound entities
- Demon entities
- Soul fragments
- Results of spirit releasement and soul integration treatment
- Results of past life regression therapy

I marked all the psychological and physical symptoms for the hundred patients in the primary and secondary symptom tables.

Treatment performed and clinical information were marked in the tables of earthbound entities, demon entities, and soul fragments.

The total number of primary and secondary symptoms treated with spirit releasement and soul integration treatment, the number of sessions, and the results were marked in the table of results of spirit releasement and soul integration therapy. I marked the same information in the table of results of past life regression therapy.

I then totaled all the numbers in each category. The conclusions that emerged from these tables were surprising, even for me. Every time I think about it, I shake my head in disbelief.

Conclusions from the Table of Presenting or Primary Psychological Symptoms

The table of presenting or primary psychological symptoms, which were the main reasons why patients came for the treatment, showed the following information.

Depression and its associated symptoms (94 patients): These were the most common primary psychological symptoms reported:

94 patients had depression.
91 patients had sleep disorders.
91 patients had chronic fatigue.
90 patients had poor concentration and memory.
43 patients had suicidal preoccupation.

Generalized anxiety disorder (87 patients): This was the second most common psychological symptom reported for which patients were seeking psychiatric treatment. These symptoms included nervousness, restlessness, irritability, and agitation.

Panic attacks (33 patients): This was the third most common symptom reported. These symptoms are often very resistant to traditional psychotherapy and medications.

Psychotic symptoms: These were the fourth most common problem reported:

24 patients had auditory hallucination.
17 patients had voices from inside the head.
7 patients had voices from outside.
9 patients had visual hallucinations.
9 patients had paranoia.
9 patients had visions of possessing entities.
10 patients had feelings of being possessed.

Spiritual or psychic symptoms: These are similar to the psychotic symptoms above, but the understanding of the reasons for them is different. In psychiatry, patients presenting these symptoms are thought to be imagining things or have lost reality. From a spiritual and psychic point of view, it can be said that most of these patients are clairvoyant, clairaudient, and clairsensient, and can see, hear, and sense real spirits other people do not beyond their five physical senses.

Symptoms of manic depression: These were the fifth most common of the symptoms reported.

18 patients had racing thoughts.
11 patients had mood swings.

Other symptoms:

14 patients had fears and phobias.
14 patients had nightmares.
11 patients had perfectionism.
10 patients had violent behavior.

9 patients had obsessive-compulsive personality.

9 patients had marital problems.

7 patients had alcoholism.

5 patients had behavioral problems.

5 patients had psychogenic amnesia.

3 patients had sexual disorders.

3 patients had bulimia.

2 patients had tics and twitches.

Table of Secondary Psychological Symptoms

In the list of secondary psychological symptoms, the major clusters and minor clusters were quite different from primary psychological symptoms.

Fears and phobias (73 patients): These were the most common psychological symptoms reported in the category of secondary symptoms. In the primary symptoms category, only 14 patients reported fears and phobias.

Psychotic symptoms or spiritual/psychic symptoms: These were the second most commonly reported symptoms. Many of these patients did not have acute symptoms of psychosis. They normally and naturally were seeing, hearing, and sensing the spirits.

21 patients had auditory hallucinations.

20 patients had visual hallucination.

15 patients had voices from outside the head.

14 patients had voices from inside the head.

12 patients had feelings of being possessed.

7 patients had tactile hallucination.

3 patients had imaginary playmates.

2 patients had paranoia.

Sexual disorders: These were the third most common symptoms reported.

14 patients reported having sexual disorders.

13 patients had marital problems.

Personality Disorders:

12 patients had perfectionism.
7 patients had obsessive-compulsive behavior.

Other Symptoms: These were reported by only a few patients.

6 patients had alcoholism.
4 patients had eating disorders.
3 patients had behavior disorders.
3 patients were using drugs.
2 patients had suicidal thoughts.
2 patients had panic attacks.
2 patient had depression.
1 patient had hyperactive disorder.
1 patient had stuttering.
1 patient had tics.
1 patient had bulimia.

Dreams

34 patients had dreams and visions of possessing spirits.
22 patients had nightmares.
20 patients had dreams of past lives.
11 patients had dreams of encounters with UFOs.
10 patients had out-of-body experiences during physical
   and emotional trauma.
9 patients had spiritual dreams.
7 patients had dreams of the future.
5 patients had out-of-body experiences during surgery.

Psychic Experiences

20 patients had psychic experiences.

Conclusions Related to Psychological Symptoms

As we look at the presenting or primary psychological symptoms, we can definitely say that almost all these patients had severe symptoms.

Depression and its associated symptoms, generalized anxiety disorder, panic attacks, psychotic symptoms, and symptoms of manic depression were the most commonly reported symptoms in the primary psychological category. They were far fewer in the secondary symptoms category.

Fears and phobias (73) were most commonly reported in secondary psychological symptoms, while only 14 patients reported fears and phobias as primary psychological symptoms.

Psychotic symptoms (or spiritual/psychic symptoms) were reported slightly more often by patients in the secondary psychological symptoms than in primary psychological symptoms.

The rest of the psychological symptoms were reported by only a few patients in both primary and secondary symptom categories.

Table of Presenting or Primary Physical Symptoms

This table showed the following:

17 patients had musculoskeletal symptoms.
    12 patients had headache.
    4 patients had arthritis.
    3 patients had aches and pain.
    3 patients had back and neck pain.
    1 patient had fibromyositis.
  8 patients had GI symptoms.
Other symptoms were reported by fewer patients.

Table of Secondary Physical Symptoms

This table showed

56 patients had musculoskeletal symptoms.
    40 patients had headaches.

31 patients had back and neck pain.

26 patients had aches and pain.

10 patients had arthritis.

32 patients had allergies.

26 patients had a weight problem.

25 patients had PMS.

19 patients had GI symptoms.

17 patients had skin condition.

17 patients had sinus problems.

13 patients had neurological symptoms.

12 patients had ear symptoms.

8 patients had eye symptoms.

4 patients had hot flashes.

2 patients had nose symptoms.

2 patients had asthma.

Conclusions Related to Physical Symptoms

When we look at the primary physical symptoms category, we can see that very few physical symptoms were reported by patients. Only 17 patients reported musculoskeletal symptoms and 8 patients reported gastrointestinal symptoms. The rest of the symptoms were reported by only one or two or no patients.

In contrast, in the secondary physical symptoms category many patients reported having physical symptoms. Again, the most commonly reported symptoms were musculoskeletal symptoms by 56 patients, then allergies by 32 patients, obesity by 26 patients, PMS by 25 patients, GI symptoms by 19 patients, skin conditions by 17 patients, sinus problems by 17 patients, neurological symptoms by 13 patients, ear symptoms by 12 patients, and the rest by only a few patients.

Headache was the most commonly reported symptom in both primary and secondary categories.

Most of these symptoms fall in the category of musculoskeletal symptoms, psychosomatic symptoms, and immune system disorders.

Table of Earthbound Entities

The following information came from the table of earthbound entities:

92 patients had earthbound spirits in them.

80 patients had more than one earthbound spirit.

12 patients had one earthbound spirit.

50 patients had spirits of their relatives with them (28 had spirits of their parents, 39 had other relatives, e.g., grandparents, uncles, aunts, siblings, children, and spouses).

22 patients had spirits of people they knew other than their relatives (such as friends and coworkers or other acquaintances).

77 patients had spirits of strangers within them.

16 patients had spirits of miscarried, aborted, or stillborn fetuses.

46 patients had human spirits who claimed to be working for Satan.

70 patients had human spirits who had been with my patients for a long time, while 35 patients had earthbound spirits who had joined my patients recently.

34 patients had human spirits who said that they had past life connections with my patients and that they had known my patients from one or many past lives and possessed them in one or more lifetimes.

66 patients had earthbound spirits who had joined them during childhood and teenage years, while 63 reported they had earthbound spirits who had joined them in adulthood.

81 patients attributed their physical and emotional symptoms to the possessing earthbound spirits.

14 patients had a past life regression that turned out to be the memories of possessing spirits and not the patients' past life.

Table of Demon Entities

The following information came from the table of demon entities:

77 patients reported having demon entities within them

71 patients reported to have more than one demon entity with them.

6 patients had one demon entity.

68 patients reported that the demon entities in them were present for a long time, while 23 patients reported that the demon entities joined them recently.

13 patients reported having demon entities who followed and attached to them in many lifetimes.

68 patients reported that their demon entities had been attached to them since childhood and teenaged years, 3 patients claimed that the demon entity attached to them while in the womb, while one reported getting an entity at birth.

58 patients reported that their demon entities attached during adulthood.

73 patients reported that their demon entities had the general purpose of creating problems and causing confusion for the patient.

26 patients reported that the demon entities in them claim to have a specific purpose, such as blocking the patients from the Light, stopping them from achieving their goals, or causing specific physical and emotional symptoms.

12 patients reported that the demon entities in them had a human soul trapped inside them.

Table of Soul Fragments

The following information came from the table of soul fragments:

59 patients reported soul fragmentation.

45 patients reported having more than one soul fragment, while 14 patients found only one soul fragment.

47 patients reported that the fragmented parts of their soul stayed in their body. Among these 47 were pure and 3 fragmented parts were holding on or attached to earthbound entities, while 8 of them were holding on to demon entities and 11 of them were trapped inside a demon entity.

24 patients reported that their fragmented soul parts left their bodies. Of these, 19 reported that their soul parts went to a family member, 11 patients reported that their soul parts went to an acquaintance, 2 patients' soul parts went to strangers, 5 patients' soul parts were just wandering around, and 12 patients' soul parts were with demons.

35 patients reported that they have foreign soul fragments of other living people. In 29 patients, these came from family members and in 17 patients they came from acquaintances.

4 patients reported mutually sharing soul parts with loved ones.

Conclusions of Tables of Earthbound Entities, Demon Entities, and Soul Fragments

As I reviewed the tables of the earthbound entities, demon entities, and soul fragments, I realized that some of the specific data presented here is much lower than it should be for several reasons.

- Because of the time factor, I did not always ask all the specific questions in detail to each entity inside my patients.
- Asking specific questions to a spirit is important to release the spirits faster; otherwise, spirits will not leave easily. But it is not necessary with each and every entity.
- Some patients have so many entities with them that it is not possible to ask each question to every one of them.
- During a session, achieving freedom from the symptoms is the primary goal; achieving thorough information is only the secondary goal.

Treatment Tables and Method of Marking the Treatment Results

In the spirit releasement therapy tables, I have included releasing earthbound, demon, and other spirits, and also locating, treating, and integrating soul fragments that belonged to patients, as well as foreign soul fragments of other living people, because they are all interconnected.

Although treating and integrating the soul fragments is an important part of the treatment, it is hard to evaluate its specific effects and the results of the treatment. So I included the results of spirit releasement and soul integration together in the spirit releasement category.

I also marked the results of how many primary and secondary symptoms were treated with spirit releasement and/or with past life regression treatment by their number to show the results accurately.

Many patients, after their presenting symptoms were relieved, were not keen on working on all the secondary symptoms. Even though they may have had the symptoms for a long time, they were not causing any severe discomfort and concern, that they could not cope with.

So the results were marked specifically as to how many of the symptoms were treated in both primary and secondary symptom categories, and how much improvement occurred.

In the number of treatment sessions, I included the number of actual hypnotherapy sessions only, excluding the history-intake sessions and other talk therapy sessions.

Spirit Releasement Therapy Tables

The table of spirit releasement therapy revealed the following information:

Average number of spirit releasement sessions done on each patient was 3.

Average number of primary symptoms treated with spirit releasement session was 4.

Average number of secondary symptoms treated with spirit releasement was 3.

Average percentage of cure of treated primary symptoms was 90%.

Average percentage of cure of treated secondary symptoms was 94%.

Past Life Regression Therapy Table

The table of past life therapy showed the following information:

Average number of symptoms treated with past life regression therapy was 2.

Average percentage of improvement with past life regressions was 80%. (The reason for these comparatively lower percentages is that patients did not stay long enough in treatment to finish it.)

Average improvement of all the treated symptoms with all the treatment modalities was 86%.

Conclusion

The most dramatic conclusion that emerged from the tables and from my experience of these treatments is that about 80% of the primary symptoms and about 30% of the secondary symptoms were caused by possessing spirits and soul fragmentation. These were relieved in just a few sessions, in most cases, sometimes in only one session.

The rest of the symptoms, which amounted to about 20% of primary symptoms and 70% of secondary symptoms, came from past lives. Even those problems that came from current life traumas had their roots in past lives.

Psychotic symptoms: Another overwhelming conclusion that comes from the tables and my experience is that most of the psychotic symptoms, such as hearing voices or seeing people or other beings that others cannot, can also be due to real spirits and not just their imagination. Demons in hell can also use patients' soul parts that are in their possession to send visions and paranoid thoughts to the patients through the connecting cords between the soul parts and the patients' soul, and patients accept them as their own.

These patients are usually clairvoyant, clairaudient, and clairsensient, and are really seeing, hearing, and feeling these spirits, but do not understand and become overwhelmed and confused. Since most of us do not see or hear beyond our five physical senses, we tend to think that they are imagining and have lost reality.

Not every person who has these gifts becomes psychotic. There are many good psychics with these gifts who understand and use them wisely. But many psychics are open for spirit entry because the boundaries of their energy fields are porous.

Personality disorders: The tables and my experience with patients also show that many personality disorders, such as obsessive-compulsive personality, perfectionism, passive-aggressive personality and other personality disorders, which are often included in the secondary-symptom category, originate in past lives. In only a small percentage of cases are they due to the attached spirits.

Physical symptoms: About 70% of the physical symptoms, which are commonly reported as secondary symptoms, come from past lives and only 30% of the physical symptoms are due to the attached entities. These symptoms are usually the musculoskeletal symptoms, psychosomatic symptoms, and immune disorders.

Looking over all the data, no matter from which angle, I see plainly that the majority of symptoms with which people struggle are caused by attachment of earthbound and demon entities, soul fragmentation and soul loss, and current and past life traumas. The data supports the case for introducing spirit releasement therapy, past life regression therapy, and soul integration therapy as extremely effective forms of treatment with patients who suffer from a variety of acute and chronic mental and physical ailments. Relief is quicker, cost is lower, and healing is complete.

Difficulties During the Treatment

During these therapies, success or failure of the treatment depends on the patients, whether they can recall the information from their subconscious minds or not and whether they can trust what is emerging from their subconscious minds. The psychiatrist or hypnotherapist acts only as a guide who helps the patients in dealing with what is surfacing from their subconscious minds. Although most of the time this approach in the treatment consistently brings dramatic results, as reported throughout this book, sometimes patients do not succeed in therapy. At times, they end up leaving the therapy before their healing is complete in spite of the improvement in their symptoms. Over the years, working with hundreds of patients, I found several reasons for their leaving:

Fear and confusion of possessing spirits (entities): When I plan to do spirit releasement, I frequently explain during the session immediately before about the therapy and what to expect. There have been times that the next session came, but the patients didn't. What happened?

As the patients listened to my explanation about earthbound and demon entities and their treatment, so did their entities. Hearing my plans, the entities became anxious and fearful, and the patients felt the effects. When the entities became anxious, they began to feel all the physical and emotional symptoms that they had prior to their own deaths. The patients, in turn, felt the symptoms of the possessing entities, such as anxiety, panic attacks, headaches, dizziness, nausea, vomiting, diarrhea, aches and pains, etc. The entities would also talk the patients out of coming for their treatment. Consequently, they would call and cancel or "forget" the appointment or develop any number of other complications that would prevent them from keeping the appointment. These symptoms can also develop in any session; it requires a great deal of discipline and determination on the part of the patients to continue the treatment and not allow the possessing spirits to control their minds and bodies.

Spirits blocking the eyes and brain: Often entities block patients' eyes and brains, preventing them from seeing and receiving the information we are seeking. At these times we are stuck. Even when I ask a question and the patients receive the information from the entities, such as the entity's name, age, etc., patients sometimes fail to trust the information, believing they are somehow making it up. This failure to trust creates a total block to the progress of treatment. If the patients keep an open mind, allow the information to come from their subconscious minds and trust it, we can succeed in spite of their visual block.

Patient's soul parts trapped in a demon: Sometimes the dark demon spirits have a soul part of the patient inside them. In this case, the angels cannot lift out the demon spirits. Because God gives us free will, if any part of the patient is touching or holding on to or trapped inside the demon, then the angels cannot lift them out. It becomes a difficult process to free the fragmented soul parts of the patient (little ones) from the demons. Sometimes these demons block the hearing of these little ones and the therapy becomes difficult with them, and in turn with the patient. Some demons have many, many soul parts of the patient trapped inside them. In these cases, it becomes a seemingly never-ending process and sometimes patients get discouraged and quit the therapy.

Infestation by multiple spirits (entities): It is rare that all the spirits can be released in one session. Almost everybody has multiple spirits. Even if we succeed in releasing several spirits in the first session, there can be others, left behind, who begin to feel anxious, frightened, and ill, and patients in turn begin to have these feelings. When they still feel sick due to the remaining entities, patients think the session has failed and they do not follow through the treatment.

Layering of spirits (entities): Another problem arises when spirits are packed in many layers, one on top of the others. This situation is not uncommon. What happens is that as entities are released from the top layer and their symptoms leave the patients, new entities from the next layer surface, bringing their own set of new symptoms. Patients then believe the therapy is not working and is making them more sick, when the fact is that these entities and their problems were already with the patients and needed to be released. But patients become discouraged and quit.

Manipulation by possessing and outside spirits (entities): Sometimes both inside and outside spirits influence patients during therapy, giving them negative thoughts and feelings about therapy and the therapist, causing them to believe the whole therapy is "hocus pocus" and not to be trusted. The entities work hard to manipulate patients and cause them to stop the treatment. They do not want to lose their hold on the patients and do not want them to get better and achieve their spiritual goals.

Influence later in therapy: Influence and interference are not only common early on in therapy, but are also common well into therapy with those patients who have learned about dark influence, but fail to recognize it when they encounter it. Therapy carries a by-product of education about God, Satan, and angels, both dark and Light. Satan is very deceiving, as are his demons. Sometimes even late in therapy, their influence invades and interferes with the process, and patients fail to recognize the signs: sudden interference with appointments, feeling sleepy and tired during the session, or having new physical or emotional symptoms and other reasons to slow the therapy and cause a breakdown in communication between the patient and the therapist.

I can almost always catch the influence, but the patients need to learn to catch it and ask the angels of the Light to remove it. Otherwise, much time in therapy is lost in dealing with unnecessary influences.

The process of spirit releasement sometimes seems to be an endless process, and it becomes discouraging for the patient and therapist. For spirit releasement to succeed, patience, discipline, and commitment must be shared between patient and therapist. Patients have to understand that the recurrence of symptoms is not due to failure of the therapy, but due to another layer of entities surfacing to magnify their symptoms—or any of a number of reasons. Total freedom from these parasitic entities is possible, but it requires mutual commitment, patience, and discipline.

Influences through the missing soul parts: Demons can insert new earthbound and demon entities, devices, and energy absorbers and negative thoughts, visions, attitudes, and behaviors inside the patients, through their missing soul parts and their connecting cords that are in possession of Satan and his demons. As a result, it is crucial to bring all those soul parts back and integrate them with patients.

New spirits and devices being pushed into the patients from other dimensions: It is done through certain points between different dimensions of similar vibrations, in spite of all the shields being in place and intact. They can create new symptoms for the patients. Angels should be requested to stay on guard at those points in this dimension and in all the other dimensions.

Past life problems: Sometimes new symptoms may arise from past life problems that surface when the overburden of the spirits is cleared up. Then the patients become aware of symptoms that are coming from past lives. The symptoms were already there, but were buried under the spirit-caused problems that needed to be resolved. To do the complete healing of the patient, these past life traumas and related problems must also be resolved and healed.

Symptoms coming from multiple past lives: Sometimes patients find multiple past lives responsible for each symptom, like in the case of Jerry in chapter 8, a patient of ulcerative colitis who had to recall traumas from more than twenty lifetimes to resolve and heal his ulcerative colitis. Although over the years I have learned many shortcuts and faster ways to heal, with some patients it still takes a long time for them to clearly understand the reasons for their problems, learn the lessons, and change their ways. Sometimes patients are not willing to spend the time needed to complete the healing and end up leaving the therapy.

Fear of finding negative lives: Sometimes patients have a fear of finding past lives when they did wrong things and hurt other people. As a result, they block those lives and cannot recall them. If somebody has such negative past lives, they are already creating a problem in their current life, whether people are aware of it or not. Through regression therapy, they can recall and resolve the physical, emotional, and mental problems coming from those negative lives and become free of them.

According to the reports of my hypnotized patients, in heaven, before entering this life, we not only plan positive and good lives, but we also plan negative lives to resolve the problems from other lives, learn the lessons we need to learn, and grow spiritually.

Soul parts lost during past life traumas: My patients report that current and past life traumas and problems create holes and weaknesses in our souls due to soul fragmentation and soul loss, which create openings in us for spirits to come in. Unless these past life problems are resolved by past life regression therapy and the holes and weaknesses are healed by retrieving and integrating all the lost soul parts, patients will continue to be influenced by the entities. Treatment will become a never-ending process and complete and thorough healing will not be possible.

It is extremely important to heal those past life problems to keep the spirits away and to have a thorough, complete, and permanent healing. This requires continued treatment. Unfortunately, many patients do not stay long enough in treatment to complete the healing needed because they feel free of their acute presenting and some secondary symptoms in just a few sessions.

Fear of becoming a psychic: During the therapy, when the possessing spirits are released session by session, then the patients are able to get in touch with their soul knowledge and become more intuitive and psychic. Some patients become afraid and end up leaving the therapy.

Patients who remain in therapy in spite of their fears recall having past lives when they were psychic and had knowledge that others did not. As a result, they were declared witches and evil, and were ultimately tortured and killed. As they were dying, they promised themselves they would never be psychic and would not have knowledge that others do not. Those fears and promises were brought back with their souls in the current life. After recalling and resolving those fears with regression therapy, they were comfortable with becoming more intuitive and receiving more soul knowledge.

Fear of seeing and communicating with angels and other spirits: Some patients are afraid of the idea of seeing and communicating with spirits, even when they are angels and other heavenly beings. Their fears open them for dark influences, which create interference and confusion during the therapy. Sometimes patients get discouraged and end up leaving the therapy.

Those who stay in therapy in spite of their fears find the source of their problems in one or more past lives, when they were clairvoyant and clairaudient and were able to see and hear the spirits that others could not. As a result, people made fun of them, declared them crazy, and sometimes tortured and killed them. During their death, they promised never to see or hear the spirits again. Those fears and promises were brought back with their souls to their current life and were creating problems during the therapy. After recalling and resolving those fears and promises with past life regression therapy, these patients were able to do the sessions and were comfortable with seeing and communicating with the spirits.

Religious beliefs: Sometimes religious beliefs can pose problems for patients. Many people do not believe in reincarnation and past lives because of their religious doctrine, and the treatment creates a conflict for them. They feel guilty about trying past life regression and sometimes quit therapy. Also, if patients equate goodness with wholeness and possession with sin, as many do, they become confused and frightened about the prospect of

589

demon possession. Many patients believe "If I have Christ within, I cannot have demons," and as a result feel that they are "protected" and are immune to possession by demon spirits. The source of this confusion is obvious and yet, time and time again, my most devout Christian patients have told me under hypnosis of having demons within themselves, in spite of their beliefs.

Some patients feel that if they have dark entities inside, they must be sinners. This is not true. It is important to note that all souls are as important to Satan as they are to God. Satan wants every soul he can get. I have learned through my patients that people with special God-given purposes, such as ministers, prophets, healers, and others, are more targeted and attacked by Satan and his demons. It is as though they are a more attractive "prize" for Satan to capture.

Inadequate spirituality: This phrase refers to an underdeveloped or undermined spirituality, a weakness of faith in one's spiritual nature and God. When this occurs, patients are easily put off by their experiences under hypnosis, or they fail to trust the information they receive. As a result, in spite of releasing spirits session after session, patients continue to be influenced by outside entities. They do not really believe or cannot accept what they have recalled and what they have experienced. They quit the therapy and continue to be infested and afflicted by the entities.

To the readers, it may seem like all of what is mentioned above is happening because of the treatment. But it is not true. These earthbound entities, demon entities, and influences through devices and energy absorbers affect all human beings whether they are in treatment or not, with symptoms that they usually accept as their own.

When patients remain long enough in treatment, a complete and thorough healing of all the psychological and physical symptoms is possible. A deep, soul-level healing can be achieved with these treatment techniques and the patients can function with their full psychological, physical, and spiritual capacity.

Failure to follow instructions and take responsibility for their healing: With this therapy, it is important for the patients to track, record, and report on their experiences in therapy as well as the changes in their lives. But patients often fail to do so. As a result, in spite of their healing, they fail to understand what was wrong and what cured them and what they can do to prevent problems in the future. They fail to learn from their experiences. Failure to follow the instructions regarding cleansing and pro-tection prayers can cause infestation by new entities and thus slow the progress and discourage the patients. This is a function of responsibility. Patients entering into this therapy, as with any therapy, must accept their own share of the responsibility for their healing. Failing to do so, laying all the responsibility on the therapist in the therapeutic process in spite of the healing of their symptoms, they gain little knowledge and understanding of their condition and fail to learn about how to prevent future infesta-tion and affliction.

Secondary gain factor: Sometimes patients experience what we call "secondary gain" from illness. When they are "sick" they receive lots of attention and, in some cases, compensatory pay. They are waited on, catered to, and fussed over. When they recover, all that stops. Some patients aren't ready to get better, to function without their secondary benefits, and as a result quit the therapy.

Not ready for a fast change: Another cause for leaving therapy early has to do with the speed and intensity of this therapy. It is fast, intense, and effective; some patients are simply not ready for a fast change. On occasion, when patients feel some relief of their symptoms, they talk themselves out of continuing.

Lack of support: Family and friends are very important factors in the success or failure of this therapy. On the one hand, a patient who may be doing well in therapy may talk about it at home and meet with discouragement or outright ridicule from family or friends who do not understand the process. They may force the patient to discontinue the therapy. On the other hand, when two members of a family or two friends enter therapy together, therapy is more successful because the two share ideas and information and do not feel as isolated or alone in therapy. Both instances emphasize the importance of educating people about the therapy and the process. The main point of my writing this book is to provide that education.

Insurance companies: Although hypnosis has been officially sanctioned by the American Medical Association since 1958 and is currently being successfully used by many medical doctors including psychiatrists, psychologists, and other therapists, most insurance companies refuse to allow and pay for hypnotherapy. As a result many patients are deprived of the treatment needed for their healing.

Hypnotherapy is a cost-effective technique. It achieves success in a much shorter length of time overall, but requires, conversely, more investment of time over the short term.

A single hypnotherapy session may take as long as three to six hours, three to six times as long as the traditional one-hour session. The number of hours required to achieve success, however, is much fewer than with traditional psychotherapy. Traditional talk therapy requires arranging eighteen weeks of one-hour-per-week treatments, or eighteen patient contact hours. No psychiatrist expects cure of a deep-seated problem in eighteen traditional patient contact hours. In contrast, six three-hour or three six-hour hypnotherapy sessions are capable of producing a cure, even for a deep-seated problem.

Traditional talk therapy can drag on for years, with patient contact hours running into the hundreds and even thousands. Hypnotherapy, while initially appearing to require more hours of treatment per patient, is actually more cost-effective because of the results. It takes comparatively little time for a patient to respond to the therapy in order to diminish the problem and improve the situation. If patients' severe symptoms can be relieved in short periods of time with extended sessions, why should we let patients suffer with their symptoms for months and years? Sometimes, when patients come to me from out of town, I have done continuous sessions for about six to eight hours a day and in some cases, just in a few days, with the patients' cooperation, we were able to relieve many of their presenting symptoms.

Cure rates for these therapies, based upon what patients have reported are much higher than for traditional talk therapy, even when talk therapy is combined with drug therapy. As evidenced by the research, I have seen severely ill patients who responded very well to these treatments. In spite of this success, many insurance companies refuse to pay for hypnotherapy.

Putting It All Together:
My Theory of Mental and Physical Illness

Here I present to you my theory of mental and physical illness, which I have derived from the information given to me by my hypnotized patients, over a period of about eleven years, and from my research. Over the years, my hypnotized patients have consistently told me that the soul is the spirit within us, an immortal energy essence of our being, a part of God that resides within us. It is our spiritual self. This soul empowers and activates the body; the body cannot live without it. When the soul leaves, the body dies; but the soul continues to survive and retains all its memories and experiences.

After the death of the physical body, the soul goes to heaven, to rest, heal, and make plans for the next life. The purpose of this cycle from heaven to birth, death, and back to heaven is to learn different lessons, grow spiritually, and perfect ourselves, so that one day we can go back to God, to our rightful place in the body of God, from where we originated.

Sometimes, spirits do not make their transition to heaven after the death of their physical bodies because of confusion, fear, anger, hate, jealousy, love, desire to take revenge, and desire for drugs, alcohol, food, cigarettes, gambling, or sex. These spirits remain on the earth plane and are called earthbound spirits. At some point they may end up entering and residing in an unsuspecting human host, whose energy field is weakened due to intense emotions such as depression, anger, fear, hate, grief, compassion, physical illnesses, surgery, or the use of drugs and alcohol. These unwanted house guests, the spiritual hitchhikers, bring their baggage of physical, mental, emotional, and spiritual problems with them, which in turn become the patients' problems.

Patients under hypnosis also report seeing black and gray blobs in them who claim to be demons. They state that they cause different types of physical, emotional, mental, and spiritual problems for the patients. These problems are often relieved by releasing the demon spirits.

My hypnotized patients consistently report that our souls and subconscious minds are one and the same. So under hypnosis, when they are recalling memories from their subconscious minds, they are in fact tapping into their soul memories. They report that everything we have ever experienced, felt, touched, smelled, seen, and heard in the current life and all our past lives and in-between lives, from the beginning of time, is recorded in our subconscious minds. No matter how dull or boring, important or unimportant, happy or unhappy, traumatic or nontraumatic, nothing is erased. We can tap in to and recall any of these memories anytime we want to and need to.

Patients under hypnosis also report that most of their current life problems and conflicts have their roots in one or more past lives. All our unresolved physical and emotional traumas and conflicts, our last thoughts, promises, and decisions from past lives are carried over with our souls from lifetime to lifetime into the current life and need to be resolved. In therapy, by recalling and resolving these unresolved traumas, conflicts, and issues from past lives, patients can be completely healed from their physical, emotional, and relationship problems.

According to my patients, our souls fragment while on earth, in the current life and in past lives, as a result of traumatic experiences.

The soul parts can remain in the body, looking and feeling the way they looked and felt at the time of the trauma, as though they were frozen in time. In traditional psychiatry they are called the "subpersonality" or the "inner child." The soul parts can also leave the body and go to different people or places, leaving holes in the soul. This situation creates weak areas in the soul and, as a result, in the body and aura, which in turn manifests in the form of physical, mental, and emotional illnesses. These holes and weaknesses in our souls and in our energy fields also open us for possession by earthbound, demon, and other entities, who occupy those empty holes in the soul and create more physical, emotional, and mental problems. Consequently, we can understand that the mental and physical illnesses are really the diseases of the soul.

In summary, we begin our journey for our spiritual development as a pure soul, a piece of God. During each life, with different emotional, mental, and physical traumas, our souls fragment and we lose pieces of them, creating the holes in them. This causes a weakness in the soul and thus in the body. These holes in our souls create the openings in our souls and bodies that are occupied by the human, demon, and other spirits. To heal the mind and body, we need to heal the soul, first by removing the foreign entities, devices, and negative energies. Then to heal these holes in the soul, we need to resolve the current and past life traumas, retrieve all the lost soul parts, and heal and close the holes, thus preventing any further infestation by outside spirits. By healing the soul, we can heal the mind and body. We can also realize that all our psychological and physical problems are some type of spiritual crisis, which can be cured by healing the spirit—the soul within.

During the whole treatment process, traditional psychotherapy and hypnotherapy are used together, whether I am working with human spirits, demon spirits, soul fragments, or present or past lives traumas.

One of the most amazing results of these sessions is the universality of the information. Although my patients have come from diverse cultural, religious, socioeconomic, and educational backgrounds, the information they receive under hypnosis is strikingly similar. Their words may differ, the expression may vary, but the information is the same, woven of common threads into the same essential themes.

There can be an alternative explanation for what is occurring in the treatment, other than what is reported by the patients. When a patient reports a past life scene and plays that past life scene out under hypnosis, it may be considered the same as psychodrama. It may also be a symbolic reenactment of an earlier problem in the current lifetime.

The idea of possession by an earthbound or a demon spirit may be seen as a symbolic gesture or a symbolic representation of the patients' subconscious or even conscious minds. Treating and dealing with these entities may be considered a method of symbolically treating the patients' subconscious or conscious mind.

Another possible explanation is that the patient may be reporting the exact facts and the psychiatrist may be dealing with the effects of actual past lives or actual possession by human or demon entities.

Whether you wish to consider these as psychodrama, as symbolic reenactment, or as actual facts is up to you. The only thing that is truly important to me is that these methods work. They relieve the patients' crippling symptoms and are fast, effective, and thorough, especially when compared with traditional psychotherapy. The extent of cure and the number of those who are cured is staggering. These numbers indicate that these methods of treatment are worthy of use by other psychiatrists, psychologists, and psychotherapists.

These therapies are not presented as substitutes for other medical and psychiatric treatments, but are to be used in conjunction with them, interwoven with these approaches into a tapestry of mental and physical health care.

✧✧✧

Logical Structure of the Universe

Over the years, I worked with different patients coming from different cultures, religious beliefs, and educational backgrounds. Under hypnosis, amazingly, most of them gave a similar description of the universe, its structure, and the beings who inhabit it.

My patients, under hypnosis, say that there is a huge Light. In this Light resides a supreme being they call "God." They describe this supreme being as a mountain of Light, a pyramid of Light or an ocean of Light and love. They call him "the one," "the all," "the whole," "the God," "all there is," etc.

Next to this supreme being there are other large souls whom they call Godheads, masters, or oversouls. They recognize these beings as religious figures in different religions of the world. Next to them there are angels and other beings of the Light. Patients say that from God descend the Godheads, also called masters or oversouls, and from them, humans and all the other souls descend. The Godheads, angels, and beings of other worlds also reside all around God.

My patients describe seeing many silver cords coming out of God and going to humans and all the other beings throughout the creation through the Godheads. Patients describe God as a powerhouse to whom all the living beings in the whole creation are connected with the silver cords.

Hypnotized patients report that between lives, we humans also reside in the Light, where we go through some type of learning and developmental process. In this Light we seem to be partially aware of who we are and what we are doing. We go through the cycle of birth, life, death, and back to the Light (heaven) again and again to learn lessons and grow spiritually toward our final aim to go back and reunite with the supreme being, God.

Many of my patients, under hypnosis, also recall their creation and what happened in the Light after they were created. They say there was a conflict and a being of the Light left and took many Light beings with it. According to my patients, these beings are really Satan and his demons, who are working on the earth opposite the purposes of the Light. They thwart the Light. To my surprise, even demons recall and give the similar information after their transformation into the Light.

Amazingly, my patients, regardless of whether they are religious, agnostic, or atheist, have repeatedly given similar accounts of the reality of the spiritual world as they see and remember it under hypnosis. I wondered if they could be recalling and describing the truth, or were they all suffering from the same delusion?

Do we really know what is the reality? What is the truth? From our earthly point of view, it seems that the earth stays still in one place and the sun comes up, crosses the heavens, and then goes down. But the fact is that the earth rotates on its axis and goes around the sun. Similarly, it appears to us that the sun must be the center of the universe. But the whole universe does not go around the sun. The sun, the center of the solar system, is but one system in the Milky Way galaxy, which in turn holds its place as one of many galaxies in the whole universe. So what seems to be real and true to us is not; and what is not, is.

We are always working backward in our logical structure. The life we live on this earth seems to be the ultimate reality. Here in this physical world it appears as if this is a real world into which we are born. We live and die in it. It seems as if we come from nowhere and we disappear under the ground to nowhere. According to my patients, the spiritual world is the real world. In reality we are spiritual beings going through a developmental process for our own purpose, and the life we live is but one step along the way.

My patients tell me that we have set up a kind of obstacle course, a series of trials or developmental steps that we must go through. Each of these steps causes us to improve and grow in our spiritual life. We cannot see this connection, but its direction is real. It is as real as gravity appears to be. We cannot see gravity; we can only see its effects. Here in our life we cannot see that spiritual connection, but we can detect the effects. Especially in my work, I have found the effects of our spiritual nature.

Here on the earth we cannot see the center of the universe. We do not know where to look. From our point of view it seems as if everything is moving away from us except our local area. Does this mean that our local area is the center of the universe? No. The center must exist, but we do not know where.

On the spiritual level my patients tell me that there is God. Where do we find God? We do not know where to look. Could we comprehend God if we saw him? I doubt it. Does it mean that God does not exist? No.

In conclusion, we can see that human perception is fallible. What we consider to be real is not; and what we believe as not real, is.

Afterthoughts

Throughout the course of this book, I have reported the information as given by my hypnotized patients and have not claimed it as my own. Having satisfied myself that I succeeded in doing so, I will now take the liberty of stepping out of the role of a reporter into the role of a commentator, whereby I would like to say some things of my own.

Those readers of the Christian faith will recognize the passage, "Ask, and you shall receive; seek, and you shall find." This book, I hope, is a nontheological affirmation of the truth of that statement. All those who ever questioned the meaning of life and death, the significance of their own existence, or the structure of the universe, should have gained some reassuring answers to those timeless questions.

Since my work began about eleven years ago, I have often wondered, why now? I have been doing hypnotherapy for twenty-five years and none of my patients before reported about past lives or spirits. And now many patients are recalling a past life or describe having spirits as the source of their problems. Many people are also able to see and communicate with heavenly beings and tap into higher knowledge. So, I began to inquire from the heavenly beings through different people under hypnosis.

According to the heavenly beings, we humans live in duality. We have a soul—which is a piece of God within us, which has all the knowledge. But, while living on earth in a body, this knowledge is being blocked, so we can go through our tests and trials and grow spiritually. It is like having a veil between our soul and body, our conscious and subconscious, or between heaven and earth.

Based on the information given by the heavenly beings, we humans have done well through our humanitarian work worldwide for the past several decades and have raised the vibrations of our planet. As a result, a part of the veil has been removed and we are more in touch with the heavenly beings and are able to tap into our past lives and other higher knowledge. If we continue to raise our planet's vibrations through our good works, more and more of the veil will be removed, allowing us to tap in to more of the higher knowledge and truth.

Why have I enjoyed this measure of success with these therapies? I have often considered this question. The best answer I have come up with is ti.at I have kept an open mind. By allowing patients to bring up information from their subconscious mind and not judging them, I was able to receive answers and knowledge that I could not have acquired in any other way. I gained a great deal of insight into the reasons for mental and physical illnesses and their treatment and prevention. I learned that we must not place parameters on our expectations based on our limited, acquired knowledge.

Drugs and Alcohol

There are some specific concerns upon which I would like to comment. The first of these concerns regards drugs and alcohol, and the devastating effects they have on individuals, on families, and on society. Although we admit and recognize the dangers of drugs, we underplay the effects of alcohol. The fact is that alcohol is as deadly and as damaging and carries consequences as far-reaching as drugs do. Perhaps because it is legal, people think alcohol is less harmful than drugs.

On the contrary, they both are progressive killers. First of all, they destroy individuals, taking away money, self-esteem, health, and jobs. They also damage relationships and break up marriages and families. Like a ripple in the water, the effects are ever-widening. Children who grow up in families torn apart by drugs and alcohol build equally sick habits and relationships based on the physical, emotional, and sexual abuse they endured. Ultimately, our society becomes weak and sick, and fails to survive. It is a perpetual, vicious problem that passes from generation to generation.

We are fed a mixed message. While we restrict our young people from drinking till the age of twenty-one, because it is so dangerous, we glamorize drinking for adults. No wedding, no party, no elegant dinner is complete without the alcohol. We associate gracious living and high society with "cocktails." All the "in" people have a wet bar and know how to mix all the fashionable drinks.

Through my patients, both dark and earthbound entities have repeatedly bragged about their ability to latch on to drug addicts and alcoholics. Sometimes only one drink can open people up by weakening their shields or energy fields. The entities have told me repeatedly that they hang around bars, just waiting for an opportunity to move in on an unsuspecting host. Once in people, entities cause arguments, fights, and family breakups and promote the desire to continue to drink. What a deal for the entities, who have nothing to lose; they get their drink and the hosts pick up the tab with loss of jobs, families, and homes.

It is time for us to take responsibility for ourselves, our families, and our society. It is time to recognize that abuse of alcohol and drugs lies in darkness, and that even for the nicest people, consuming drugs and alcohol creates an open invitation for dark influence.

How We Treat Each Other

Another concern I have is how we treat each other. If we visualize God as a huge gem, the Godheads are like the facets on the edge of the gem, reflecting energy and Light. This collective energy around God is referred to by my hypnotized patients as the Christ consciousness. Each Godhead in this Christ consciousness is the focal figure of a major world religion, such as Jesus, Buddha, Shiva, Vishnu, Mohammed, and all the others. My patients, under hypnosis, describe Jesus as the Christian religion's Godhead or Christ, Vishnu and Shiva as the Hindu Christ, Buddha as the Buddhist Christ, Mohammed as the Moslem Christ, etc.

We all descend from and are all linked to one of these Godheads through a silver cord. That cord is our link through our Godhead to God. All Godheads are connected to each other; they are a continuous energy field immediately surrounding God. In this way, we are all linked to a Godhead, all the Godheads are linked to each other and to God, and in turn we are all linked to each other. We are all joined as pieces of God. If we can imagine God as one body, then we are like different cells and parts of that body of God. When any part of that body hurts, the whole body hurts. Similarly, when we hurt any other person, we hurt ourselves as well. We must treat each other with love and care to preserve the whole. When we speak to others with love, it can penetrate through the depths of their darkness and reach deep inside, into their souls. Love is the most powerful resource in the universe. When we give love to others, we also receive it and, as it moves back and forth, it grows and provides the healing for everybody involved. Only love can heal and it is the only thing that really matters.

The Law of Cause and Effect

Many of the world religions teach the law of cause and effect: "Every action has a reaction"; "As you sow, so shall you reap"; "What you send around, comes around." All these statements underscore the boomerang aspect of human interaction. Our actions and behavior create consequences. Indeed, what we send around comes around, individually, as a society, as a nation, in this life and hereafter. Every action creates energy that returns to us in a similar way. Our good deeds will have positive effects on our lives, while our negative actions will have negative consequences for us.

On a much greater scale "as you sow, so shall you reap" has some staggering ramifications. Under the guise of freedom of speech, of expression, of the press, of comedy, some of our news media, recording artists, writers, and producers of television shows and motion pictures send out some frightening messages to people. Children model what they see. They absorb without discrimination. What measurable effect do all the movies and television programs that are ridden with violence, nudity, and illicit sex have on our children and our society?

Though our youth are a major concern, "copycat" behavior knows no age restrictions. Multiple murders, brutal rapes, and suicides can be committed, and aberrant sex is practiced in direct response to some movies, television shows, and song lyrics. These facts present a challenge to those writers and producers of radio, T.V., movie, and the music industry who have such an astounding effect on our society. They can make or break the society. The choice is theirs; it will have positive or negative consequence for our society and for them, depending on their actions.

Choices we make have far-reaching ramifications. Our words and actions reflect who we are. Whatever we do and say affects others in a ripple effect. We must acknowledge that no matter how we strive to rationalize our actions, the results and consequences of those actions remain the same. Pain is pain, no matter the reason. Rationalization for our actions may help us feel better for the moment, but the long-range damage is done to everyone concerned, including ourselves. It is as though, once we set the cosmic wheel in motion, it goes where it goes and we cannot change that. Consequently, it pays to think about where our actions will lead before we criticize, judge, and act in a negative way toward others.

During past life regression therapy, I have seen the effects of "as you sow, so shall you reap." Many of my patients have found the source of their physical and emotional problems in one or more past lives when they hurt others through their actions. Now in this life they are suffering with problems similar to those they caused others in their past lives.

Foregiveness

The importance of forgiveness is something I should emphasize. The world is full of anger and hurt. When we are hurt, it is easy to become angry and resentful. These feelings, unresolved, grow quickly into bitterness and vengefulness—we desire the opportunity to "pay back." There is another avenue of response open to us: that of forgiveness. Most religions teach about the power of forgiveness. When we forgive, we free ourselves from anger, hate, resentment, and a desire to take revenge; thus we heal ourselves. Those we forgive are also healed, as our forgiveness releases them from guilt and anguish.

While treating patients with these therapies, I have seen the healing and regenerative power of forgiveness. During a past life regression therapy, a patient who is able to forgive a person who hurt him or her often reports being completely free from that problem. Even the other person who hurt the patient in that past life and is also here with the patient in the current life, heals without ever coming for treatment.

It is critical that we understand and remember that we are all interconnected. When we hurt someone else, we hurt ourselves. What we do affects all those we touch. When we generate anger, hate, hurt, or any other negative feelings or behaviors, we affect many people, far more than we realize. When we give or receive forgiveness, those scars heal. It is only through forgiveness that we can ensure our healing; thus the energy of the universe remains positive and in balance. Positive energy heals—not only the person who generates it, but also all the souls it touches.

Power of Prayers

Another thing I want to emphasize is the importance and power of prayer in our day-to-day living. What I have found time after time from my hypnotized patients is that all prayers are heard, no matter how superficial. Sometimes they are not answered right away or the way we want because there is a lesson to be learned from whatever is going on in our lives. The answer depends upon our plan. God granted us free will to learn the lessons and grow spiritually, but, like the angels, God does not invade or interfere with our free will. Asking for God's help is an exercise of our free will. God is all-knowing, but will not intervene unless we ask.

As mentioned before, through our silver cords passes all communication between us and God. When we pray, our prayers ascend through our cords to God. God hears and answers all our prayers through this "cosmic umbilical cord." As with a telegraph, information is always flowing through this cord, whether we are aware of it or not. I am thoroughly convinced that it is very important to pray for protection and guidance daily. While individual prayers are important, group prayers have incredible impact. It is very important for families to pray both individually and together for protection and guidance for themselves and for all the people in their lives. Praying for other people sometimes is more powerful, maybe because it is selfless.

With prayers, we can also transform the demons into the Light and send them to heaven. Thus, we have fewer problems to deal with. They are also part of the same body of God. They are the lost souls and need our prayers and help for their transformation.

As controversial as the subject is, prayers are especially important in schools. Through prayers in schools, our kids can remain clear of all the dark influences that plague them. When we pray, a column of Light and love floods to us and oursurroundings from God. As we know, the demon entities are afraid of Light and cannot come close to it. If we can keep our children and schools filled and illuminated with the Light through prayers, they can be protected from negative, dark influences. It is important to remember that where there is no Light, darkness will rule. It is particularly important that we teach our children these protection techniques, not out of fear, but out of awareness. We must keep our children clear of dark influences and thereby keep them away from drugs, alcohol, violence, and other self-destructive and antisocial behaviors. This way we can build a loving and peaceful society. Through prayers, we can block the dark influences and even transform the dark beings and illuminate and heal our world. Prayers are our open line to God. God will protect us and guide us and will listen and answer our prayers. But we must ask.

Meditation

Another thing I want to stress is the importance of meditation in our daily lives. Light beings, through different patients, have consistently advised us to meditate daily. When we pray, we speak to God; but when we meditate, we allow God to speak to us and guide us. Through meditation we can also get in touch with our soul, that piece of God that is in each of us and is a storehouse of all the knowledge there is. It is our inheritance; through meditation we all can tap into that knowledge, which no books, no teachers, and no science can teach us.

Religious Conflicts and Wars

An additional concern is the fact that throughout history people have quarreled and waged wars on one another in the name of religion. This is just as true now as it has ever been. Even within major religions, there are points of contention great enough to cause divisions within the denominations, all in the name of God and in defense of religious beliefs.

The dark entities in my patients have frequently bragged about making one religion fight with another, and about causing wars in the name of God. They actually laugh at our frailty and ignorance as we fall in with their schemes. Like puppeteers, they pull our strings and we respond.

Light beings through my hypnotized patients have repeatedly told us that scriptures of all the religions are gifts from God. But they also have subtle influences from Satan and his demons. Because the scriptures were received by humans and written with human hands, they were also subject to human errors. Demons often brag about influencing humans to change the words, and consequently the meaning, in the translations. Over the ages, all the scriptures have endured much dark influence. As readers, we must use our judgment in accepting those things that feel right and set aside what does not feel quite right.

When we believe, "My religion is the only correct religion, and the religious figure in whom I believe is the only one who is real," we are bringing into our beliefs our ego and arrogance, which have no place in the truth. As mentioned throughout the book, we are all linked to God through our Godheads. All Godheads work in perfect harmony with God and with one another to help humanity, why then can we not live and work harmoniously with each other, worshiping one God, and believing in all the Godheads?

It is time for us to quit listening to Satan and his demons. It is time for us to recognize the dark influence at the core of all our strife, within ourselves, our families, our communities, our nation, our religions, and the world. It is time for one worldwide religion, which believes in one God and all the masters and for one world in which every person contributes prayerfully to the good of us all.

Crimes

After reading this book, probably many of you will not be able to intellectually buy into the concept of Satan and his demons and how they may be behind all the pain and suffering in our families, societies, nations, and our world. I know; I had a hard time accepting what was coming from my patients' subconscious minds. But the reports were consistent from patient to patient, who were coming from different cultures, nationalities, religions, and educational backgrounds, regardless of whether they were religious, agnostic, or atheist.

What if it is true? Can it explain Hitler, Jeffrey Dahmer, Jim Jones, the serial killers, rapists, gangsters, wars, and every type of evil in our world? Can it provide an explanation for the breakdown of our families and societies? Can it give us new insights into mental and physical illness?

Demons in my patients have often bragged about their tremendous success in making us believe that they do not exist. They work hard to keep us from finding the truth about them, because if we know that they do exist, then we can resist their influences and find different ways to free ourselves from them and their influences.

What if they are real? Then can we have understanding and solutions to most of our problems? Can we free ourselves, our society, our nation, and our world from dark influences through education, prayers, and treatment? I believe we can, but because of our fear of Satan and his demons and because we cannot perceive them with our five physical senses, we have a tendency not to believe in them. During treatment, what impressed me the most was that, under hypnosis, my patients have consistently reported that with the help of God and his angels, we can be more powerful than Satan and his demons. They have only as much power as we give them. The issue here is: should we feel we are right with our beliefs and with our limited knowledge, or should we keep our minds open and search for the truth?

Capital Punishment

This also leads us to another important problem we are facing in our society: the issue of capital punishment. Just think what could have made those criminals commit those horrible, inhuman crimes. It has to be human and dark spirits. So even if we get rid of them physically through death, are we really free of them? I doubt it. Because of the dark influences, their spirits probably have difficulty going to the Light. So there is a fairly good possibility of them remaining on the earth plane and possessing somebody else and pushing their hosts to commit the same or worse crimes. So can we really be free of those criminals by killing them? And when we kill them, does it not make us murderers, too? It is something to think about.

Faith and Trust in God

Working with these therapies and with heavenly beings through patients for over eleven years, I have learned a great deal about having faith and trust in God. Faith and trust in God literally form pillars of communication between us, our higher selves, the Godhead, and God. They are extremely important in our daily lives, especially during tragedies, losses, and the hardships.

During these times, most of us conclude that God is punishing us because he does not love us or because we did something wrong. It is extremely important to know that God is loving and caring. He does not judge or punish us, no matter what we have done.

It is crucial to know that every tragedy, every loss, every sickness and suffering we are going through in our lives, we ourselves have chosen and planned very carefully in heaven before entering into this life. Through pain and suffering, we learn the lessons and grow spiritually. God does not interfere with them because if he does, then he will hinder our spiritual growth and evolvement. Those with a great deal of faith and trust in God can literally step beyond the material world and understand that many painful events that they are going through are for their lessons and spiritual growth. They try to learn the lessons and move on without much complaining.

As our faith and trust in God grow, fear cannot enter into the picture. Instead of complaining and being unhappy about a situation, we need to ask and continue to ask in our prayers, "What do I need to learn from this?" In time, we will be given the understanding about it. Prayers and meditations are important elements in building our faith and trust in God. It is important to talk to God as in prayers and important to listen to him as in meditation. As we work on these concepts, they become stronger. As our faith and trust in God grow, we grow in love. When we begin to understand that we ourselves planned many of these events, we appreciate and obtain an inner peace and harmony. We begin to focus on the positive rather than on the negative and become happy and peaceful people, no matter what happens around us.

Strong faith and trust in God can bring us closer to God and enlighten us and those around us. The stronger our faith, the more we are protected from the dark influences. Our faith and trust in God can carry us through pain and suffering and can literally transport and transcend us beyond.

Love and Grace of God

Through this work over the years, the greatest knowledge I have received is about God, our creator. He is all-knowing, all-seeing, and all-powerful. He is pure love and Light. There is no judgment, no condemnation, and no punishment ever by God, no matter what we have done. He understands that we live in duality and our real spiritual knowledge is blocked from us, while we live on earth and go through our tests and trials for our spiritual growth. He understands our hurt, pain, and even our anger and resentment toward him and does not judge or punish us for it. Our anger does not faze him. He understands the reasons for our feelings and loves us just the same.

His love, Light, and grace are always pouring on us steadily, like a waterfall, through our connecting cords. He is constantly bathing, embracing, and healing us with his love and Light. He assigns his angels to protect us and help us while on earth. He allots us our heavenly guides from birth, to take care of us, guide us, and provide us love, support, and the knowledge we need. They are his gifts to us. His love, Light, and grace are provided to every soul constantly. He never shuts us off, never leaves us alone, and never rejects us. It is we, with the help of the dark beings, who choose to reject and shut him off by shutting off the flow of his Light and love, but he continues to work around it.

He animates us, motivates us, and helps us to exist here. He listens to and answers our prayers. Sometimes he may not answer right away or in the way we want, because we have some lessons to learn from whatever is going on in our life. He gives us free will and as a result he will not intrude and interfere with our life unless we ask for help. But he is always ready to help us when we ask. He can heal us, balance us, transform us, and enlighten us. He can do anything for us. I see the results of his love and Light daily in my office.

Prayers and meditation are the keys to the heart of God. He is always present in our lives. Let us together reach out for him, open our hearts for his unconditional love, and just watch him create the miracles for us and our planet. His love is limitless, powerful, and simply awesome.

As I consider what has been written in these pages and how the book came to be, I realize that I have some very intense aspirations regarding it. The most compelling wish is that even if readers are intellectually unable to buy in to what they have read, their souls will remember what happens after the death of the physical body and different choices they have. By having this knowledge, at the moment of physical death I hope their souls will look to the Light and follow it home to the Light.

My second hope is that in reading and discussing the knowledge found in this book, we not only inform and educate ourselves, but also those internal and external entities that my patients insist are always there; I hope they can also find their way home to the Light, too.

We have only tapped the tip of the iceberg. There is so much we do not yet know about the human mind and its capacity to heal. The possibilities are limitless. We need to do more research in a variety of settings for a variety of illnesses and see if we get the same results. But more important, let us push the limits of these amazing therapies: who really knows where the healing stops? God knows, and he will tell. But only if we ask.

Glossary

Angels: Heavenly beings who have never been human. Their purpose is to guard and protect us throughout our earthly lives. Everybody has at least one guardian angel. Angels' help must be asked for. They will not invade or interfere with our free will.

Aura: An invisible electromagnetic energy field emanating from all living things, e.g., humans, animals, and plants, and reflecting the health and emotions of a being. It shields and protects us from outside negative influences, including earthbound, demon, and other entities.

Automatic Writing: Writing achieved by spirits, using and controlling the hand of a person. It is performed using a pen, pencil, or typewriter.

Channeling: Manifestation and information generated by a spirit from the higher planes through the physical body of a living person. It can be in the form of speaking, writing, healing, or a form of art, e.g., painting, playing musical instruments, etc.

Clairaudience: Psychic ability to hear beyond normal hearing.

Clairsensient: Psychic ability to sense beyond normal senses.

Clairvoyance: Psychic ability to see beyond normal sight.

Cleansing: The process of removing all the negative energies, entities, devices, and anything else that is not a part of us from our bodies, auras, cords, and souls and then healing and filling us with the white Light. It is often achieved with the help of the angels.

Dark Entity: Used interchangeably with demon entity.

Demons: The Light beings, tricked by Lucifer (Satan) to leave heaven and God and go with him. They were turned into dark entities by Satan. They are trained and instructed to possess and influence people on earth and the whole creation, negatively. Angry, frightened, and subversive, they are Satan's dark angels who are afraid of the Light.

Discarnate/disembodied: Terms that literally mean the spirit that left the body. *Discarnate* and *disembodied* are used interchangeably.

Earthbound: A state in which a spirit remains on the earth plane after the death of the physical body, because it has failed to make the transition to the Light (heaven).

Entity/Spirit: The immortal essence of a person, which does not die with the death of the physical body. *Entity*, *spirit*, and *soul* are used synonymously in this book.

Exorcism: A religious rite to expel possessing demon spirits from a living person, a place, or an object.

Exorcist: A specialist, often a Catholic priest, who is trained to use religious ritual to exorcize a possessing demon entity from a person, a place, or an object.

Extrasensory perception (ESP): The ability to perceive and interpret knowledge, happenings, or presence beyond the five physical senses.

God: An all-knowing, all-seeing, all-powerful parent force from which we all originated, to which we are all still connected by a silver cord, and to whom we all will ultimately return. Under hypnosis, my patients identify him as a mountain of Light, a pyramid of Light, or an ocean of Light and love. They call him "the one," "the whole," "the all," "the light," "the God," "all there is," etc.

Hypnosis: A state of focused concentration in which we set aside our constantly chattering conscious mind so we can contact the subconscious mind, which is the storehouse for memories, feelings, and knowledge and is open to suggestions, to questions, and to make changes that affect conscious behavior, attitudes, and feelings.

Hypnotic Regression: The accessing of prior memories and experiences from current or past lives from the subconscious mind for therapeutic purposes under hypnosis.

Induction: The process through which a hypnotic state is achieved, usually by relaxation techniques.

Influence: Interference with people's thinking, behavior, actions, attitude, and physical and mental health by Satan, his demons, and earthbound spirits. These influences can be from inside or outside. They influence directly by entering a person or indirectly through spiritual devices and energy absorbers created by Satan and his demons.

Karma: An ancient concept, best described by the popular phrases: "As you sow, so shall you reap," "Every action has a reaction," "What you send around, comes around," etc. It has to do with the consequences of our present or past actions in this life or future lives. A positive or negative "payback."

Light Beings: Souls that reside in heaven, e.g., God, Godheads, angels, spirit guides, humans between lives, and all the other beings.

Masters, Godheads or Oversouls: Terms that are used interchangeably. Collectively they refer to the energy immediately next to and surrounding God, which is often described by my hypnotized patients as Christ consciousness. Part of it consists of seven or more sections, called Godheads, oversouls, or masters for our planet. They are like God, but they are not "the God." These Godheads also represent religious figures of different religions of the world. Each of us descends from one of these Godheads; we are connected to them with silver cords. This silver cord is our link to God through our Godhead.

Medium: A psychically sensitive person who can communicate and channel information from spirits of other planes.

Metaphysics: What lies beyond the realm of physics, sometimes referred to as the occult. Metaphysics is concerned with higher planes, astrology, reincarnation, auras, spirits, possession, etc.

Near-death Experience: Literally being clinically dead for a short time and reversed with or without medical intervention. Frequently glimpses of the existence beyond life occur in near-death experiences.

Ouija Board: A board on which the alphabet, "yes," "no," and numbers are printed. Using a small, heart-shaped pointer, called a planchet, spirits spell out messages through a person who touches the planchet.

Out-of-Body Experience (OBE): An experience in which the soul leaves the physical body through the silver cord, and returns the same way when it is ready. It is also called astral projection or soul travel.

Past-life Regression Therapy: A type of psychotherapy in which a patient is regressed to a former lifetime to resolve a current life problem.

Possession/Attachment: Interchangeable terms that refer to a state in which an entity (spirit) attaches or inhabits a person.

Psychic: A person who perceives information from sources other than those received through the five physical senses.

Reincarnation: The rebirth of the soul in another body repeatedly in order to learn lessons and evolve spiritually.

Repression: Selective forgetting of emotionally painful experiences. Repression is of a protective nature and can happen at any age. Hypnotherapy is usually the method of uncovering and resolving the repressed memories.

Satan/Devil: An evil being who is chief of all the demons and other evil beings under his control. My hypnotized patients describe him as a fallen angel, Lucifer, who rebelled and left God and the Light, and took many angels and other beings of the Light with him, who turned into negative energy and became the demons.

Séance: A meeting of people in which spirit contact is made through a medium for the purposes of communication.

Shaman: An individual who uses spiritual techniques in order to heal people. Also called "medicine man" or "witch doctor."

Silver Cord: A spiritual energy, a cord or line that connects our souls to God. It is usually seen as a silvery, efflorescent cord or tunnel, depending on whether it is perceived from without or within. We receive our guidance from God through this cosmic "umbilical cord." Through it passes all communication to and from God, as prayers. Like an open line or a telegraph, messages are always moving through it, although we may be unaware or unwilling to acknowledge them.

Patients report that during near-death experiences they traveled through their cords, which they describe as tunnels to heaven. We also go to the Light through our silver cord during our sleep to plan future events and to learn from the higher beings.

Soul: A creative, vital, and immortal energy essence, a part of God that dwells within each of us and is still connected to God by a silver cord. It empowers our body, which cannot function without it. During death, the body dies, but the soul continues with all its memories, feelings, and attitudes. According to my hypnotized patients, the soul and the subconscious mind are one and the same; when we are dealing with our subconscious mind under hypnosis, we are really dealing with our soul.

Spirit Guides: The Light beings who have chosen to guide and protect us in this life. These are often confused with angels. Guides differ from angels in that they have been human before and have lived on the earth. Perhaps we have known them, perhaps not. Everybody has at least one guide and sometimes more than one. In most cases our guides are connected to the same Godhead as we are.

Spirit Releasement Therapy: Releasing earthbound, demon, and other spirits from a patient in a therapeutic situation. The spirits are treated as the secondary patients. They are not cast out, but sent to the Light (heaven) after some therapy.

Although I have always used the term "spirit releasement," because it describes the treatment process, William Baldwin, Ph.D. has trademarked this term.

Subconscious: The part of the mind that functions just below the conscious level. The subconscious mind and the soul in reality are one and the same and house all our memories and knowledge.

Telepathy: Psychic transmission and reception of thoughts.

Trance: A state in which there is reduced conscious awareness. It can range from light to deep. It can be hypnotic or nonhypnotic.

Transformation of the Demon: A process in therapy whereby a demon is isolated, made to realize its true identity, and directed to focus on its inner Light until it is changed to a being of pure Light and sent back to heaven.

White Light: An energy, an emanation that comes from God. In this book Light is used synonymously for God, heaven, and an emanation or a Light coming from heaven and from God.

God Smiled and the World Shined

And God watched it all, and smiled,
Knowing it was good.
And the Light bathed us,
And we drank it, thirsty as a newborn babe.

And we knew in that moment we were the Light's,
And the Light was ours.
And together we were God's, and God was ours.
And we are all one and the same.
And in that moment God smiled,
And the world sparkled and shined.

—Jane

Let me reaffirm that no lay person should attempt to use any of these techniques without proper training, as they deal with very powerful and often very painful emotions and memories that the untrained person is not equipped to handle. This is not a "how-to manual for lay readers."

If you are interested in finding someone who can assist you, either with therapy or perhaps with training, you may contact the International Association for Regression, Research, and Therapies (IARRT). It is located at Post Office Box 20151, Riverside, CA 92516. The phone number is 951-784-1570.

Bibliography

Past Life Therapy

Dethlefsen, Thorwald. *Voices from Other Lives*. New York: M. Evans & Co., Inc., 1977.

Finkelstein, Adrian, M.D. *Your Past Lives and the Healing Process*. Farmingdale, N.Y.: Coleman Publishing, 1985.

Fiore, Edith, Ph.D. *You Have Been Here Before*. New York: Ballantine Books, 1978.

Goldberg, Bruce, D.D.S. *Past Lives, Future Lives*. New York: Ballantine Books, 1988.

Hickman, Irene, D.O. *Mind Probe-Hypnosis*. Kirksville, Mo: Hickman Systems, 1983.

Kelsey, Dennys, and Joan Grant. *Many Lifetimes*. New York: Ballantine Books, 1987.

Lucas, Winafred, Ph.D. *Regression Therapy: A Handbook for Professionals*, Vol. 1, Crest Park, Calif.: Deep Forest Press, 1993.

Moody, Raymond, M.D. *Coming Back: A Psychiatrist Explores Past-Life Journeys*. New York: Bantam, Doubleday, Dell Publishing Group, 1990.

Netherton, Morris, Ph.D., and Nancy Shiffrin. *Past Lives Therapy*. New York: Ace Books, 1978.

Schlotterbeck, Karl. *Living Your Past Lives: The Psychology of Past Life Regression*. New York: Ballantine Books, 1987.

Sutphen, D. *You Were Born Again To Be Together*. New York: Simon & Schuster, 1976.
———. *Past Lives, Future Loves*. New York: Simon & Schuster, 1978.

Wambach, Helen, Ph.D. *Life Before Life*. New York: Bantam Books, 1979.

——. *Reliving Your Past Lives: The Psychology of Past-Life Regression*. New York: Ballantine Books, 1978.

Weiss, Brian L., M.D. *Many Lives, Many Masters*. New York: Simon and Schuster, 1988.
——. *Through Time into Healing*. New York: Simon & Schuster, 1992.
——. *Only Love Is Real: A Story of Soulmates Reunited*. New York: Warner Books, 1997.

Whitton, Joel, M.D., and Joe Fisher. *Life between Life: Scientific Explorations into the Void Separating One Incarnation from the Next*. New York: Doubleday, 1980.

Williston, Glen, and Judith Johnstone. *Discovering Your Past Lives*. Northampton, England: Thorsons Publishing Group, 1983.

Woolger, Roger, Ph.D. *Other Lives, Other Selves*. New York: Doubleday, 1987.

Past Life Experience and Research

Bernstein, Morey. *The Search for Bridey Murphey*. New York: Doubleday, 1956.

Bolduc, Henry L. *The Journey Within: Past Life and Channeling*. Independence, Mo.: Adventures Into Time, 1993.

Cerminara, Gina. *Many Mansions: The Edgar Cayce Story on Reincarnation*. New York: Nal/Dutton, 1988.
——. *Many Lives, Many Loves*. Marina del Rey, Calif.: DeVorss & Co., 1981.
——. *World Within*. Virginia Beach, Va.: A.R.E. Press, 1985.

Chadwich, Gloria. *Discovering Your Past Lives*. Chicago: Contemporary Books, Inc., 1988.

Clow, Barbara. *Eye of the Centaur: A Visionary Guide into Past Lives*. Sante Fe, N.M.: Bear & Company, 1990.

Cranston, Sylvia, and Carey Williams. *Reincarnation: A New Horizon in Science, Religion and Society*. Pasadena, Calif.: Theosophical University Press, 1993.

Ebon, Martin. *Reincarnation in the Twentieth Century*. New York: NAL/Dutton, 1979.

Fisher, Joe. *The Case for Reincarnation*. New York: Carol Publishing Co., 1992.

Glaskin, G. M. *Windows of the Mind: The Christos Experiment*. London: Wildwood House, 1974.

Grant, Joan. *Far Memory*. Alpharetta, Ga.: Ariel Press, 1995.
———. *Winged Pharaoh*. Alpharetta, Ga.: Ariel Press, 1985.

Guirdham, Arthur, M.D. *The Cathars and Reincarnation*. London: Neville Spearman, 1970.
———. *We Are One Another*. London: Neville Spearman, 1974.

Hall, Manley P. *Reincarnation: The Cycles of Necessity*. Los Angeles: Philosophical Research Society, Inc., 1978.
———. *Past Lives and Present Problems*. Los Angeles: Philosophical Research Society, Inc., 1978.

Lenz, Frederick. *Lifetimes: True Accounts of Reincarnation*. New York: Bobbs-Merrill, 1979.

MacGregor, Geddes. *Reincarnation in Christianity*. Wheaton, Ill.: Theosophical Publishing House, 1989.

MacLaine, Shirley. *Out on the Limb*. New York: Bantam Books, 1986.

McClain, Florence. *A Practical Approach to Past Life Regression*. St. Paul, Minn.: Llewellyn Publishers, 1985.

Rieder, Marge. *Mission to Millboro*. Los Angeles: Authors Unlimited, 1991.

Rogo, D. Scott. *The Search for Yesterday: A Critical Examination of the Evidence of Reincarnation*. Englewood Cliffs, N.J.: Prentice Hall, 1985.

Smith, Robert C., and Charles T. Cayce. *You Can Remember Your Past Life*. New York: Warner Books, 1989.

Steiger, Brad. *Your Future Lives*. Atglen, Pa.: Schiffer Publishing, Ltd., 1988.

Steiger, Brad, and Francie Steiger. *Discover Your Past Lives*. Atglen. Pa.: Schiffer Publishing, Ltd., 1987.

Steiger, Brad, and Lorin Williams. *Other Lives*. Phoenix: Esoteric Publication, 1985.

Steiner, Rudolf. *Reincarnation and Immortality*. Hudson, N.Y. Garber Communications Inc., 1970.

Stevenson, Ian, M.D. *Twenty Cases Suggestive of Reincarnation*. New York: American Society for Psychical Research, 1966.
———. *Twenty Cases Suggestive of Reincarnation*. Charlottesville, Va.: University Press of Virginia, 1974.

———. *Children Who Remember Previous Lives: A Question of Reincarnation*. Charlottesville, Va.: University Press of Virginia, 1987.
———. *Xenoglossy: A Review and Report of a Case*. Charlottesville, Va.: University Press of Virginia, 1974.
———. *Unlearned Language: New Studies in Xenoglossy*. Charlottesville, VA.: University Press of Virginia, 1984.

Talbot, Michael. *Your Past Lives*. New York: Fawcett Book Group, 1989.

Van Auken, John. *Past Lives, Present Relationships: How Karma Affects You and Your Relationships*. Virginia Beach, Va.: Inner Vision Publishing Co., 1985.

Spirit Possession

Allison, Ralph, M.D. *Mind in Many Pieces*. New York: Rawson, Wade, 1980.

Baldwin, William, Ph.D. *Spirit Releasement Therapy: A Technical Manual*. Terra Alta, W.Va.: Human Potential Foundation Press, 1993.

Chaplin, Annabel. *The Bright Light of Death*. Marina del Rey, Calif.: DeVorss and Co., 1977.

Crabtree, Adam. *Multiple Man: Explorations in Possession and Multiple Personality*. New York: Prager Publishers, 1985.

Fiore, Edith, Ph.D. *The Unquiet Dead*. New York: Doubleday, 1987.
———. "Freeing Statement in Relationships by Resolution of Entity Attachments." *The Journal of Regression Therapy*, Vol. 3, No. 1, (1988).

Friesen, James G., Ph.D. *Uncovering the Mystery of MPD*. Nashville, Tenn.: Thomas Nelson, Inc., 1991.

Guirdham, Arthur, M.D. *The Psychic Dimensions of Mental Health*. Wellingborough, Northamptonshire, U.K.: Thurstone Press, 1982.
———. *Obsession: Psychic Forces and Evil in the Causation of Disease*. London: Neville Spearman, 1972.

Hickman, Irene, D.O. *Remote Depossession*. Kirksville, Mo.: Hickman Systems, 1994.

Lucas, Winafred, Ph.D. *Regression Therapy: A Handbook for Professionals, Vol. 2*. Crest Park, Calif.: Deep Forest Press, 1993.

Maurey, Eugene, *Exorcism*. Chicago: Midwest Books, 1989.

McAll, K. *Healing the Family Tree*. London: Sheldon, 1982.

Naegeli-Osjord, Hans, M.D. *Possession and Exorcism*. Oregon, Wis.: New Frontiers Center, 1988.

Peck, M. Scott, M.D. *People of the Lie: The Hope for Healing Human Evil*. New York: Simon & Schuster, 1983.

Wickland, Carl, M.D. *Thirty Years among the Dead*. Hollywood, Calif.: Newcastle, 1974.

Wilson, C. W. M., M.D., Ph.D. *Entity Possession: A Causative Factor in Disease*. Scotland: Psionnic Medicine, 1987.

Prenatal and Birth Experiences

Chamberlain, David. *Babies Remember Birth*. Los Angeles, Calif.: Jeremy P. Tarcher, Inc., 1986.

Cheek, David, M.D. "Techniques for Eliciting Information Concerning Fetal Experience." Paper presented at the meeting of the Society for Clinical and Experimental Hypnosis, Los Angeles, Calif, 1977.
———. "Maladjustment Patterns Apparently Related to Imprinting at Birth." *The American Journal of Clinical Hypnosis*, Vol. 18, 2 (1975).

Findeisen, Barbara. "Rescripting for Pre- and Perinatal and Early Childhood Regression Work." *The Journal of Regression Therapy*, Vol. 3, 1, (1988).

Gabriel, Michael, and Marie Gabriel. *Voices from the Womb*. Santa Rosa, Calif.: Aslan Publishing, 1992.

Givens, Alice. "The Alice Givens Approach to Prenatal and Birth Therapy." *The Journal of Pre- and Perinatal Psychology* Vol. 1, 3 (1987).

Lucas, Winafred. Ph.D. *Regression Therapy: A Handbook for Professionals*, Vol. 2, Crest Park, Calif.: Deep Forest Press, 1993.

Orr, Leonard, and Sandra Ray. *Rebirthing in the New Age*. Berkeley, Calif.: Celestial Arts, 1977.

Rank, Otto. *The Trauma of Birth*. New York: Robert Brunner Publishers, 1952.

Verney, Thomas. *The Secret Life of the Unborn Child*. New York: Delta Publishing Co., 1981.

Wambach, Helen. *Life Before Life*. New York: Bantam Books, 1979.

Other Related Books

Abrams, J. *Reclaiming the Inner Child*. Los Angeles: Jeremy P. Tarcher, 1990.

American Psychiatric Association. *Diagnostic and Statistical Manual of Mental Disorders*. 4th ed,. rev. *DSM IV*. Washington, D.C., 1994.

Beahrs, J. *Unity and Multiplicity: Multilevel Consciousness of Self in Hypnosis, Psychiatric Disorder, and Mental Health*. New York: Brunner/Mazel, 1982.

Bernstein, Morey. *The Search for Bridey Murphy*. Garden City, N.Y.: Doubleday & Company, 1965.

Bradshaw, J. *Homecoming: Reclaiming and Championing Your Inner Child*. New York: Bantam, 1990.

Brittle, G. *The Devil in Connecticut*. New York: Bantam, 1983.

Burnham, Sophy. *A Book of Angels*. New York: Ballantine Books, 1990.

Carroll, Lee. *Kryon, Book I: The End Time (New Information for Personal Peace)*. Del Mar, Calif.: The Kryon Writings, 1993.
———. *Kryon, Book II: Don't Think Like a Human*. Del Mar, Calif.: The Kryon Writings, 1994.
———. *Kryon, Book III: Alchemy of the Human Spirit. (A Guide to Human Transition into the New Age.)* Del Mar, Calif.: The Kryon Writings, 1995.

Cheek, David B., M.D. *Clinical Hypnosis: The Application of Ideomotor Techniques*. Needham Heights, Mass.: Allyn and Bacon, Inc., 1993.

Compton's Encyclopedia, 1988 ed., s.v. "mental illness."

Denning, Hazel M., Ph.D. *True Hauntings: Spirits with a Purpose*. St. Paul, Minn.: Llewellyn Publications, 1996.

Denning, M., and O. Phillips. *Psychic Self-Defense and Well-Being*. St. Paul. Minn.: Llewellyn Publications, 1980.

Dunner, David L., M.D. *Current Psychiatric Therapy*. Philadelphia: W.B. Saunders Co., 1993.

Eadie, Betty J., *Embraced by the Light*. Carson City, Nev.: Goldleaf Press, 1992.

Evans-Wentz, W. Y. *The Tibetan Book of the Dead*. Oxford: Oxford University Press, 1960.

Finch, W. J. *The Pendulum and Possession*. Rev. ed. Sedona, Ariz.: Esoteric Publications, 1975.

Freedman, Alfred M., M.D., and Harold I. Kaplan, M.D., ed. *Comprehensive Textbook of Psychiatry*. Baltimore: The Williams and Wilkins Co., 1967.

Fremantle, F., and Trungpa, C. *The Tibetan Book of the Dead*. Boulder, Colo.: Shambhala, 1975.

Gallup, G. *Adventures in Immortality*. New York: McGraw-Hill, 1982.

Grof, Stanislav, M.D. *Realms of the Human Unconscious*. New York: E. P. Dutton, 1976.
———. *Ancient Wisdom and Modern Science*. Albany, N.Y.: State University of New York Press, 1984.
———. *Beyond the Brain*. Albany, N.Y.: State University of New York Press, 1985.

Grof, Stanislav, and Christina Grof. *Beyond Death*. London and New York: Thames & Hudson, 1980.

Harman, W. "Survival of Consciousness after Death: A Perennial Issue Revisited." In *Consciousness and Survival*, edited by J. S. Spong. Sausalito, Calif.: IONS, 1987.

Harner, M. *The Way of the Shaman*. New York: Harper & Row, 1974.

Hewitt, William W. *Hypnosis: A Power Program for Self Improvement, Changing Your Life, and Helping Others*. St. Paul, Minn.: Llewellyn Publications, 1987.

Hilgrad, E. R. *Divided Consciousness: Multiple Controls in Human Thought and Action*. New York: John Wiley, 1977.

Hodson, Geoffrey. *The Brotherhood of Angels and Men*. Wheaton, Ill.: The Theosophical Publishing House, 1982.

Hoyt, O. *Exorcism*. New York: Franklin Watts, 1978.

Hunt, S. *Ouija: The Most Dangerous Game*. New York: Harper & Row, 1985.

Kaplan, H. I., and B.J. Sadock. *Modern Synopsis of Comprehensive Textbook of Psychiatry/IV*, 4th ed. Baltimore: Williams & Wilkins, 1985.
———. *Comprehensive Textbook of Psychiatry IV*, Vol. 2. 5th ed. Baltimore: Williams and Wilkins, 1989.
———. *Synopsis of Psychiatry*. 6th ed. Baltimore: Williams & Wilkins, 1994.

Kardec, A. *The Spirits' Book*. London: Psychic Press, 1898.

Kenny, M.G. "Multiple Personality and Spirit Possession." *Psychiatry*, 44, 4 (1981): 337—58.

Kubler-Ross, Elisabeth. *On Death and Dying*. New York: Macmillan, 1969.
———. *Living with Death and Dying*. New York: Macmillan, 1981.

Larson, B. *Satanism: The Seduction of America's Young*. Nashville, Tenn.: Thomas Nelson, 1989.

LeCron, Leslie M., Ph.D. *The Complete Guide to Hypnosis*. New York: Harper Collins Publishers, 1973.

Lewis, G. R. "Criteria for the Discerning of Spirits." In *Demon Possession*, edited by J. Warwick Montgomery, 346-63. Minneapolis: Bethany Fellowship, Inc., 1976.

MacLaine, Shirley. *Going Within: A Guide for Inner Transformation*. New York: Bantam Books, 1990.

Martin, M. *Hostage to the Devil*. New York: Bantam Books, 1976.

Meek, G. *After We Die, What Then?* Franklin, N.C.: Metascience, 1980.

Michels, Robert, et. al., ed. *Psychiatry*, Vol. 1, Rev. ed. Philadelphia: J. B. Lippincott Co., 1993.

Monroe, Robert *Journeys out of the Body*. New York: Doubleday, 1971.
———. *Far Journeys*. Garden City, New York: Doubleday/Dolphin, 1985.

Montgomery, J.W., ed. *Demon Possession*. Minneapolis: Bethany Fellowship, Inc., 1976.

Montgomery, R. *Strangers among Us*. New York: Ballantine Books, 1979.

Moody, Raymond, Jr., M.D., J.D. *Life After Life*. Covington, Ga.: Mockingbird, 1975.
———. *The Light Beyond*. NewYork: Bantam Books, 1989.
———. *Reunions: Visionary Encounters with Departed Loved Ones*. New York: Willard Books, 1993.

Morse, Melvin, M.D., and Paul Perry. *Closer to the Light: Learning from the Near-Death Experiences of Children*. New York: Fawcett Book Group, 1997.

Putnam, F., M.D. *Diagnosis and Treatment of Multiple Personality Disorder*. New York: Guilford, 1989.

Ring, Kenneth. *Life at Death*. New York: Quill, 1980.
———. *Heading toward Omega*. New York: Quill, 1984.

Ritchie, George G., M.D. *Return from Tomorrow*. Waco, Texas: Chosen Books, 1978.

Saggant, W. *The Mind Possessed*. New York: Penguin, 1973.

Snow, C., Ph.D. *Mass Dreams of the Future*. New York: Doubleday, 1989.

Spiegel, H., and D. Spiegel, M.D. *Trance and Treatment*. New York: Basic Books, 1978.

Steiger, Brad, and Francie Steiger. *The Star People*. New York: The Berkley Publishing Group, 1981.

Stein, Diane. *Essential Reike: A Complete Guide to an Ancient Healing Art*. Freedom, Calif.: The Crossing Press Inc., 1995.

Sutphen, Dick *Lighting and Light Within*. Malibu, Calif.: Valley of the Sun, 1987.
———. *Unseen Influences*. New York: Pocket Books, 1982.

Swedenborg, Emanuel *Heaven and Hell*. Translated by G.F. Dole. New York: Swedenborg Foundation, 1979. Original work published in 1758.

Van Dusen, W. *The Presence of Other Worlds*. New York: Swedenborg Foundation, 1974.

Van Auken, John. *Past Lives.*, Virginia Beach, Va.: Inner Vision 1984.
———. *Born Again and Again.*, Virginia Beach, Va.: Inner Vision, 1989.

Whitfield, C. L. *Healing the Child Within*. Deerfield Beach, Fla.: Health Communications, 1987.

Woodward, Mary Anne. *Scars of the Soul: Holistic Healing in the Edgar Cayce Readings*. Columbus, Ohio.: Brindabella Books, 1985.